# Physical Regulation of Skeletal Repair

Published by the

American Academy of
Orthopaedic Surgeons

# Physical Regulation of Skeletal Repair

*Edited by*
Roy K. Aaron, MD
Professor of Orthopaedics
Brown Medical School
Providence, Rhode Island

Mark E. Bolander, MD
Professor of Orthopaedics
Mayo Clinic College of Medicine
Rochester, Minnesota

*Workshop*
Aspen Wye River Conference Center, Queenstown, MD
September 2003

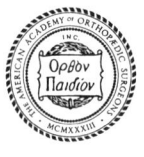

*Supported by the*
American Academy of Orthopaedic Surgeons
  and the
National Institute of Arthritis and Musculoskeletal and Skin Diseases

*Supported in part by grants from*
NASA
EBI, L.P.
Smith and Nephew Inc.
OrthoLogic Corp.
IGEA, S.R.L.
The Whitaker Foundation

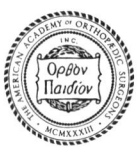

*Published by the*
American Academy of Orthopaedic Surgeons
6300 North River Road
Rosemont, Illinois 60018

American Academy of Orthopaedic Surgeons

# Physical Regulation of Skeletal Repair

American Academy of Orthopeadic Surgeons

The material presented in *Physical Regulation of Skeletal Repair* has been made available by the American Academy of Orthopaedic Surgeons for educational purposes only. This material is not intended to present the only, or necessarily best, methods or procedures for the medical situations discussed, but rather is intended to represent an approach, view, statement, or opinion of the author(s) or producer(s), which may be helpful to others who face similar situations.

Some drugs or medical devices demonstrated in Academy courses or described in Academy print or electronic publications have not been cleared by the Food and Drug Administration (FDA) or have been cleared for specific uses only. The FDA has stated that it is the responsibility of the physician to determine the FDA clearance status of each drug or device he or she wishes to use in clinical practice.

The FDA has expressed concern about potential serious patient care issues involved with the use of polymethylmethacrylate (PMMA) bone cement in the spine. A physician might insert the PMMA bone cement into vertebrae by various procedures, including vertebroplasty and kyphoplasty. Orthopaedic surgeons should be alert to possible complications.

PMMA bone cement is considered a device for FDA purposes. In October 1999, the FDA reclassified PMMA bone cement as a Class II device for its intended use "in arthroplastic procedures of the hip, knee, and other joints for the fixation of polymer or metallic prosthetic implants to living bone." Some bone cements have recently received marketing clearance for the fixation of pathologic fractures of the vertebral body using vertebroplasty or kyphoplasty procedures. Orthopaedic surgeons should contact their manufacturer for the FDA-clearance status. The use of a device for other than its FDA-cleared indication is an off-label use. Physicians may use a device off-label if they believe, in their best medical judgment, that its use is appropriate for a particular patient (eg, tumors).

The use of PMMA bone cement in the spine is described in Academy educational courses, videotapes, and publications for educational purposes only. As is the Academy's policy regarding all of its educational offerings, the fact that the use of PMMA bone cement in the spine is discussed does not constitute an Academy endorsement of this use.

Furthermore, any statements about commercial products are solely the opinion(s) of the author(s) and do not represent an Academy endorsement or evaluation of these products. These statements may not be used in advertising or for any commercial purpose.

All rights reserved. No part of this publication may be reproduced, stored in a retrieval system, or transmitted, in any form, or by any means, electronic, mechanical, photocopying, recording, or otherwise, without prior written permission from the publisher.

Some of the authors or the departments with which they are affiliated have received something of value from a commercial or other party related directly or indirectly to the subject of their chapter.

First Edition
Copyright © 2005
by the American Academy of Orthopaedic Surgeons
ISBN 0-89203-363-0

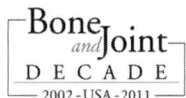

American Academy of Orthopaedic Surgeons

## American Academy of Orthopaedic Surgeons
### Board of Directors, 2005

Stuart L. Weinstein, MD
*President*

Richard F. Kyle, MD
*First Vice President*

James H. Beaty, MD
*Second Vice President*

Edward A. Toriello, MD
*Treasurer*

Robert W. Bucholz, MD

James H. Herndon, MD

Gordon M. Aamoth, MD

Oheneba Boachie-Adjei, MD

Frances A. Farley, MD

Kristy Weber, MD

Frank B. Kelly, MD

Dwight W. Burney III, MD

Matthew S. Shapiro, MD

Mark C. Gebhardt, MD

Andrew N. Pollak, MD

Joseph C. McCarthy, MD

Leslie L. Altick

William L. Healy, MD

Karen L. Hackett
(*Ex-Officio*), FACHE, CAE

### Staff

Mark Wieting, *Chief Education Officer*

Marilyn L. Fox, PhD, *Director, Department of Publications*

Lynne Roby Shindoll, *Managing Editor*

Gayle Murray, *Associate Senior Editor*

Mary Steermann, *Manager, Production and Archives*

Sophie Tosta, *Assistant Production Manager*

Karen Danca, *Production Assistant*

Courtney Astle, *Production/Database Associate*

COVER ILLUSTRATION:
The clinical practice of orthopaedics empirically creates a variety of biophysical environments in attempts to optimize skeletal repair. These include internal fixation with plates and rods of varying flexibility; external fixators of varying stiffness; dynamized fixation; and a number of weight-bearing, bracing, and rehabilitative regimens. The cover figure illustrates fracture healing in two different mechanical environments: the fracture fixed with a rigid plate experiences minimal mechanical strain and is healing by direct osteonal repair, whereas the fracture subject to motion is healing by endochondral ossification. In both cases, extracellular matrix synthesis and gene expression are being regulated by the physical environment.

American Academy of Orthopaedic Surgeons

# Contributors and Participants

Roy K. Aaron, MD
Professor of Orthopaedics
Brown Medical School
Providence, Rhode Island

Peter Augat, PhD
Institute of Orthopaedic Research and
 Biomechanics
University of Ulm
Ulm, Germany

Mark E. Bolander, MD
Professor of Orthopaedics
Mayo Clinic College of Medicine
Rochester, Minnesota

Pier Andrea Borea, PhD
Department of Clinical and
 Experimental Medicine
Molecular and Cellular Pharmacology
 Unit
University of Ferrara
Ferrara, Italy

Mathias P. G. Bostrom, MD
Department of Orthopaedics
Hospital for Special Surgery
New York, New York

Barbara D. Boyan, PhD
Professor and Price Gilbert, Jr Chair in
 Tissue Engineering
Department of Biomedical Engineering
Georgia Institute of Technology
Atlanta, Georgia

Elisabeth H. Burger, PhD
Professor
Department of Oral Cell Biology
ACTA-VU
Amsterdam, The Netherlands

Ruggero Cadossi, MD
Director
Department of Research and
 Development
IGEA
Carpi, Italy

Elena Cattabriga, PhD
University of Ferrara
Ferrara, Italy

Edmund Y. S. Chao, PhD
Emeritus Staff
Department of Orthopaedic Surgery
Johns Hopkins University
Baltimore, Maryland
and
Department of Orthopaedics
Mayo Clinic/Mayo Foundation
Rochester, Minnesota

Deborah McK. Ciombor, PhD
Co-Director, Duffy Cell Biology
 Laboratory
Associate Director, Center for
 Restorative and Regenerative
 Medicine
Department of Orthopaedics
Department of Molecular
 Pharmacology, Physiology, and
 Biotechnology
Brown Medical School
Providence VA Medical Center
Providence, Rhode Island

Lutz Claes, PhD
Professor and Chairman
Institute of Orthopaedic Research and
 Biomechanics
University of Ulm
Ulm, German

Dennis M. Cullinane, PhD
Assistant Professor
Department of Biology
Fairfield University
Fairfield, Connecticut

Michael A. DiMicco, PhD
Postdoctoral Associate
Center for Biomedical Engineering
Massachusetts Institute of Technology
Cambridge, Massachusetts

Randall L. Duncan, PhD
Associate Professor
Department of Orthopaedic Surgery
Indiana University School of Medicine
Indianapolis, Indiana

Xian Fan, MD
Senior Research Associate
Department of Medicine
Emory University School of Medicine/VAMC
Decatur, Georgia

Milena Fini, MD
Laboratorio di Chirurgia Sperimentale
Instituto Ortopedico Rizzoli
Bologna, Italy

Jean C. Gan, PhD
Senior Scientist
Department of Research
EBI, L.P.
Parsippany, New Jersey

Damian C. Genetos, PhD
Department of Orthopaedic Surgery
University of California School of Medicine
Davis, California

Stefania Gessi, PhD
University of Ferrara
Ferrara, Italy

Allen Goodship, BVSc, PhD, MRCVS
Professor
Royal Veterinary College
Institute of Orthopaedics and Musculoskeletal Science
University College London
London, United Kingdom

Alan J. Grodzinsky, ScD
Professor of Electrical, Mechanical, and Biological Engineering
Director, MIT Center for Biomedical Engineering
Electrical, Mechanical, and Biological Engineering Departments
Massachusetts Institute of Technology
Cambridge, Massachusetts

Farshid Guilak, PhD
Professor
Director of Orthopaedic Research
Department of Surgery
Duke University Medical Center
Durham, North Carolina

Michael Hadjiargyrou, PhD
Associate Professor
Department of Biomedical Engineering
SUNY, Stony Brook
Stony Brook, New York

Eun Hee Han, BS
Undergraduate Student Researcher
Department of Bioengineering
University of California, San Diego
La Jolla, California

Sue J. Harris, PhD
Project Leader
Department of Clinical Therapies, Research, and Development
Smith and Nephew Orthopaedics
Memphis, Tennessee

R. Bruce Heppenstall, BSc, MD, MA, FACS
Professor and Vice Chair of Clinical Affairs
Department of Orthopaedic Surgery
University of Pennsylvania
Philadelphia, Pennsylvania

Valeria Iannotta, MSc
University of Ferrara
Ferrara, Italy

Nozomu Inoue, MD, PhD
Associate Professor
Department of Orthopaedic Surgery
Johns Hopkins University
Baltimore, Maryland

Jameel Iqbal, BSc
Endocrinology Assistant
Department of Endocrinology
Mount Sinai School of Medicine
New York, New York

Stefan Judex, PhD
Assistant Professor in Biomedical
   Engineering
Department of Biomedical Engineering
SUNY, Stony Brook
Stony Brook, New York

Travis J. Klein, MS
Graduate Student Researcher
Department of Bioengineering
University of California, San Diego
La Jolla, California

Jenneke Klein-Nulend, PhD
Professor
Department of Oral Cell Biology
Academic Center of Dentistry
   Amsterdam (ACTA)
Vrije Universiteit
Amsterdam, The Netherlands

Joseph M. Lane, MD
Hospital for Special Surgery
New York, New York

Christoph H. Lohmann, MD
Professor of Orthopaedics
Department of Orthopaedics
University of Eppendorf
Hamburg, Germany

Mary J. MacDougall, PhD
University of Alabama
Birmingham, Alabama

Leo Massari, MD
Dipartimento di Scienze Biomediche
University of Ferrara
Ferrara, Italy

Joan McGowan, PhD
NIAMS/NIH
Bethesda, Maryland

Rainer H. Meffert, MD
Department of Trauma, Hand, and
   Reconstructive Surgery
University of Münster
Münster, Germany

Stefania Merighi, PhD
University of Ferrara
Ferrara, Italy

Marjolein C.H. van der Meulen, PhD
Sibley School of Mechanical &
   Aerospace Engineering
Cornell University
Ithaca, New York

Peter J. Nijweide, PhD
Department of Cell Biology
School of Medicine, University of
   Leiden
Leiden, The Netherlands

Isao Ohnishi, MD, PhD
Department of Orthopaedic Surgery
University of Tokyo
Tokyo, Japan

Regis J. O'Keefe, MD, PhD
University of Rochester School of
   Medicine
Rochester, New York

Cecilia Pancaldi, PhD
University of Ferrara
Ferrara, Italy

Javad Parvizi, MD
Assistant Professor
Department of Orthopaedic Surgery
Rothman Institute
Philadelphia, Pennsylvania

Richard Pearce
Research and Development Department
Smith and Nephew Inc.
Memphis, Tennessee

Solomon Pollack, PhD
University of Pennsylvania
Philadelphia, Pennsylvania

Neill M. Pounder, BSc, PhD
Senior Research Project Manager
Department of Clinical Therapies,
   Research, and Development
Smith and Nephew Orthopaedics
Memphis, Tennessee

Yi-Xian Qin, PhD
Associate Professor
Department of Biomedical Engineering
SUNY, Stony Brook
Stony Brook, New York

Bahman Rafiee, MD
Resident
Department of Radiology
Temple University Hospital
Philadelphia, Pennsylvania

A. Hari Reddi, PhD
Orthopaedic Research Labs
University of California, Davis
Sacramento, California

Clinton T. Rubin, PhD
Professor and Chair
Department of Biomedical Engineering
State University of New York
Stony Brook, New York

Janet Rubin, MD
Professor
Department of Medicine
Emory University School of Medicine
Veterans Affairs Medical Center
Atlanta, Georgia

Jack Ryaby
Smith and Nephew Inc.
Memphis, Tennessee

James T. Ryaby, PhD
Senior Vice President Research and
    Clinical Affairs
Chief Technology Officer
OrthoLogic Corporation
Tempe, Arizona

Robert L. Sah, MD, ScD
Professor and Vice-Chair
Department of Bioengineering
University of California, San Diego
La Jolla, California

Barry Sands
Clinical Research and Regulatory
    Affairs
EBI, L.P.
Parsippany, New Jersey

Tannin A. Schmidt, MS
Graduate Student Researcher
Department of Bioengineering
University of California, San Diego
La Jolla, California

Victor Schneider, MD
Bioastronautics Research Division
NASA HQ
Washington, DC

Barbara L. Schumacher, BS
Staff Research Associate IV
Department of Bioengineering
University of California, San Diego
La Jolla, California

Zvi Schwartz, DMD, PhD
Full Professor
Department of Periodontics
School of Dental Medicine, Hebrew
    University
Jerusalem, Israel

Lori A. Setton, PhD
Associate Professor
Department of Biomedical Engineering
Duke University
Durham, North Carolina

William J. Sharrock, PhD
National Institute of Arthritis and
    Musculoskeletal and Skin Diseases
NIH/DHHS
Bethesda, Maryland

Bruce J. Simon, PhD
Director of Research
EBI, L.P.
Parsippany, New Jersey

R. Lane Smith, PhD
Professor, Research
Department of Orthopaedic Surgery
Stanford University School of
    Medicine
Stanford, California

Jon Szafranski, PhD
Biological Engineering Division
Massachusetts Institute of Technology
Cambridge, Massachusetts

Nora Szasz, PhD
Massachusetts Institute of Technology
Cambridge, Massachusetts

Francesco Traina, MD
Divisione di Ortopedia
Instituto Ortopedico Rizzoli
Bologna, Italy

Gian Carlo Traina, MD
Dipartimento di Scienze Biomediche
University of Ferrara
Ferrara, Italy

Stephen B. Trippel, MD
Department of Orthopaedic Surgery
Indiana University Medical Center
Indianapolis, Indiana

Charles H. Turner, PhD
Professor
Department of Biomedical Engineering
Indiana University School of Medicine
Indianapolis, Indiana

Katia Varani, PhD
University of Ferrara
Ferrara, Italy

Michael S. Voegtline, PhD
Staff Research Associate III
Laboratory Manager
Department of Bioengineering
University of California, San Diego
La Jolla, California

Teresa Wu, MD
Chief Resident and Clinical Instructor
Stanford University
Division of Emergency Medicine,
    Department of Surgery
Stanford Hospitals and Clinics
Palo Alto, California

Mone Zaidi, MD, PhD
Director Mount Sinai Bone Program
Professor of Medicine and
    Endocrinology
Department of Endocrinology
Mount Sinai School of Medicine
New York, New York

# Table of Contents

Preface · xv

## Section 1: Biophysical Regulation of Clinical Bone Healing

1   Clinical Results of Physical Techniques for Skeletal Repair    3
*James T. Ryaby, PhD*

2   Mechanical Regulation of Bone Healing    17
*Allen Goodship, BVSc, PhD, MRCVS*

3   Pulsed Low-Intensity Ultrasound for Fracture Healing:    27
A Review of Clinical and In Vivo Evidence
*R. Bruce Heppenstall, MD*

4   Electric and Magnetic Stimulation of Bone Repair:    39
Review of the European Experience
*Ruggero Cadossi, MD, Gian Carlo Traina, MD, Leo Massari, MD*

*Consensus Panel 1: Evaluation of Biophysical Regulation of*    53
*Clinical Bone Healing*

## Section 2: Biophysical Regulation of Bone Healing in Animal Models

5   Bone's "Preferred Strain History" Provides Insight into    61
a Proposed Common Pathway for the Stimulation of
Bone Formation by Distinct Biophysical Signals
*Clinton T. Rubin, PhD, Yi-Xian Qin, PhD, Michael Hadjiargyrou, PhD, Stefan Judex, PhD*

6   Mechanical Regulation of Bone Repair    77
*Lutz Claes, PhD, Peter Augat, PhD*

7   Pulsed Low-Intensity Ultrasound and Fracture Healing:    85
A Proposed Mechanism of Action
*Javad Parvizi, MD, Sue J. Harris, PhD, Neill M. Pounder, PhD*

8   Pulsed Electromagnetic Fields on Osteotomy Healing    97
and Normal Bone Turnover
*Edmund Chao, PhD, Isao Ohnishi, MD, Bahman Rafiee, MD, Rainer Meffert, MD, Teresa Wu, MD, Dennis Cullinane, PhD, Bruce Simon, PhD, Nozomu Inoue, MD, PhD*

*Consensus Panel 2: Evaluation of Biophysical Regulation of*    111
*Bone Healing in Animal Models*

## Section 3: Biophysical Regulation of Skeletal Cells and Tissues

| | | |
|---|---|---|
| 9 | Biophysical Regulation of Cell and Tissue Function<br>*Alan J. Grodzinsky, ScD, Jon Szafranski, MS,*<br>*Michael DiMicco, PhD, Nora Szasz, PhD* | 119 |
| 10 | Mechanical Regulation of Osteocyte Function<br>*Jenneke Klein-Nulend, PhD, Peter J. Nijweide, PhD,*<br>*Elisabeth H. Burger, PhD* | 131 |
| 11 | Mechanical Signals Repress Osteoclast Formation In Vitro<br>*Janet Rubin, MD, Xian Fan, MD* | 143 |
| 12 | Chemomechanical Coupling in Articular Cartilage: IL-1α and TGF-β$_1$ Regulate Chondrocyte Synthesis and Secretion of Proteoglycan 4<br>*Tannin A. Schmidt, MS, Barbara L. Schumacher, BS, Eun Hee Han, BS,*<br>*Travis J. Klein, MS, Michael S. Voegtline, PhD, Robert L. Sah, MD, ScD* | 151 |
| | *Consensus Panel 3: Evaluation of Biophysical Regulation of Skeletal Cells and Tissues* | 163 |

## Section 4: Biophysical Regulation of Growth Factor Synthesis

| | | |
|---|---|---|
| 13 | Stimulation of Growth Factors by Physical Agents: An Intermediary Mechanism of Action<br>*Deborah McK. Ciombor, PhD* | 173 |
| 14 | Mechanical Loading and Growth Factor Effects on Connective Tissue Metabolism<br>*R. Lane Smith, PhD* | 185 |
| 15 | EMF Regulates Growth Factor Synthesis by Osteoblasts<br>*Barbara D. Boyan, PhD, Bruce J. Simon, PhD, Jean C. Gan, PhD, Mary J.*<br>*MacDougall, PhD, Christoph H. Lohmann, MD, Zvi Schwartz, DMD, PhD* | 201 |
| 16 | The Role of Genetics in Skeletal Mechanotransduction<br>*Charles H. Turner, PhD* | 209 |
| | *Consensus Panel 4: Evaluation of Biophysical Regulation of Growth Factor Synthesis* | 217 |

## Section 5: Transduction of Biophysical Signals

| | | |
|---|---|---|
| 17 | Transduction of Physical Signals in Articular Cartilage<br>*Farshid Guilak, PhD, Lori A. Setton, PhD* | 225 |
| 18 | Common Cellular Signaling Mechanisms for Mechanotransduction<br>*Jameel Iqbal, BS, Mone Zaidi, MD, PhD, FRCP* | 241 |
| 19 | Calcium Signaling in Osteoblasts in Response to Mechanical Stimulation<br>*Randall L. Duncan, PhD, Damian C. Genetos, PhD* | 247 |

**20** Effect of Low Frequency Electromagnetic Fields on  259
A$_{2A}$ and A$_3$ Adenosine Receptors in Human Neutrophils
*Pier Andrea Borea, PhD, Katia Varani, PhD, Stefania Gessi, PhD,
Stefania Merighi, PhD, Valeria Iannotta, MSc, Elena Cattabriga, PhD,
Cecilia Pancaldi, PhD, Ruggero Cadossi, MD*

*Consensus Panel 5: Evaluation of Transduction of*  269
*Biophysical Signals*

Index  277

# Preface

Bone and cartilage cells exist in a complex biophysical environment defined in large part by mechanical strain relative to the nature of the extracellular matrix. Although mechanical strain is the most obvious of physical forces, it affects the overall physical environment of tissues, including pH, $pO_2$, hydrostatic pressure, fluid flow, osmotic pressure, and electrokinetic phenomena. Mechanical loading produces gradients in fluid pressure and ion flow, resulting in electrokinetic events such as streaming potentials. These strain-related events can be modulated by cyclic loading and by alterations in extracellular matrix composition or charge, thus constituting a signaling mechanism that reflects both the mechanical environment and the state of the extracellular matrix. The physical environment exerts regulatory influences on gene expression and the synthesis of structural proteins, including those constituting the extracellular matrix, and signaling and regulatory proteins, including growth factors. The physical environment, therefore, has an overall influence on morphogenesis, particularly chondrogenesis and endochondral bone formation.

The American Academy of Orthopaedic Surgeons' Physical Regulation of Skeletal Repair workshop explored basic and clinical information on the regulation of skeletal repair by biologically active physical agents, including mechanical strain, ultrasound, and electrical energy. Physical agents increase the synthesis and organization of extracellular matrix in bone repair and stimulate gene expression for structural extracellular matrix proteins. They also stimulate gene expression and synthesis of several signaling proteins, including growth factors, coincident with the stimulation of repair. Stimulation of growth factors is most likely an intermediary mechanism of action of physical agents. The workshop explored biophysical agents and related technologies for their relevance to repair of cartilage and bone. Workshop participants approached this information from clinical, physiological, and cellular perspectives and identified areas in which further investigation is needed.

*Roy K. Aaron, MD*
*Mark E. Bolander, MD*

# Section One
## Biophysical Regulation of Clinical Bone Healing

# Chapter 1
# Clinical Results of Physical Techniques for Skeletal Repair

*James T. Ryaby, PhD*

## Introduction

The development of physical techniques for stimulation of bone repair is based on the discovery of the electric properties of bone tissue in the 1950s. The first study on bone piezoelectric properties was conducted in Japan by Fukada and Yasuda[1] in 1954. They measured an electric potential upon deformation of dry bone, motivating several research groups in the United States to verify these findings. In the 1960s, groups directed by Bassett and associates[2,3] at Columbia University and Brighton[4] at the University of Pennsylvania, among others, reported on the generation of electric potentials in wet bone upon mechanical deformation.[5] The overall synthesis of these observations led to the hypothesis that mechanical and electric signals originating during loading of bone provided an explanation for Wolff's law. Separation of the relative contributions of the individual components (mechanical and strain-generated electric potentials) has been a challenging problem with no clear solution to date.

Since this initial discovery, electric, electromagnetic, and ultrasonic fields have been under investigation for the past 30 years as potential noninvasive stimulation techniques for fracture healing and bone repair in general. The physical mechanisms of interaction of electric and electromagnetic fields are not completely known; however, one well-accepted biologic transductive mechanism is the stimulation of endogenous growth factor production.[6-8] Even though each electric, electromagnetic, and ultrasonic field system is unique in its respective signal parameters, this stimulation of growth factor synthesis is a common and reproducible experimental finding among these various physical stimulation techniques.

In preclinical studies, various physical stimulation techniques—such as acoustic, electric, electromagnetic, laser, mechanical, ultrasonic, and vibratory—have shown effects on bone and musculoskeletal repair using a variety of animal models.[9-15] The application of these experimental findings led to preclinical evaluation and eventual development of therapeutic devices based solely on electric, electromagnetic, and ultrasonic stimulation; the other physical stimuli described above have not yielded commercial medical devices to date.

The first therapeutic device was based on an implanted, electrode-based, direct current technique. This was followed by the development of noninvasive technologies using electric, electromagnetic, and ultrasonic fields. In the United States, applications of these technologies have resulted in Food and Drug Administration (FDA-) approved applications for treatment of fractures (nonunions and fresh fractures) and spinal fusion.[16] Orthopaedic clinical indications—such as treatment of osteonecrosis,[17,18] osteoarthritis,[19] and tendinitis[20]—have also shown effectiveness; however, these are not FDA-approved indications in the United States at the present time. This chapter will review these FDA-approved technologies and the important prospective clinical trials demonstrating their clinical efficacy and utility.

For electric and electromagnetic stimulation techniques, three different approaches are currently in use: capacitive coupling, direct current, and electromagnetic stimulation.[16] Capacitively coupled electrical fields (CCEF) use 60-kHz sinusoidal electric fields that induce electric fields of approximately 7 $\mu A/cm^2$ at the skin surface. Direct current (DC) uses implanted electrodes delivering a current of approximately 20 $\mu A$. The third technique, electromagnetic induction, includes two types of devices based on their respective electromagnetic signals. The first technology uses pulsed electromagnetic fields (PEMF), which induce an electric and magnetic field in tissue of approximately 20 $\mu A/cm^2$. The second inductive coupling technique, combined magnetic fields (CMF), uses a specific combination of DC and alternating current magnetic fields that are believed to tune specifically to ion transport processes.[21] The remaining physical technique, ultrasonic stimulation, generates mechanical forces associated with the acoustic wave and radiation pressure;[22] it also generates acoustic streaming, which may in fact provide more of a micromechanical input than any streaming potential input.[23]

## Prospective, Controlled Clinical Studies

The initial application of physical stimulation techniques is for nonunion fracture repair. As stated above, various techniques exist for physical stimulation, with specific signal parameters, device configurations, and prescribed daily treatment times. Clinical evaluation conducted under FDA investigational device exemptions evaluating the benefit of these techniques set the foundation for controlled studies on nonunion healing. The important precedents set by these studies include the use of large, multicenter, prospective clinical trials; blinded radiographic panel assessment, and no surgical intervention for 3 months prior to study enrollment.[16]

The first system developed for clinical treatment of nonunions was direct current stimulation with implanted electrodes, which produces a localized electric current (E field) between electrodes inserted at the fracture site. This technique was developed concurrently by Brighton and associates[24] in the United States and Patterson[25] in Australia. The success rates for nonunion treatment in these prospective clinical studies ranged from 78% to 86% respectively (data not shown). The mode of action of direct current stimulation is the subject of an excellent monograph by Black.[26]

The first noninvasive system developed in the United States uses PEMF and was developed by Bassett, Pilla, and Ryaby (the author's father).[27,28] Clinical studies evaluating the efficacy of PEMF showed that 64% to 87% of nonunions healed in different studies. In one prospective series by Bassett and associates,[29] 127 tibial diaphyseal delayed unions or nonunions were exposed to PEMF for 10 hours per day, and 87% healed with a median healing time of 5.2 months. A follow-up multicenter, prospective study by Heckman and associates[30] showed a success rate of 64% in a series of 149 patients who had undergone PEMF treatment. Stratification of the data showed that, in the responsive population, 85% healed within 3 to 6 months after treatment initiation. Clinical studies using PEMF are the subject of comprehensive reviews by Bassett,[31] Gossling and associates,[32] and Hinsenkamp.[33]

The noninvasive CCEF technique developed by Brighton and Pollack[34] uses disk electrodes coupled to the skin via a conductive gel with a recommended daily treatment time of 24 hours per day. The first nonunion study reported an overall efficacy of 77% with a mean time to healing of 23 weeks in a series of 22 nonunions. This study included 17 recalcitrant nonunions that failed to heal with bone graft or prior electric stimulation (the technology is not specified but believed to be PEMF).

The CMF technique was first evaluated as a treatment for fracture nonunions in the mid 1990s.[35] The CMF technique employs an external pair of coils oriented parallel to one another, which produces two parallel low-energy magnetic fields. The alternating magnetic field is a sinusoidal wave of 76.6 Hz and amplitude of 40 µT peak to peak, with the static field set at 20 µT.[16] The clinical study protocol provided for one 30-minute treatment per day with the CMF device until nonunions healed or for a maximum of 9 months. The results noted by the blinded radiographic review panel showed that 51 nonunions healed (61%) and 33 nonunions did not heal (39%), with a mean healing time of 5.8 months (Table 1). Stratification of tibial nonunions (Fig. 1) demonstrated healing in 31 of 41 nonunions, representing an efficacy rate of 76%. These results show that CMF demonstrates clinical efficacy with one 30-minute per day treatment time for fracture nonunions.

Ultrasonic field stimulation of nonunions has also received FDA approval based on a retrospective series conducted in Germany (Table 1). Since ultrasound previously had been approved for fresh fractures in the United States based on double-blind clinical trials (described below), the nonunion approval was based on less rigorous data and was not prospective. Therefore, it is not possible to compare the ultrasonic technique to any of the electric or electromagnetic-based techniques for nonunion treatment.

## Prospective, Placebo-controlled, Randomized, Double-blind Studies

### Nonunions and Fresh Fractures

The use of electric, electromagnetic, or ultrasonic fields for nonunion treatment is viewed with some skepticism in the US orthopaedic community. It should be appreciated, however, that rigorous placebo-controlled, double-blind trials have been conducted both inside and outside the United States to assess the beneficial effects of physical stimulation on bone healing (Table 2). Randomized trials in orthopaedics have been recently recommended,[36] and it is important to underscore the fact that the first use of ran-

Section One   Biophysical Regulation of Clinical Bone Healing

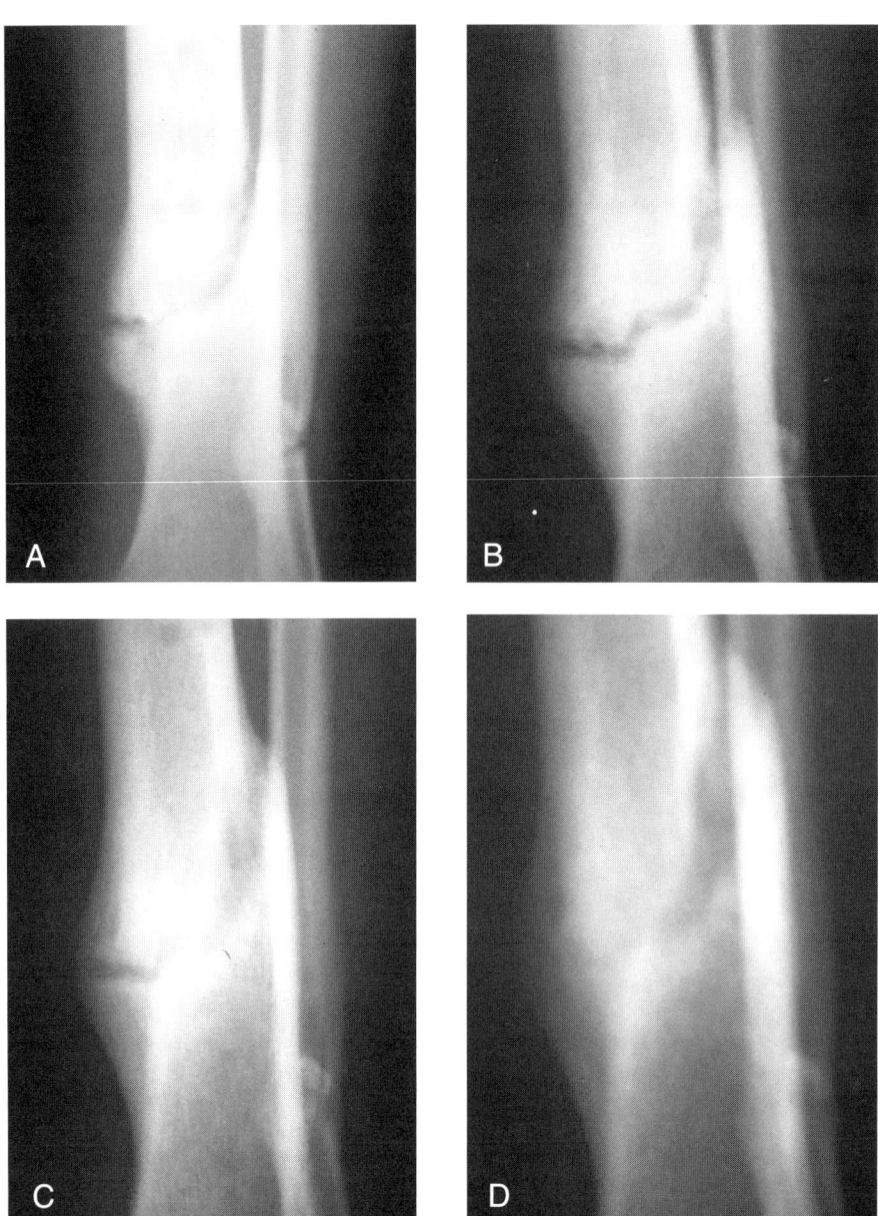

**Figure 1** Radiographic progression of healing of tibial nonunion treated with CMF. **A,** Nonunion at diagnosis, 24 months postfracture. **B,** Nonunion followed for 3 months prior to study entry, showing no progression to healing (criteria as described in references 29 and 30). **C,** Nonunion after 3 months of CMF stimulation. **D,** Nonunion after 6 months of treatment, assessment of moderate to complete healing. (*Radiographs courtesy of the late Howard Rosen, MD, New York, NY.*)

**Table 1 Summary of Nonunion Indications Based on FDA Summary of Safety and Effectiveness Data**

|  | EBI | Orthofix | EBI (Biolectron) | Orthologic | Smith and Nephew (Exogen) |
|---|---|---|---|---|---|
| **Technology** | PEMF | PEMF | CCEF | CMF | Pulsed Ultrasound |
| **Study Population** | Nonunion | Nonunion | Nonunion | Nonunion | Nonunion |
| **Clinical Trial** | Prospective | Prospective | Prosepctive | Prospective | Retrospective |
| **No. Patients** | 115 | 120 | 79 | 84 | 74 |
| **No. Investigators** | 20 | 70? | 16 | 16 | 54 |
| **Enrollment Criteria Verification** | Investigator | Investigator | Investigator | Panel | Investigator |
| **Efficacy Evaluation** | Investigator | Investigator/Panel | Investigator/Panel | Panel | Investigator |
| **Efficacy Rate (%)** | 63.5 | 72 | 50 | 61 | 86 |
| **Long-term follow-up** | Yes | Yes | Yes | Yes | No |
| **Change after long-term follow-up** | Downgraded | Downgraded | Downgraded | No Change | ? |
| **FDA Approval Date** | 1979 | 1986 | 1986 | 1994 | 1998 |
| **Daily Treatment Time** | 8 to 10 hours | Minimum 3 hours | Recommended 24 hours | 30 minutes | 20 minutes |

domized, controlled studies in orthopaedics was in the evaluation of physical stimulation techniques.

The first successful prospective, placebo-controlled, randomized, double-blind trial was performed by Borsalino and associates[37] in 1988. The Italian experience on use of physical stimulation in orthopaedics is the subject of a chapter by Cadossi in this book; accordingly, these studies will not be summarized here.

The first placebo-controlled, randomized, double-blind trial on the effect of PEMF on delayed union healing was reported by Sharrard[38] in 1990. Patients with tibial delayed unions (51 total) were randomized to receive either active or placebo devices with a treatment time of 12 hours per day for 12 weeks. Blinded radiographic assessment was conducted by the treating orthopaedic surgeon and a musculoskeletal radiologist. The active device

**Table 2 Selected Prospective, Placebo-controlled, Randomized, Double-blind Trials Performed to Assess Efficacy of Physical Stimulation Techniques**

| Author | Year | Method | Indication |
|---|---|---|---|
| Borsalino et al[37] | 1988 | PEMF | Femoral osteotomies |
| Sharrard[38] | 1990 | PEMF | Delayed union |
| Mooney[52] | 1990 | PEMF | Spinal fusion |
| Ieran et al[58] | 1990 | PEMF | Venous ulcers |
| Stiller et al[59] | 1992 | PEMF | Venous ulcers |
| Mammi et al[60] | 1993 | PEMF | Tibial osteotomies |
| Scott and King[39] | 1994 | CCEF | Nonunion |
| Heckman et al[44] | 1994 | Ultrasound | Tibial fractures |
| Kristansen et al[45] | 1997 | Ultrasound | Distal radius fractures |
| Goodwin et al[53] | 1999 | CCEF | Spinal fusion |
| Linovitz et al[55] | 2002 | CMF | Spinal fusion |
| Simonis et al[40] | 2003 | PEMF | Tibial nonunion |

had a significant effect on healing, with the treating surgeon's assessment more significant than that of the radiologist. According to the orthopaedic surgeon, 45% of the active device patients healed compared with only 14% of placebo patients, a statistically significant difference. This study concluded that progress to union is significantly affected by electromagnetic stimulation, although no complete data on solid or functional union were provided.

The first prospective, placebo-controlled, randomized, double-blind study on nonunions was reported by Scott and King[39] in the United Kingdom. Stimulation with CCEF for 24 hours per day showed that 60% of the active device patients healed in a mean time of 21 weeks compared with none in the placebo device group, a statistically significant effect.

Recently, another randomized, double-blind clinical trial on electric treatment of tibial nonunions was reported by Simonis and associates.[40] The entry criteria were strict and provided for an elegant study, with each nonunion surgically treated with an oblique fibular osteotomy and unilateral external fixator. Patients were then randomized to either an active or placebo electromagnetic field device. The electromagnetic field signal used in this study is not FDA approved in the United States. Thirty-four nonunions were enrolled in this trial; 89% of the active group showed bony union compared with 50% in the placebo group, a statistically significant difference.

The use of ultrasound for fresh fracture healing was developed by Xavier and Duarte[41,42] in Brazil, who showed in preclinical and clinical studies a beneficial effect on fracture healing; these studies were followed in the United States by Pilla and associates.[43] These efforts led to the development of the technique currently used in the United States. The first study of this technique, by Heckman and associates,[44] assessed the efficacy of pulsed ultrasound on fresh fracture healing in 67 closed or grade I open fractures. Clinical and radiographic evaluation demonstrated a significant reduction in healing time, from 154 days in the placebo group to 96 days in the ultrasound group. Kristiansen and associates[45] investigated ultrasonic effects on distal radius fracture healing. Ultrasonic stimulation decreased the fracture healing time from 98 days in the placebo group to 61 days in the ultrasound-treated group. The major limitation of this study is the clinical literature describing Colles fracture healing times to be approximately 45 to 60 days, essentially the same as those of the ultrasound-treated group. Therefore, in the clinical setting, the usefulness of ultrasound on distal radius fracture healing is unclear.

One recent prospective, placebo-controlled, randomized, double-blind study by Larsson and associates[46] in Sweden investigated the use of ultrasound to enhance the healing of intramedullary fixed fractures. Patients with tibial fractures treated by static locked intramedullary nailing were randomized to receive active or placebo devices. In contrast to previous findings, active device patients showed only a slight increase in healing time as assessed by the radiologist. The orthopaedist's assessment noted no difference between active and placebo patients. The authors concluded that there was no effect of ultrasound on fracture healing in this study, a conclusion that contradicts those of previous studies on the pulsed ultrasound device. It should be noted, however, that a key difference in this study was the limitation of ultrasound to the first 75 days of healing in comparison to its continuous use throughout healing in the studies by Heckman and associates[44] and Kristiansen and associates.[45]

The clinical studies summarized here clearly show, in prospective, placebo-controlled, randomized studies, that physical stimulation techniques have a profound effect on bone repair. It should be appreciated, however, that there is a variation in efficacy dependent on anatomic site, that the daily treatment time varies for the different physical stimulation techniques, that use of physical stimulation may not be compatible with some internal fixation techniques,[46] and that to date there are no well-controlled studies on the effectiveness of physical stimulation used in conjunction with concurrent bone grafting. In summary, these trials on fracture repair and nonunions have all demonstrated the effectiveness of various forms of electric, electromagnetic, and ultrasonic stimulation devices. Additional indications for these devices remain to be further defined.

## Spinal Fusion

Double-blind clinical trials have also demonstrated therapeutic efficacy of electric and electromagnetic fields for treatment of spinal fusions. This finding has recently been supported by the publication of a meta-analysis by a Japanese statistical team.[47] Initially, the use of bone growth stimulation in spinal fusion was limited to surgically implantable DC stimulation devices, as reported by Dwyer and associates[48] in 1974. Following this report was the randomized study by Kane[49] in 1988, which used an implantable DC stimulator. This device uses electrodes that are surgically placed lateral to the fusion site and powered by a battery pack to deliver a current of 20 $\mu A/cm^2$. There were three components to this report, with the key component (and the only component reviewed here) being the randomized trial. This study comprised 59 patients, both male and female, 28 control and 31 with the DC stimulation device. The stimulated group healed with a percentage of 81% compared with 54% in the control group, a statistically significant increase.

The major limitations in this study were the lack of a placebo control, no blinding, and no information on the fusion technique or use/type of instrumentation. The study also had a high dropout rate; only 59 patients out of 99 enrolled patients were included in the data analysis, with no intent-to-treat analysis. Therefore, it is difficult to reach a conclusion on the real effectiveness of DC stimulation, although several subsequent studies have been performed with more rigorous protocols.[50,51]

The first use of a noninvasive electromagnetic technology was the study by Mooney,[52] who reported on the use of PEMF for stimulation of interbody fusions in 1990. This was a multicenter, prospective, placebo-controlled, randomized, double-blind trial, and analysis was ultimately performed on 195 patients with a mean age of 38 years. Patients were fitted with electromagnetic coils in a brace and instructed to use the electromagnetic device for a minimum of 8 hours per day for 12 months. An additional strength of this study was the use of a confirmatory reading of fusion success by a blinded radiologist. The overall patient population showed a significant effect; active device patients fused at 83% compared with 65% of placebo patients. Stratification of the fusion success data into consistent users ($\geq$ 8 hours/day) and inconsistent users ($<$ 4 hours/day) showed an important difference; this was the first report showing a true dose response to PEMF stimulation. In the 117 patients who were consistent users, the active device patients achieved a fusion success rate of 92% compared with the placebo success rate of 68%, a statistically significant difference. Patients who used the device inconsistently had the same success rate in the active and placebo groups, 65% and 61% respectively. There were some limitations in this study, including use of both instrumented and noninstrumented techniques as well as autograft, allograft, or combined autograft/allograft.

The second noninvasive technology for stimulation of spinal fusion is CCEF, as reported by Goodwin and associates[53] in 1999. The study design was a multicenter, prospective, placebo-controlled, randomized, double-blind trial that reported on 179 patients with a mean age of 43 years. The daily device treatment time was 24 hours per day using two electrodes placed laterally 10 cm apart at the fusion site. This study used a blinded radiographic and clinical review, and the study end point was 9 months. The results showed that 85% of the active device patients fused compared with 65% of the placebo patients, a statistically significant difference. Limitations of the study included use of both instrumented and noninstrumented technique, variation in daily treatment time (average patient use was 16 hours/day), and type of graft (autograft, allograft, or a combination). The one puzzling outcome was that the noninstrumented patient population fused at a higher success rate than the instrumented patients, which was unexpected in reference to the literature.[54]

The third noninvasive technology for adjunctive stimulation of spinal fusion is CMF, as reported by Linovitz and associates.[55] The clinical study conducted was a prospective, placebo-controlled, randomized, double-blind trial on lumbar spinal fusion. Patients had one- or two-level fusions (between L3 and S1) without instrumentation, with either autograft alone or in combination with allograft. The CMF device uses a single posterior coil with one

30-minute treatment per day. The primary end point was assessment of fusion at 9 months, based on radiographic evaluation by a blinded panel consisting of the treating physician, a musculoskeletal radiologist, and a spine surgeon. The difference in this panel evaluation was that the blinded panel could overrule the treating surgeon's assessment of fusion. This is the largest study to date, with 201 patients evaluated. Among all active device patients, 64% healed at 9 months compared with 43% of placebo device patients, a statistically significant difference. This was the first study to stratify by gender. The results showed a statistically significant increase in fusion success in females, with 67% of the active device females fused compared with 35% of the placebo device females.

A comparison of the different physical stimulation devices for spinal fusion is provided in Table 3. The major differences are the need for surgical implantation and explantation for the DC device and patient compliance regarding use of the noninvasive devices. The implantable DC stimulator does not pose a compliance issue provided that the electrodes are not in contact with internal fixation. The noninvasive devices require the patient to comply with the treatment protocol, which can vary from 30 minutes per day for CMF to a recommended 24 hours per day for CCEF.

**Table 3 Comparison of FDA-approved Technologies for Stimulation of Lumbar Spine Fusion**

|  | Orthofix Spinal Stim Lite (McKinney, TX) | Biolectron/ EBI Spinalpak (Parsippany, NJ) | Orthologic Spinalogic (Tempe, AZ) |
| --- | --- | --- | --- |
| **Technology** | PEMF | CCEF | CMF |
| **Reference** | 52 | 53 | 55 |
| **Device Type** | External, noninvasive | External, noninvasive | External, noninvasive |
| **Percent Change** | 18 | 20 | 21 |
| **Active** | 83 | 85 | 64 |
| **Placebo** | 65 | 65 | 43 |
| **Clinical Trial** | Double-blind, placebo-controlled | Double-blind, placebo-controlled | Double-blind, placebo-controlled |
| **Study Population** | Instrumented/ noninstrumented fusions | Instrumented/ noninstrumented fusions | Noninstrumented fusions |
| **Study Population Age (years)** | 38 | 45 | 58 |
| **FDA Approval Date** | 1990 | 1999 | 1999 |
| **Daily Treatment Time** | Minimum 2 hours | Recommended 24 hours | 30 minutes |

To date, there are no studies on any of the electric/electromagnetic field technologies with fusion cages, nor are there studies comparing the benefits of the devices using an outcome instrument such as the Oswestry score. Regardless, the above well-controlled studies do provide strong support for the adjunctive use of electric/electromagnetic fields in spinal fusion.

## Additional Clinical Applications

Publications have recently described effects of physical stimulation techniques on Charcot neuroarthropathy. The first was a clinical trial that assessed the effect of CMF as a treatment for Charcot neuroarthropathy.[56] This trial was a prospective, randomized pilot study on acute phase 1 Charcot patients, with 10 patients in the control group and 11 patients in the CMF group. Patients were followed weekly and treated until consolidation, with a CMF treatment time of 30 minutes per day. Statistical analysis of this initial cohort revealed a statistical benefit in the CMF treatment group. Subsequently, an additional 10 patients were enrolled in the CMF treatment group. The final results showed that the mean time to consolidation in the control group was 23 weeks compared with 11 weeks in the CMF group, a statistically significant difference. The authors concluded that the CMF treatment significantly accelerated the process of consolidation in this study. The second article, a case report study by Strauss and Gonya,[57] described the effect of ultrasound on ankle arthodesis in two patients with severe Charcot neuroarthropathy. Both patients healed after treatment with ultrasound, demonstrating that even these difficult conditions may be amenable to treatment with physical stimulation techniques.

Well-conducted placebo-controlled, randomized, double-blind trials have also been performed on venous ulcer healing in humans,[58,59] although the regulatory status is unknown at the present time.

## Discussion and Conclusions

Many unanswered questions remain regarding the clinical applications of electric, electromagnetic, and ultrasonic fields. When are these biophysical technologies indicated? Are there subgroups of patients (based on, for example, age, gender, fracture type, or risk factors) that benefit more than others? How do the outcomes compare with those of standard surgical procedures (for example, how does nonunion treatment with physical stimulation compare with treatment with bone graft)?

To answer these remaining questions, several approaches could be implemented in the design of future clinical studies. Outcome studies could be performed, randomizing patients in two- or three-arm clinical trials comparing different treatment regimes to biophysical stimulation. Well-designed prospective registry studies with clinical monitoring (akin to Phase 4 drug studies) may be useful in expansion of clinical indications where FDA-approved indications already exist. For example, this approach might include an expansion of the indications of electric/electromagnetic field techniques to all spinal fusions, not the current limitation to lumbar fusion only.

In conclusion, electric, electromagnetic, and ultrasonic devices have been demonstrated to positively affect the healing process in fresh fractures, delayed unions and nonunions, osteotomies, and spinal fusions. These outcomes have been validated by well-designed and statistically powered placebo-controlled, randomized, double-blind clinical trials. Physical stimulation technologies provide an important tool in a comprehensive orthopaedic treatment program. The discovery of additional orthopaedic applications of physical stimulation depends on continuation of basic, preclinical, and clinical research.

# References

1. Fukada E, Yasuda I: On the piezoelectric effect of bone. *J Phys Soc Japan* 1957;12: 121-128.
2. Bassett CAL, Becker RO: Generation of electric potentials in bone in response to mechanical stress. *Science* 1962;137:1063-1064.
3. Bassett CAL, Pawluk RJ: Electrical behavior of cartilage during loading. *Science* 1974;814:575-577.
4. Friedenberg ZB, Brighton CT: Bioelectric potentials in bone. *J Bone Joint Surg Am* 1966;48:915-923.
5. Grodzinsky AJ, Lipshitz H, Glimcher MJ: Electromechanical properties of articular cartilage during compression and stress relaxation. *Nature* 1978;275:448-450.
6. Fitzsimmons RJ, Ryaby JT, Mohan S, Magee FP, Baylink DJ: Combined magnetic fields increase IGF-II in TE-85 human bone cell cultures. *Endocrinology* 1995;136: 3100-3106.
7. Fitzsimmons RJ, Ryaby JT, Magee FP, Baylink DJ: IGF-II receptor number is increased in TE-85 cells by low-amplitude, low-frequency combined magnetic field (CMF) exposure. *J Bone Min Res* 1995;10:812-819.
8. Ryaby JT, Fitzsimmons RJ, Khin NA, et al: The role of insulin-like growth factor in magnetic field regulation of bone formation. *Bioelectrochem Bioenerg* 1994;35:87-91.
9. Augat P, Claes L, Suger G: In vivo effect of shock waves on the healing of fractured bone. *Clin Biomech* 1995;10:374-378.
10. Lavine LS, Grodzinsky AJ: Electrical stimulation of repair of bone. *J Bone Joint Surg Am* 1987;69:626-630.
11. Otter MW, McLeod KJ, Rubin CT: Effects of electromagnetic fields in experimental fracture repair. *Clin Orthop* 1988;355:90-104.
12. Yaakobi T, Maltz L, Oron U: Promotion of bone repair in the cortical bone of the tibia in rats by low energy laser (He-Ne) irradiation. *Calcif Tiss Int* 1996;59:297-300.
13. Kenwright J, Richardson JB, Cunningham JL, et al: Axial movement and tibial fractures: A controlled randomised trial of treatment. *J Bone Joint Surg Br* 1991;73:654-659.
14. Rubin CT, Bolander M, Ryaby JP, Hadjiargyrou M: The use of low-intensity ultrasound to accelerate the healing of fractures. *J Bone Joint Surg Am* 2001;83:259-270.
15. Usui Y, Zerwekh JE, Vanharanta H, Ashman RB, Mooney V: Different effects of mechanical vibration on bone ingrowth into porous hydroxyapatite and fracture healing in a rabbit model. *J Orthop Res* 1989;7:559-567.

16. Ryaby JT: Clinical effects of electromagnetic and electrical fields on fracture healing. *Clin Orthop* 1998;355:205-215.

17. Aaron RK, Lennox D, Bunce GE, Ebert T: The conservative treatment of osteonecrosis of the femoral head: A comparison of core decompression and pulsing electromagnetic fields. *Clin Orthop* 1989;249:209-218.

18. Steinberg ME, Brighton CT, Corces A, et al: Osteonecrosis of the femoral head: Results of core decompression and grafting with and without electrical stimulation. *Clin Orthop* 1989;249:199-208.

19. Zizik TM, Hoffman KC, Holt PA, et al: The treatment of osteoarthritis of the knee with pulsed electrical stimulation. *J Rheumat* 1995;22:1757-1761.

20. Binder A, Parr G, Hazelman B, Fitton-Jackson S: Pulsed electromagnetic field therapy of persistent rotator cuff tendonitis: A double blind controlled assessment. *Lancet* 1984;1:695-697.

21. Diebert MC, McLeod BR, Smith SD, Liboff AR: Ion resonance electromagnetic field stimulation of fracture healing in rabbits with a fibular ostectomy. *J Orthop Res* 1994;12:878-885.

22. Hill CR (ed): *Physical Principles of Medical Ultrasonics.* New York, NY, Halstead Press, 1986.

23. Rubin CT, Bolander M, Ryaby JP, Hadjiargyrou M: The use of low-intensity ultrasound to accelerate the healing of fractures. *J Bone Joint Surg Am* 2001;83:259-270.

24. Brighton CT, Friedenberg ZB, Mitchell EI, Booth RE: Treatment of nonunion with constant direct current. *Clin Orthop* 1977;124:106-123.

25. Patterson D: Treatment of nonunion with a constant direct current: A totally implantable system. *Orthop Clin North Am* 1984;15:47-59.

26. Black J: *Electrical Stimulation: Its Role in Growth, Repair, and Remodeling of the Musculoskeletal System.* New York, NY, Praeger, 1987.

27. Bassett CAL, Pawluk RJ, Pilla AA: Augmentation of bone repair by inductively coupled electromagnetic fields. *Science* 1974;184:575-577.

28. Hinsenkamp M, Ryaby J, Burny F: Treatment of non-union by pulsing electromagnetic fields: European multicenter study of 308 cases. *Reconstr Surg Traumatol* 1985;19:147-156.

29. Bassett CAL, Mitchell SN, Gaston SR: Treatment of ununited tibial diaphyseal fractures with pulsing electromagnetic fields. *J Bone Joint Surg Am* 1981;63:511-523.

30. Heckman JD, Ingram AJ, Lloyd RD, Luck JV, Mayer PW: Nonunion treatment with pulsed electromagnetic fields. *Clin Orthop* 1981;161:58-66.

31. Bassett CAL: Fundamental and practical aspects of therapeutic uses of pulsed electromagnetic fields (PEMFS). *Crit Rev Biomed Eng* 1989;17:451-529.

32. Gossling HR, Bernstein RA, Abbott J: Treatment of ununited tibial fractures: A comparison of surgery and pulsed electromagnetic fields. *Orthopedics* 1992;16:711-717.

33. Hinsenkamp M: Treatment of non-unions by electromagnetic stimulation. *Acta Orthop Scand* 1982;196:63-79.

34. Brighton CT, Pollack SR: Treatment of recalcitrant nonunion with a capacitively coupled electric field. *J Bone Joint Surg Am* 1985;67:577-585.

35. Longo JA: The management of recalcitrant nonunions with combined magnetic field stimulation. *Orthop Trans* 1998;22:408-409.

36. Laupacis A, Rorabeck CH, Bourne RB, Feeny D, Tugwell P, Sim DA: Randomized trials in orthopaedics: Why, how, and when? *J Bone Joint Surg Am* 1989;71:535-543.

37. Borsalino G, Bagnacani M, Bettati E, et al: Electrical stimulation of human femoral intertrochanteric osteotomies: Double blind study. *Clin Orthop* 1988;237:256-263.

38. Sharrard WJW: A double-blind trial of pulsed electromagnetic fields for delayed union of tibial fractures. *J Bone Joint Surg Br* 1990;72:347-355.

39. Scott G, King JB: A prospective double blind trial of electrical capacitive coupling in the treatment of non-union of long bones. *J Bone Joint Surg Am* 1994;76:820-826.

40. Simonis RB, Parnell EJ, Ray PS, Peacock JL: Electrical treatment of tibial non-union: A prospective, randomized, double blind trial. *Injury* 2003;34:357-362.

41. Xavier CAM, Duarte L: Estimulaca ultra-sonica de calo osseo: Applicaca clinica. *Rev Brasil Orthop* 1983;18:73-80.

42. Duarte LR: The stimulation of bone growth by ultrasound. *Arch Orthop Trauma Surg* 1983;101:153-159.

43. Pilla AA, Mont MA, Nasser PR, et al: Non-invasive low-intensity pulsed ultrasound accelerates bone healing in the rabbit. *J Orthop Trauma* 1990;4:246-253.

44. Heckman JD, Ryaby JP, McCabe J, Frey JJ, Kilcoyne RF: Acceleration of tibial fracture-healing by non-invasive, low-intensity pulsed ultrasound. *J Bone Joint Surg Am* 1994;76:26-34.

45. Kristiansen TK, Ryaby JP, McCabe J, Frey JJ, Roe LR: Accelerated healing of distal radial fractures with the use of specific, low-intensity ultrasound: A multicenter, prospective, randomized, double-blind, placebo-controlled study. *J Bone Joint Surg Am* 1997;79:961-973.

46. Emami A, Petren-Mallmin M, Larsson S: No effect of low-intensity ultrasound on healing time of intramedullary fixed tibial fractures. *J Orthop Trauma* 1999;13:252-257.

47. Akai M, Kawashima N, Kimura T, Hayashi K: Electrical stimulation as an adjunct to spinal fusion: A meta-analysis of controlled clinical trials. *Bioelectromagnetics* 2002;23:496-504.

48. Dwyer AF, Yau AC, Jeffcoat KW: The use of direct current in spine fusion. *J Bone Joint Surg Am* 1974;56:442-446.

49. Kane WJ: Direct current electrical bone growth stimulation for spinal fusion. *Spine* 1988;13:363-365.

50. Meril AJ: Direct current stimulation of allograft in anterior and posterior interbody fusions. *Spine* 1994;19:2393-2398.

51. Tejano NA, Puno R, Ignacio JMP: The use of implantable direct current stimulation in multilevel fusion without instrumentation. *Spine* 1996;21:1904-1908.

52. Mooney V: A randomized double blind prospective study of the efficacy of pulsed electromagnetic fields for interbody lumbar fusions. *Spine* 1990;15:708-715.

53. Goodwin CB, Brighton CT, Guyer RD, Johnson JR, Light KI, Yuan HA: A double blind study of capacitively coupled electrical stimulation as an adjunct to lumbar spinal fusions. *Spine* 1999;24:1349-1357.

54. Zdeblick TD: A prospective, randomized study of lumbar fusion: Preliminary results. *Spine* 1993;18:983-991.

55. Linovitz R, Pathria M, Bernhardt M, et al: Combined magnetic fields accelerate and increase spine fusion: A double-blind, randomized, placebo controlled study. *Spine* 2002;27:1383-1389.

56. Hanft JR, Goggin JP, Landsman A, Surprenant M: The role of combined magnetic field bone growth stimulation as an adjunct in the treatment of neuroarthropathy/Charcot joint: An expanded pilot study. *J Foot Ankle Surg* 1998;37:510-515.

57. Strauss E, Gonya G: Adjunct low intensity ultrasound in Charcot neuroarthropathy. *Clin Orthop* 1998;349:132-138.

58. Ieran M, Zaffuto S, Bagnacani M, Annovi M, Moratti A, Cadossi R: Effect of low frequency pulsing electromagnetic fields on skin ulcers of venous origin in humans: A double-blind study. *J Orthop Res* 1990;8:276-282.

59. Stiller MJ, Pak GH, Shupack JL, Thaler S, Kenny C, Jondreau L: A portable pulsed electromagnetic field (PEMF) device to enhance healing of recalcitrant venous ulcers: A double-blind, placebo-controlled clinical trial. *Br J Dermatol* 1992;127:147-154.

60. Mammi GI, Rocchi R, Cadossi R, Traina GC: Effect of PEMF on the healing of human tibial osteotomies: A double blind study. *Clin Orthop* 1993;288:246-253.

# Chapter 2

# Mechanical Regulation of Bone Healing

*Allen Goodship, BVSc, PhD, MRCVS*

## Mechanical Regulation of Skeletal Architecture

Each bone in the skeleton has the ability to optimize mass and architecture in response to changes in mechanical demand. This process of functional adaptation can occur in localized regions of the skeleton, within a limb, or even at specific locations within individual bones.

The genetic template of each individual bone provides the basic shape and proportions. This basic pattern, however, is modified and refined by the functional loading patterns sustained throughout life, with abnormal loading inducing a related abnormal morphology. Changes in biologic environment also influence the form of the skeleton. Chalmers and Ray[1] performed a classic experiment in which the cartilage precursor of a mouse femur from the developing fetus was transplanted into the spleen. The cartilage precursor developed through the process of endochondral ossification to form a skeletal element is recognizable as a femur but lacking the refinements present in the femora that develop in the normal location and are subjected to the mechanical stimuli occurring during development. Thus, the processes of ossification and subsequent modeling of the bone are regulated by both genetic and functional mechanical influences. Fell[2] also showed in isolated chick limb buds that some anatomic features developed in culture and others did not, again suggesting the dual influences of genetics and environment in the regulation of normal bone development.

In the postnatal skeleton, mechanical regulation influences both modeling and subsequent remodeling of the skeleton during growth and development. Bone as a connective tissue is distributed by the actions of bone cell populations in removing and depositing bone matrix. These are complex processes involving both cell-to-cell and cell-to-matrix interactions. The modeling and remodeling processes are extremely sensitive to mechanical regulation in addition to biologic mediators.

Experimental and clinical studies have enhanced the understanding of these processes. The imposition of an osteogenic mechanical signal results in rapid matrix and cellular events. The ability of investigators to quantify one direct mechanical influence on the skeleton, namely deformation, using strain gauges has paved the way to perturb the mechanical environment in a quantifiable manner and observe the response to determine the role and mechanisms of mechanical influences on bone adaptation. Mechanical strain and such related events as streaming potentials elicit responses in the resident osteocytes and, via cell signaling, processes the lining cells, osteoblasts, and osteoclasts in a coordinated manner to reestablish an optimal organization of bone tissue to withstand the magnitude and distribution of the applied loads.

Studies on the mechanical regulation of intact bone have shown that potent osteogenic mechanical stimuli comprise short daily periods of cyclical deformation, high rates of deformation, and diverse strain distributions. Recently it has been shown that strain magnitudes significantly lower than physiologic levels can provide an osteogenic stimulus when applied at a frequency of around 30 Hz.[3]

## Mechanical Modulation of Indirect Bone Repair

The outcome of indirect bone repair can range from a near-scarless restoration of both tissue and structural integrity, through delayed union and nonunion, to the formation of a synovialized pseudarthrosis. The time to attain bone union may also vary. These outcomes can be influenced by the mechanical conditions pertaining during the various stages of the repair process. Understanding the interactions between mechanical influences and biologic processes may provide new strategies for the controlling of fracture repair. Part of the repair process in bone following fracture resembles the processes of development; therefore, it is reasonable to assume that similar regulatory processes may be active in healing.

The mechanical environment at the fracture site is the result of a combination of the mechanical properties of the fixation device and the loads applied to the limb as a consequence of muscle action, weight bearing, and fracture geometry. Following fracture, normal loading of the limb is reduced and further reduction in localized mechanical stimuli occurs as a consequence of fracture fixation, with the fixation device providing a load-sharing system. The compliance of the fixation device in combination with functional loading and the geometry of the fracture site determine interfragmentary movements, and, as healing progresses, a complex heterogeneous temporal and spatial arrangement of tissues develops. The levels of load applied to the stabilized fracture and the material properties of any interfragmentary tissues will influence the general interfragmentary strains and the complex local strain distributions within the specific tissue types of the differentiating callus between the bone fragments. Measurement of the tissue-specific strains within the tissues of the differentiating callus is complex, and attempts have been made to determine these values indirectly using computer modeling to predict the stresses and strains within heterogeneous callus and provide insight into the mechanical regulation of tissue differentiation. Many of these studies use models where input values are provided from in vivo experimental and clinical observations.[4-6] The geometry of the fracture or osteotomy site may also influence both the magnitude and distribution of strains that occur with any given method of fixation. Perren[7] indicated that, in rigid fixation of fractures with good reduction, any small gaps between the bone fragments could generate very high levels of strain if the fixation was not absolutely rigid. This concept was evaluated in vivo by examining healing in an osteotomy subjected to a gradient of initial strain, and results showed that the lower strain fields facilitated bone union compared with high strain fields.[8]

## Device-related Mechanical Regulation of Indirect Bone Repair

The stiffness of a fixation device and the stability of fixation can modify the loads applied to the limb and the progression of the repair process. High levels of fixation stiffness result in higher levels of applied loading to the limb than when lower stiffness fixation is applied. However, high stiffness fixation also reduces the level of interfragmentary motion when compared with a similar lower stiffness fixation device. In a controlled study, the lower stiffness frame, although reducing loads applied to the limb in the early stages of repair, effected an increased rate of repair. Conversely, the high stiffness device inhibited the progression of bone healing, possibly reducing interfragmentary movement in the early stages of repair.[9] In another study, interfragmentary movement was measured in a standard model in which the fixator compliance was high in one group and low in the other; the levels of displacement were significantly different in the initial period of healing. This cyclical deformation of the early callus resulted in an increased progression of healing compared with the high compliance group.[10]

Using a rigid fixation system in which the axial displacement induced by weight bearing was 0.06 mm in an osteotomy gap of 0.6 mm, Claes and associates[11] showed that the healing of a transverse osteotomy was enhanced by dynamization. A defined displacement activated by weight bearing of 0.15 mm to 0.34 mm was permitted in the dynamized group and compared with the control nondynamized group.

The degree of fixation compliance and the size of an osteotomy gap can also affect the progression of tissue differentiation in terms of the distribution of tissue types in the cascade of callus differentiation. Claes and associates[12] observed that large interfragmentary displacements could engender callus proliferation yet inhibit union. An increased osteotomy gap size also reduced the rate of healing, and a combination of large gap size and large interfragmentary displacements could result in nonunion. These data need analysis in terms of absolute levels of strain within the osteotomy gap, as small gaps with movement can engender very high tissue strains. Claes and associates[13] compared two groups of sheep in which a similar fixator was used to produce displacements of 1 mm and 0.2 mm with an osteotomy gap of 2 mm. At the end point of 9 weeks, there was a greater amount of fibrocartilage and a reduced amount of bone within the larger displacement group. Thus, the small difference in level of interfragmentary motion had modulated the progression of indirect bone repair. In this model, the greater interfragmentary strain resulting from functional loading of the limb had reduced the formation of bone.

## Mechanical Regulation of Bone Repair Using Imposed Controlled Mechanical Stimulation

Studies have been performed to test the hypothesis that short periods of cyclical mechanical deformation could be used to modulate the process of indirect bone repair in a given mechanical environment. Using a single-sided rigid external fixator with constant geometry, investigators applied various regimens of cyclical interfragmentary movement for a short period each day, and varying magnitudes of displacement, amounts of force, and rates of movement were explored. For each variable, three levels of magnitude were compared. The regimens were applied at the onset of healing of a 3-mm mid-diaphyseal ovine tibial osteotomy. It appears that, despite the short-term stimulation superimposed on normal functional loading, the patterns of healing were significantly altered by the different regimens of applied micromotion. The applied mechanical signals could enhance the progression of repair compared with unstimulated controls. Certain regimes of short periods of applied stimulation enhanced repair, whereas others inhibited repair compared with unstimulated controls.[14-16] The data obtained indicate the potential to regulate the process of indirect bone healing through controlled mechanical stimulation. This has implications not only for management of bone repair but also for in vivo tissue engineering of skeletal tissues, structures, and organs.

Other studies also indicate the sensitivity of indirect bone repair to mechanical conditions. In a similar model, Wolf and associates[17] observed that callus proliferation was related to the magnitude of interfragmentary displacement. These authors implied an optimal interfragmentary displacement of 0.5 mm but could not show a statistically significant effect. They concluded that externally applied mechanical stimulation may have a role in stimulation of healing in patients prevented from normal weight bearing, avoiding a delayed union. Augat and associates[18] were unable to demonstrate significant effects of imposed cyclical micromovement when applied using a flexible external fixator. These studies are difficult to compare directly because the models and characterization of frame stiffness, functional input, and applied dosage differ. Studies should be performed on standard calibrated models to identify the specific characteristics of mechanical modulation of indirect bone repair.

To refine the magnitude of imposed cyclical deformation as a function of time, researchers applied a programmed micromovement regime involving incremental reduction in displacement magnitude to the ovine tibial osteotomy model. Compared with the optimal displacement magnitude from the previous study, this programmed regimen resulted in significant enhancement of the progression of indirect bone repair.[19]

Rubin and McLeod[3] studied the effects of imposed mechanical stimulation using extremely low strain magnitudes at specific frequencies around 30 Hz on osteogenesis in bone repair. Stimulation using the ovine tibial osteotomy external fixation model and a regimen of 250 µm displacement at 30 Hz was applied for a short period each day directly to the fixator. The functional loading for the remainder of each day resulted in interfragmentary displacements on the order of 1 mm. Compared with the unstimulated controls, there was an enhancement in the progression of healing, particularly in the formation of periosteal callus. This resulted in a significantly greater torsional stiffness.[20] In other studies using a resonance technique to apply interfragmentary displacements of 20 µm at 20 Hz, researchers found no statistically significant overall effect, although they did report 11%

greater callus in the stimulated group compared with controls.[21] Chen and associates[22] used a rabbit radius model to evaluate the effects of different frequencies of mechanical vibration on the repair of a fracture of the radius. They found that all vibration stimuli enhanced repair compared with the nonstimulated control. The most effective vibration frequencies were 25 Hz and 50 Hz. Interestingly, application of a vibration resonance stimulus of 25 Hz enhanced bone formation and ingrowth into porous implants and increased callus formation in a fracture model.[23] These data suggest a frequency-dependent relationship with displacement magnitude, again resembling the effects seen in intact bone. Additionally, osteogenic mechanical stimulation appears to influence the periosteal callus and may be acting on the process of intramembranous ossification.

## Transduction Mechanisms

Perhaps the greatest challenge in both understanding and applying the mechanical regulation of bone repair is the identification of the mechanotransduction pathways. The complex nature of the repair process in bone and the apparent sensitivity of the different tissues to mechanical regulation imply a number of potential transduction mechanisms. These may range from direct mechanical stimulation of the various cell populations, to strain-related events such as induction of streaming potentials and fluid shear stresses, to matrix effects to which the various cells respond.

Direct deformation of cells has been shown to influence both proliferation and cell metabolism in vitro.[24] Zhuang and associates[25] showed an association between applied mechanical stimulation and both osteoblast proliferation and transforming growth factor-beta (TGF-$\beta$) production. Neidlinger-Wilke and associates[26] demonstrated that the response of bone cells to direct strain in vitro was modulated in skeletal conditions, such as osteoporosis, in which osteoblasts responded to in vitro cyclical strain with reduced proliferation and TGF-$\beta$ synthesis compared with osteoblasts from normal subjects. Mechanical stresses can also regulate gene expression for extracellular matrix constituents.[27] Dynamic fluid pressures have been shown to regulate chondrogenesis in vitro.[28] The cells may also respond to fluid shear stresses and the electric effects of streaming potentials as ionic fluids flow within both the cells and matrix as a consequence of mechanical deformation of skeletal structures.[29,30] The effect of high rate micromotion could therefore be a direct effect of strain at the cellular level or, alternatively, mediated indirectly as a consequence of fluid movement and streaming potentials. The effect of high strain rates on the viscoelastic properties of fracture callus could also alter the strains induced in the fragment ends and associated cell signaling to periosteal cells and periosteal callus formation.

The transduction pathway of mechanical strain in bone has been shown to involve the prostaglandins.[31] Inhibitors of prostaglandin synthesis such as indomethacin, which blocks both constitutive and inducible cyclooxygenases, down-regulate the adaptive response of bone to mechanical stimulation.[32,33] The prostaglandins also play a role in bone repair. The effects of mechanical stimulation using applied cyclical interfragmentary micromotion involve the presence of endogenous prostaglandins. Different regimens of micromotion were shown to be associated with different levels of prostaglandins in the callus at a very early stage of the repair process.[34]

Recently it has been found that mechanical strain in intact bone acts via the estrogen receptor, and thus this receptor provides a common pathway for mechanical and hormonal activation of bone cells.[35,36] Estrogen receptor mRNA has also been found in fracture callus[37] and thus could represent part of the transduction pathway for mechanical modulation of bone healing. Furthermore, evidence suggests that estrogen receptors are only found in the callus tissues present in the early stages of healing, not those in the latter stages.[38] This may also be related to the importance of imposing the correct mechanical stimulus in the early stages of repair. Thus, manipulation of estrogen-related pathways also has the potential to modulate the progression of bone healing.

Further studies are needed to investigate effects of mechanical stimulation with inhibition or overexpression of the suggested mediators of mechanical stimulation, using a mechanically defined model of bone repair. Determining the levels of mediators associated with specific doses of mechanical input at defined stages of the repair process would also assist in unraveling the complex transduction pathways.

## Time-related Application of Mechanical Regulation of Indirect Bone Repair

Some of the putative mediators of mechanotransduction are present in the very early stages of healing at levels associated with specific regimens of mechanical stimulation, again suggesting the importance of early mechanical regulation of repair. Some studies in which mechanical stimulation was applied later in the healing period have shown either no effect when applied at 4 weeks[39] or a destruction of the forming callus when a regimen shown to be stimulatory in the early stages was applied 6 weeks postosteotomy. Both studies were conducted using a 3-mm ovine tibial osteotomy model.[16] Coutts and associates[40] reported a transient beneficial effect of a delay of 2 weeks in plate fixation of osteotomies in terms of bone formation and progression of healing. These observations suggest an important role of interfragmentary motion in the early stages of repair. The role of mechanical stimulation in relation to timing may concur with some methods of biologic stimulation— for example, a single application of TGF-$\beta$ preoperatively induced subsequent healing of the defect in a rodent critical defect model with controlled mechanical environment.[41] The normal presence of TGF-$\beta$ in the early phase of fracture repair has been shown to be stimulated by and persists under the influence of mechanical forces in distraction osteogenesis.[42] Lewinson and associates[43] recently reported the early activation of gene expression for c-Fos and c-Jun with expression retained in preosteoblasts and osteoblasts in an ovine distraction osteogenesis model. Recent mathematical modeling studies also imply a benefit of early moderate loading and the adverse effects of late excessive loading on progression of bone healing.[44]

## Clinical Application of Mechanical Regulation of Fracture Repair

Following experimental studies, the principles of mechanical regulation of bone repair by imposed mechanical stimulation regimens have also been investigated in human clinical fractures. Application of micromotion from an early stage of repair enhanced the rate of healing. The application of a mechanical stimulus increased the rate of healing with respect to an objective end point of fracture.[45,46] Another trial in human patients was performed by Kershaw and associates[47] in which the magnitude of interfragmentary motion was determined in the early stages of healing and found to be in the order of 0.6 mm. This was then increased by 50% using an externally attached actuator. A significant reduction in healing time was obtained using micromotion applied in the early stages of the healing process.

## Future Studies

The varied responses reported in different studies, although indicating general effects of mechanical regulation of bone repair, have not defined the mechanical characteristics and optimal times for application in terms of dose and stage of repair that could be used to enhance or inhibit bone healing. There is a need for standardization of models to allow a more valuable and productive elucidation of mechanical regulation of bone repair and identification of transduction mechanisms. Because repair is both influenced by biologic factors and sensitive to mechanical influences, these conditions must be controlled and defined in a model to allow the assessment of regulatory mechanical stimuli. The appropriate dose, duration, and timing of treatment are in need of further definition.

The restoration of mechanical and structural integrity also requires improved understanding of tissue responses and new technology for monitoring and imaging tissue responses. Such studies will not only improve the management of fractures but also have implications for the engineering of connective tissues for repair and replacement of skeletal structures.

## References

1. Chalmers J, Ray RD: The growth of transplanted fetal bones in different immunological environments. *J Bone Joint Surg Br* 1962;44:149-164.

2. Fell HB: Skeletal development in tissue culture, in Bourne GH (ed): *The Biochemistry and Physiology of Bone*. New York, NY, Academic Press, 1956.

3. Rubin CT, McLeod KJ: Promotion of bony ingrowth by frequency-specific, low-amplitude mechanical strain. *Clin Orthop* 1994;298:165-174.

4. Carter DR, Blenman PR, Beaupre GS: Correlations between mechanical stress history and tissue differentiation in initial fracture healing. *J Orthop Res* 1988;6:736-748.

5. Carter DR, Beaupre GS, Giori NJ, Helms JA: Mechanobiology of skeletal regeneration. *Clin Orthop* 1998;355:S41-S55.

Section One   Biophysical Regulation of Clinical Bone Healing

6. Claes LE, Heigele CA: Magnitudes of local stress and strain along bony surfaces predict the course and type of fracture healing. *J Biomech* 1999;32:255-266.

7. Perren SM: Physical and biological aspects of fracture healing with special reference to internal fixation. *Clin Orthop* 1979;138:175-196.

8. Cheal EJ, Mansmann KA, DiGioia AM, Hayes WC, Perren SM: Role of interfragmentary strain in fracture healing: Ovine model of a healing osteotomy. *J Orthop Res* 1991;9:131-142.

9. Goodship AE, Watkins PE, Rigby HS, Kenwright J: The role of fixator frame stiffness in the control of fracture healing: An experimental study. *J Biomech* 1993;26:1027-1035.

10. Goodship AE, Cunningham JL, Lawes TJ: Sensitivity of endochondral fracture repair to interfragmentary motion levels modulated by biofeedback mechanism. *Trans 44th Annual Meeting.* Rosemont, IL, Orthopaedic Research Society, 1998.

11. Claes LE, Wilke HJ, Augat P, Rubenacker S, Margevicius KJ: Effect of dynamization on gap healing of diaphyseal fractures under external fixation. *J Orthop Trauma* 1995; 5:351-364.

12. Claes L, Wolf S, Augat P: Mechanical modification of callus healing. *Chirurg* 2000; 71:989-994.

13. Claes L, Eckert-Hubner K, Augat P: The effect of mechanical stability on local vascularization and tissue differentiation in callus healing. *J Orthop Res* 2002;20:1099-1105.

14. Goodship AE, Kenwright J: The influence of induced micromovement upon the healing of experimental tibial fractures. *J Bone Joint Surg Br* 1985;67:650-655.

15. Kenwright J, Goodship AE: Controlled mechanical stimulation in the treatment of tibial fractures. *Clin Orthop* 1989;241:36-47.

16. Goodship AE, Cunningham JL, Kenwright J: Strain rate and timing of stimulation in mechanical modulation of fracture healing. *Clin Orthop* 1998;355:S105-S115.

17. Wolf S, Janousek A, Pfeil J, et al: The effects of external mechanical stimulation on the healing of diaphyseal osteotomies fixed by flexible external fixation. *Clin Biomech* 1998;13:359-364.

18. Augat P, Merk J, Wolf S, Claes L: Mechanical stimulation by external application of cyclic tensile strains does not effectively enhance bone healing. *J Orthop Trauma* 2001; 15:54-60.

19. Clasbrummel B, Muhr G, Goodship AE: Time-dependent mechanical stimulation of enchondral fracture healing in the sheep. *Biomed Tech* 1997;42:521-522.

20. Goodship AE, Lawes TJ, Rubin CT: Low magnitude high frequency mechanical stimulation of endochondral bone repair. *Orthop Trans* 1997;22:234.

21. Wolf S, Augat P, Eckert-Hubner K, Laule A, Krischak GD, Claes LE: Effects of high-frequency, low-magnitude mechanical stimulus on bone healing. *Clin Orthop* 2001; 385:192-198.

22. Chen LP, Han ZB, Yang XZ: The effects of frequency of mechanical vibration on experimental fracture healing. *Zhonghua Wai Ke Za Zhi* 1994;32:217-219.

23. Usui Y, Zerwekh JE, Vanharanta H, Ashman RB, Mooney V: Different effects of mechanical vibration on bone ingrowth into porous hydroxyapatite and fracture healing in a rabbit model. *J Orthop Res* 1989;7:559-567.

24. Neidlinger-Wilke C, Wilke HJ, Claes L: Cyclic stretching of human osteoblasts affects proliferation and metabolism: A new experimental method and its application. *J Orthop Res* 1994;12:70-78.

25. Zhuang H, Wang W, Tahernia AD, Levitz CL, Luchetti WT, Brighton CT: Mechanical strain-induced proliferation of osteoblastic cells parallels increased TGF-beta 1 mRNA. *Biochem Biophys Res Commun* 1996;229:449-453.

26. Neidlinger-Wilke C, Stalla I, Claes L, et al: Human osteoblasts from younger normal and osteoporotic donors show differences in proliferation and TGF beta-release in response to cyclic strain. *J Biomech* 1995;28:1411-1418.

27. Chiquet M: Regulation of extracellular matrix gene expression by mechanical stress. *Matrix Biol* 1999;18:417-426.

28. Mukherjee N, Saris DB, Schultz FM, Berglund LJ, An KN, O'Driscoll SW: The enhancement of periosteal chondrogenesis in organ culture by dynamic fluid pressure. *J Orthop Res* 2001;19:524-530.

29. MacGinitie LA, Wu DD, Cochran GV: Streaming potentials in healing, remodeling, and intact cortical bone. *J Bone Miner Res* 1993;8:1323-1335.

30. Knothe-Tate ML, Steck R, Forwood MR, Niederer P: In vivo demonstration of load-induced fluid flow in the rat tibia and its potential implications for processes associated with functional adaptation. *J Exp Biol* 2000;203:2737-2745.

31. Zaman G, Suswillo RF, Cheng MZ, Tavares IA, Lanyon LE: Early responses to dynamic strain change and prostaglandins in bone-derived cells in culture. *J Bone Miner Res* 1997;12:769-777.

32. Pead MJ, Lanyon LE: Indomethacin modulation of load-related stimulation of new bone formation in vivo. *Calcif Tissue Int* 1989;45:34-40.

33. Norrdin RW, Jee WS, High WB: The role of prostaglandins in bone in vivo. *Prostaglandins Leukot Essent Fatty Acids* 1990;41:139-149.

34. Goodship AE, Norrdin R, Francis M: The stimulation of prostaglandin synthesis by micromovement in experimental leg-lengthening, in Turner-Smith AR (ed): *Micromovement in Orthopaedics.* Cambridge, England, Oxford University Press, 1993, pp 291-295.

35. Jessop HL, Sjoberg M, Cheng MZ, Zaman G, Wheeler-Jones CP, Lanyon LE: Mechanical strain and estrogen activate estrogen receptor alpha in bone cells. *J Bone Miner Res* 2001;16:1045-1055.

36. Ehrlich PJ, Noble BS, Jessop HL, Stevens HY, Mosley JR, Lanyon LE: The effect of in vivo mechanical loading on estrogen receptor alpha expression in rat ulnar osteocytes. *J Bone Miner Res* 2002;17:1646-1655.

37. Boden SD, Joyce ME, Oliver B, Heydemann A, Bolander ME: Estrogen receptor mRNA expression in callus during fracture healing in the rat. *Calcif Tissue Int* 1989;45:324-325.

38. Monaghan BA, Kaplan FS, Lyttle CR, Fallon MD, Boden SD, Haddad JG: Estrogen receptors in fracture healing. *Clin Orthop* 1992;280:277-280.

39. Hente R, Cordey J, Rahn BA, Maghsudi M, von Gumppenberg S, Perren SM: Fracture healing of the sheep tibia treated using a unilateral external fixator: Comparison of static and dynamic fixation. *Injury* 1999;30:A44-A51.

40. Coutts RD, Woo SL, Boyer J, et al: The effect of delayed internal fixation on healing of the osteotomized dog radius. *Clin Orthop* 1982;163:254-260.

41. Harrison LJ, Cunningham JL, Stromberg L, Goodship AE: Controlled induction of a pseudarthrosis: A study using a rodent model. *J Orthop Trauma* 2003;17:11-21.

42. Yeung HY, Lee KM, Fung KP, Leung KS: Sustained expression of transforming growth factor-beta 1 by distraction during distraction osteogenesis. *Life Sci* 2002;71: 67-79.

43. Lewinson D, Rachmiel A, Rihani-Bisharat S, et al: Stimulation of fos- and jun-related genes during distraction osteogenesis. *J Histochem Cytochem* 2003;51:1161-1168.

44. Bailon-Plaza A, van der Meulen MC: Beneficial effects of moderate, early loading and adverse effects of delayed or excessive loading on bone healing. *J Biomech* 2003; 36:1069-1077.

45. Richardson JB, Cunningham JL, Goodship AE, O'Connor BT, Kenwright J: Measuring stiffness can define healing of tibial fractures. *J Bone Joint Surg Br* 1994; 76:389-394.

46. Kenwright J, Richardson JB, Cunningham JL, et al: Axial movement and tibial fractures: A controlled randomised trial of treatment. *J Bone Joint Surg Br* 1991;73:654-659.

47. Kershaw CJ, Cunningham JL, Kenwright J: Tibial external fixation, weight bearing, and fracture movement. *Clin Orthop* 1993;293:28-36.

# Chapter 3

# Pulsed Low-Intensity Ultrasound for Fracture Healing: A Review of Clinical and In Vivo Evidence

*R. Bruce Heppenstall, MD*

## Introduction

Ultrasound exists in a number of different product formats, ranging from surgical excision using high-intensity focused ultrasound, through medium intensity physiotherapy ultrasound, to low-intensity, short-burst ultrasound for diagnostic imaging. Many parameters besides intensity can vary in an ultrasound signal, including the ultrasonic carrier frequency, signal modulation, pulse frequency, pulse duration, pulse profile, duty cycle, beam profile, beam uniformity, mechanical index, and degree of acoustic impedance matching of the transducer to tissue.

Casual use of the phrase therapeutic ultrasound can lead to confusion between physiotherapy ultrasound and fracture repair ultrasound. This confusion presumably accounts for the findings of Busse and Bhandari[1] who reported that some orthopaedic surgeons and physiotherapy students believe therapeutic ultrasound to be contraindicated or harmful to healing bone, which indeed is true for physiotherapy ultrasound.

Only one type of ultrasound has approval for sale in the United States for the treatment of fractures and other osseous defects. This ultrasound signal consists of 1.5 MHz ultrasound wave pulsed at 1 kHz with a 20% duty cycle at an intensity of 30 mW/cm$^2$ SATA (spatial average temporal average) applied for 20 minutes per day. When tested in water, the devices deliver a broadly collimated beam with a high degree of spatial uniformity, low mechanical index, and high impedance matching. This combination will hereafter be referred to as PLIUS (pulsed low-intensity ultrasound).

PLIUS is widely used within the clinical community to accelerate healing of fresh fractures, to minimize delayed healing, and to stimulate healing of established nonunions. This chapter reviews the clinical and in vivo evidence available for this technology and focuses on controlled clinical and in vivo studies either reported in peer reviewed journals, submitted to the Food and Drug Administration (FDA) as part of the approval process, or presented at clinical research conferences with peer review acceptance procedures. A substantial body of case review work also exists, and although these findings shed important light on potential new areas for controlled study investigation, they have not been included. Also excluded, for brevity, are studies on mandibular fractures, distraction osteogenesis, osteoporosis, and spinal fusion.

Three review reports cover different aspects of the technology. Rubin and associates[2] produced a comprehensive review of the history, clinical evidence, and basic science evidence for ultrasound as of 2001. Warden and associates[3] reviewed similar evidence in the context of the clinic as well as various phases of the repair process, and Busse and associates[4] conducted a systematic review and meta-analysis of clinical evidence.

## Early Work

In the 1950s, Corradi and Cozzolino[5,6] used continuous wave rather than pulsed ultrasound and demonstrated enhancement of callus formation, first in a rabbit model and then in a small clinical study. Also using continuous wave ultrasound, Reuter and associates[7,8] achieved similar positive effects. Dyson and Brookes[9] used a 500 mW/cm$^2$ pulsed signal to demonstrate accelerated fracture healing, as did Klug and associates[10] with a 200 mW/cm$^2$ signal. Duarte,[11] building on this earlier work, investigated a range of signals with varying ultrasound frequencies, but all were pulsed and of low intensity. He demonstrated 28% acceleration in cortical bridging in a controlled rabbit osteotomy model. Pilla and associates[12] conducted a large controlled study of PLIUS in 139 rabbits with midshaft fibular osteotomies. They demonstrated that the actively treated group achieved a torsional strength equivalent to intact bone at day 17 as opposed to day 28 for the control group.

## Device Safety

A number of studies and evaluations of PLIUS were submitted as part of the premarket approval (PMA) process.[13] The toxicology studies demonstrated no pathologic, histologic, or hematologic changes in vital organs of animals with fractures treated by PLIUS. An independent university-based medical expert in ultrasound concluded that the maximum temperature rise under a worst-case scenario would be less than 1°C, which is considered insignificant. It was also concluded that the specifics of the beam profile would make nonthermal effects such as transient cavitation highly unlikely. Subsequent PMA supplements[14] also demonstrated that the benefits of ultrasound in fracture repair were not affected by the presence of a metallic internal fixation device, that there were no untoward effects on tissue histology in the presence of metallic implants, and that the stability and structural integrity of pins or screws subjected to PLIUS were unchanged. Additionally, in vivo temperature changes were measured in bone with a 20-minute application of PLIUS. In the presence of an intramedullary rod, a temperature elevation of 0.15°C was observed. In the absence of a rod, there was no detectable temperature change.

# Initial Pivotal Studies of Clinical Effect in Fresh Fractures

The pivotal investigations on PLIUS in fresh fractures were reported by Heckman and associates[15] and Kristiansen and associates.[16] These prospective, placebo-controlled, randomized, double-blind, multicenter studies were two of the first examples of such rigorously designed studies reported in the orthopaedic literature.

Heckman and associates[15] examined 67 closed or grade I open cortical tibial fractures. Their study demonstrated that PLIUS treatment induced a 38% acceleration in achieving the prospectively defined primary end point of a combination of clinical and radiographic healing with PLIUS treatment (96 ± 4.9 days in the active group versus 154 ± 13.7 days in the control group; $P < 0.0001$). Radiographic healing was defined as three out of four cortices bridged as judged by the blinded principal investigator. Various alternative end points were also assessed and are summarized in Table 1.

The second pivotal study, by Kristiansen and associates,[16] included 61 conservatively treated cancellous radial fractures with the prospectively defined primary end point of a combination of clinical and radiographic healing (in this case four out of four cortices bridged as judged by the blinded principal investigator). Again it was demonstrated that PLIUS treatment accelerated healing by 38% (61 ± 3.4 days in the active group versus 98 ± 5.2 days in the control group; $P < 0.0001$). Statistically significant accelerations were also seen for a range of intermediate assessments including first, second, third, or fourth cortex bridged (22%, 23%, 34%, and 39%

**Table 1 Primary and Secondary Healed Fracture End Points for Closed or Grade I Open Tibial Fractures Treated With PLIUS or a Placebo (Heckman et al[15])**

|  | Days After Fracture Active | Days After Fracture Placebo | Percentage Acceleration Versus Placebo | P value ANOVA |
|---|---|---|---|---|
| **Clinical Healing** | 86 ± 5.8 | 114 ± 10.4 | 25 | 0.01 |
| **3 Cortices Bridged** | | | | |
| Blinded Principal Investigator | 89 ± 3.7 | 148 ± 13.2 | 40 | 0.0001 |
| Blinded Independent Radiologist | 102 ± 4.8 | 190 ± 18.3 | 46 | 0.0001 |
| **4 Cortices Bridged** | | | | |
| Blinded Principal Investigator | 114 ± 7.5 | 182 ± 15.8 | 37 | 0.0002 |
| Blinded Independent Radiologist | 136 ± 9.6 | 243 ± 18.4 | 79 | 0.0001 |
| **Endosteal Healing** | | | | |
| Blinded Principal Investigator | 117 ± 8.5 | 167 ± 13.9 | 30 | 0.002 |
| Blinded Independent Radiologist | 171 ± 13.6 | 271 ± 19.6 | 37 | 0.0001 |

respectively) and percentage organized trabecular bridging at weeks 5, 6, 8, 10, 12, and 16 (325%, 208%, 180%, 106%, 67%, and 35% respectively).

It is also interesting to note the impact of PLIUS on the rate of delayed union or nonunion. Figures 1 and 2 show the cumulative heal rate for tibial fractures[15] and distal radius fractures[16] respectively. Cook and associates[17] used a 150-day definition of delayed union and determined that there was a statistically significant difference ($P < 0.003$) in delayed union rate (active group 6% versus control group 36%). If 6 months were to be taken as a reasonable definition of nonunion for such fractures, then all of the active group were healed at that time whereas more than 20% of the control group had not healed, suggesting a positive effect of PLIUS on reducing the incidence of nonunion. The cumulative percentage of distal radius fractures healed at various time points (Fig. 2) again allows for an assessment of impact on the rate of delayed union or nonunion. For example, at the 120-day time point, 97% of the active group had healed versus 84% of the control group.

Kristiansen and associates[16] also assessed how PLIUS affected fracture reduction during healing. The subset of fractures that were satisfactorily reduced after presenting with at least 10° of negative volar angulation (15 active and 17 control) were analyzed. The active group demonstrated less ultimate loss of reduction compared with the placebo group (20% versus 43% respectively; $P < 0.01$), less time to loss of reduction stopping (12 days versus 25 days), and higher incidence of reduction being maintained to the degree achieved at surgery (7 versus 3).

In these pivotal studies, long-term follow-up of all patients able to be contacted confirmed that all fractures remained healed, with the duration of follow-up a minimum of 2 years for tibial fractures and an average of 6 years for distal radius fractures.

In a separate analysis of data from these two studies, Cook and associates[17] demonstrated that the acceleration in healing due to PLIUS was significantly greater in the subset of people who smoked versus nonsmokers (41% versus 26% respectively in the tibial study, and 51% versus 34% respectively in the radial study). Remarkably, the heal time for smokers in the active group was lower than that for the placebo-treated nonsmokers and similar to that for the actively treated nonsmokers. The conclusions drawn from these data include the statement that PLIUS mitigates the delayed healing effects of smoking. It could be argued that PLIUS is particularly suited to fractures that have a risk of delayed healing due to factors related to a patient's general health and lifestyle.

## In Vivo Evidence of Bone Quality

Clearly there is no opportunity in clinical studies to analyze bone quality histologically, but numerous preclinical studies have been conducted, and these indicate that the acceleration of bone healing induced by PLIUS has no negative impact on the quality of bone. In vivo studies in rat fracture models[18-20] confirmed the earlier work in rabbits[12] in which PLIUS accelerated fracture healing, as evidenced by increased mechanical properties at the fracture site. Wang and associates[18] and Yang and associates[21] also demonstrated some

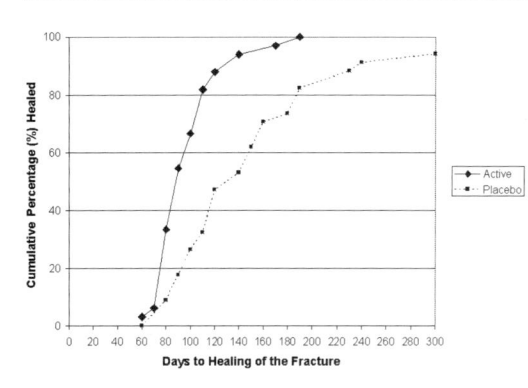

**Figure 1** Cumulative heal rate of clinically and radiographically healed closed or grade I open tibial fractures treated with PLIUS and with a placebo. *(Reproduced with permission from Heckman JD, Ryaby JP, McCabe J, Frey JJ, Kilcoyne RF: Acceleration of tibial fracture healing by noninvasive, low-intensity pulsed ultrasound. J Bone Joint Surg Am 1994;76:26-34.)*

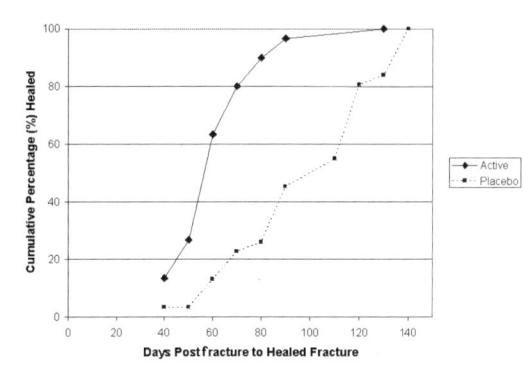

**Figure 2** Cumulative percentage of distal radius fractures that healed with active PLIUS and with a placebo. *(Reproduced with permission from Kristiansen TK, Ryaby JP, McCabe J, Frey JJ, Roe LR: Accelerated healing of distal radial fractures with the use of specific low-intensity ultrasound. J Bone Joint Surg Am 1997;79:961-973.)*

sensitivity in healing profile to the specifics of the signal parameters, testing ultrasound frequency and intensity respectively. Through histologic analysis and micro CT, Azuma and associates[19] were able to determine that fracture healing in the PLIUS-treated group, although accelerated, was typical of normal bone healing. Their investigation showed an impact at early, middle, and late stages of fracture healing with maximum impact achieved when treatment was applied throughout the healing process. Their analysis suggested PLIUS-induced cellular reactions at each phase of fracture healing from inflammation through to endochondral ossification. Spadaro and Albanese[22] looked at the impact of PLIUS on the epiphyseal region of the tibia and femur in immature rats. Experiments were done both with intact bones and after surgical periosteal abrasion to the femur. No significant difference was seen in bone length or bone mineral density, indicating that physeal bone growth is less sensitive to PLIUS than fracture repair. This finding suggests that treatment of a fracture in the vicinity of a growth plate may be appropriate.

Takikawa and associates[23] studied the impact of PLIUS in a hypertrophic nonunion model, demonstrating 50% resolution in the active group versus 0% in the control group at 6 weeks. Analysis by micro CT and histology again suggested no abnormalities in the resultant healed or healing callus.

## Subsequent Fresh Fracture Clinical Evidence

Two single-center, prospective, placebo-controlled, randomized, double-blind studies, each approximately half the size of the initial pivotal studies, have investigated the impact of PLIUS on surgically treated tibial fractures. The first of these, by Emami and associates,[24] used inclusion criteria similar to that of Heckman and associates[15] but treated with closed reduction and a reamed, statically locked intramedullary nail. The primary end point of radiographic healing (three out of four cortices bridged) showed no statistically significant difference between the active group and control group, but data indicated a trend toward slower healing in the active group. Discussing the contrast between the results of this study and those seen by Heckman and associates,[15] the authors considered factors that may have affected the outcome. These included differences in loading between nailed and casted fractures, the presence of metal, the length of treatment (treated until healed in the Heckman study but only 75 days in Emami's study), and the low incidence of smokers. No definitive conclusion could be reached as to why the data between these studies were in disagreement.

The second study on tibial fractures[25] (single-center, prospective, placebo-controlled, randomized, double-blind) investigated the impact of PLIUS on open, comminuted, and segmental fractures of varying severity treated with either reamed, locked intramedullary nails (closed diaphyseal or Gustillo I and II open) or external fixation (Gustillo IIIA and metaphyseal). An acceleration of at least 40% was seen for the actively treated group in all clinical and radiographic assessments (Table 2).

DXA measurement of bone mineral content at the fracture site was consistently higher in the active group and reached statistical significance at weeks 6, 15, 18, and 21. Plasma bone-specific alkaline phosphatase activity (a good measure of osteoblastic activity) was also measured and again was generally higher in the active group, reaching significance at weeks 12, 18, and 27. An interesting observation from the radiographs is that fracture callus appearance was independent of whether the cortex was at the side where the transducer was placed or the side directly opposite.

The effect of PLIUS on fractures of types of bone besides long bone has also been clinically studied. A single-center, prospective, placebo-controlled, randomized, double-blind study of 40 scaphoid fractures[26] demonstrated a statistically significant 31% acceleration in the primary end point of clinical plus radiographic healing (active 43 days; control 62 days; $P < 0.01$) and a 41% improvement in percentage of trabecular bridging at 6 weeks (active 81%, control 55%, $P < 0.05$). A smaller (n = 20) single-center, prospective, placebo-controlled, randomized, double-blind study of Jones' fractures[27] showed that all actively treated fractures healed within 56 days whereas only 60% of placebo-treated fractures had healed by 87 days and 20% remained unhealed after 140 days. In addition, the actively treated group reached pain-free status 31 to 70 days earlier than the placebo group and on average took only half the rehabilitation time.

**Table 2 Clinical and Radiographic Healed Fracture End Points for Complex Tibial Fractures Treated With PLIUS or a Placebo (Leung et al[25])**

|  | PLIUS Treatment | Placebo Treatment | Acceleration Compared With Placebo | P Value (two-sided Student's *t*-test) |
|---|---|---|---|---|
| Time to full weight bearing (weeks) | 9.3 ± 2.1 | 15.5 ± 3.0 | 40% | < 0.05 |
| Time to removal of external fixator (weeks) | 9.9 ± 3.8 | 17.1 ± 8.5 | 42% | < 0.05 |
| Time to 3 cortices bridged (weeks) | 11.5 ± 3.0 | 20 ± 4.0 | 43% | < 0.05 |

The study by Rue and associates[28] showed no statistically significant difference in time to become asymptomatic from (mainly) tibial stress fractures, although after discounting the delay in diagnosis and delay in treatment (when there was no active or control treatment), there was a 13% trend to faster healing in the active group (27.5 ± 11.6 active; 31.5 ± 13.2 control). The variability in outcome (see above SDs), the difficulty in diagnosis (only 10 out of 47 fractures were diagnosed by bone scan), and the subjectivity of outcome measure make the suggested acceleration statistically insignificant with this size of study (n = 47). To declare the difference between the mean healing rates of the active and control groups statistically significant, patient groups of approximately 150 per side would be needed.

Frankel[29] reviewed the status of a postmarket surveillance registry after 3,737 completed treatments, classifying fractures by the time at which PLIUS treatment started. For the fresh fracture subset (treatment started within 90 days; n = 2,040), high success rates were seen for all bones regardless of the superficiality of the fracture site or the type of primary fracture management (eg, 94% for femur and 93% for tibia). High success rates were also seen for some disease or comorbidity states that might normally be expected to reduce treatment efficacy, such as diabetes mellitus or infection.

## The Role of PLIUS in Fresh Fracture Treatment

One testable hypothesis that suggests itself is that maximum clinical impact of PLIUS use will be in those situations in which normal healing may be expected to be compromised or at risk, whether by fracture characteristics, primary fracture management technique, patient illness, medication or substance abuse, or some combination of these factors. The data fit this hypothesis while also allowing for alternatives.

Several studies demonstrated acceleration of fracture healing and suggested a reduction in incidence of complications, delayed union, or nonunion. The indications studied either could be described as hard-to-heal fractures by definition[25-27] or demonstrated increased magnitude of effect for higher-risk patient groups.[17] Registry information in a range of bones and with a range of primary fracture management techniques demonstrates equally high success rates with concomitant disease states and medication use that might be expected to reduce effectiveness.

In the only study that showed no acceleration,[24] a number of possible reasons were discussed for this result. It was suggested that this outcome may be due to load shielding because of the presence of intramedullary nails, but this possibility has been contradicted by the complex tibial fracture study.[25] That same study, coupled with the nonunion evidence (see below), supports ultrasound's ability to be effective in treatment alongside metal implants including reamed intramedullary nails. Cook and associates[17] showed significant acceleration even in the nonsmoking group, implying that the lack of smokers in the study by Emami and associates[24] is not the single cause. In vivo evidence shown by Azuma and associates[19] suggests the importance of treatment throughout healing, although Emami and associates[24] note no difference in healing response during the time that the fractures were being stimulated. The small size of the study, along with the resultant possibility of type II or beta error, also needs to be considered; however, the explanation that best fits the above hypothesis is that the fixation technique used in this study is already optimal for such relatively simple fractures with no comorbidities.

## Nonunion and Delayed Union

Controlled clinical studies to evaluate stimulation devices for the treatment of nonunions have been limited by either the ethical unacceptability of placebo-controlled studies or the confounding nature of surgical treatment as a control arm. For these reasons, every stimulation device has used self-controlled study data. While it is recognized that this situation is not ideal, certain factors in the study design make such studies clinically meaningful.

A common approach informed three studies submitted to the FDA[14] as the basis for established nonunion approval. Nonunion fractures had to have been established for a minimum time and had to have not undergone recent surgery in order to rule out the possibility of spontaneous healing from that treatment. In addition, the only change in treatment at the PLIUS start date had to be the application of the device. Table 3 summarizes the results of the three prospective self-paired studies.

A total of 409 nonunion fractures averaged greater than 21 months since fracture date and greater than 15 months since any prior surgery, which would classify them as established nonunions unlikely to heal spontaneously. With no other change in treatment, these fractures resolved at a success rate of more than 80% when stimulated with PLIUS.

Nolte and associates,[30] reporting on the Netherlands study, confirmed the 86% success rate and showed the average healing time to be around 5 months. Patients had previously undergone an average of 1.4 failed surgical procedures. Although the small numbers in this study make stratification imprecise, high success rates were seen with atrophic and oligotrophic nonunions (80% and 92% respectively) where some biologic deficiency may contribute to the original nonunion. Additionally, the application of PLIUS to hyper-

**Table 3 Summary Data of Nonunion Studies Presented to the FDA**

| | Fracture Inclusion Criteria Defined Within the Protocol | | Fracture Characteristics of Included Patient Cohort | | Outcome | |
|---|---|---|---|---|---|---|
| | Fracture age (months) | Time since last surgery (months) | Fracture age (months) | Time since last surgery (months) | Number of fractures | Success rate (%) |
| Netherlands study[30] | 6 | 3 | 14.0 | 12.2 | 29 | 868 |
| Germany study[31] | 8 | 4 | 31.0 | 24.2 | 67 | 85 |
| US study[32] | 9 | 3 | 20.0 | 14.2 | 313 | 80 |
| Average | | | 21.3 | 15.7 | | 81.2 |

trophic nonunions, which might usually be considered as requiring revised treatment to correct fracture instability, was successful in 80% of cases. Success was seen for a range of bones, all types of typical primary fracture management, and across all patient age ranges. Mayr and associates[31] supported the effectiveness of PLIUS across the different types of nonunions in their study of 100 delayed and nonunion fractures. The self-paired study defined delayed unions as 120 to 240 days old (n = 64) and nonunions as greater than 240 days old (n = 36). At least 90 days had passed since any prior treatment change, and the only change at the start date of the study was the use of PLIUS. Both delayed unions and nonunions resolved at an 86% success rate, with an 83% success rate in atrophic nonunions (n = 84) and a 100% success rate in hypertrophic nonunions (n = 16).

The German data reaffirmed the Nolte analysis but with larger patient numbers. In this case, patients had an average of 1.5 prior surgeries, but PLIUS showed high success rates for a range of bones, all types of nonunion, all typical primary fracture management techniques, and all patient age ranges. Fracture types included closed, open, arthrodesis, and osteotomy. Of note is the fact that the fractures that did not heal averaged over 8 years in fracture age and were predominantly scaphoid fractures with a long history of failed surgery.

Frankel and Mizuno[32] reviewed the above evidence along with prescription registry data from the United States and Japan. Their analysis of the US study data supported the findings reported in the Dutch and German studies. Stratification of the US 1,546-patient nonunion registry also demonstrated that, for patients with risk factors that may impair fracture healing, such as substance abuse, diabetes mellitus, vascular problems, or steroid use, there was no significant change in PLIUS efficacy. Frankel[29] provided further insight into the US patient registry by stratifying the data to include early delayed unions (91 to 150 days) and late delayed unions (151 to 269 days) in addition to fresh fractures and nonunions (270 days or greater). Again, high success rates were achieved for all bones regardless of fracture age, but there was a trend toward higher success rates and faster healing with earlier intervention.

Data from one of the largest cohorts of patients treated with PLIUS has been presented by Duarte (LR Duarte, University of Sao Paulo, Brazil, unpublished data presented at the Société Internationale de Chirurgie Orthopédique et de Traumatologie annual meeting, 1996). A total of 380 nonresponding delayed and nonunions averaging 14 months old were treated with PLIUS with an 85% success rate across a range of bones.

Collectively, these analyses have shown PLIUS to be effective at resolving all types of nonunions of all ages, with a wide range of fracture types and primary fracture management techniques. The body of evidence also demonstrates equally high success rates for deep bones and superficial bones in that healing rates in the femur are comparable with those in the tibia or metatarsal. Romano and associates[33] and Pigozzi and associates[34] have since added to the literature, reporting on prospective longitudinal studies in infected nonunions and pseudarthrosis respectively, suggesting high success rates in both situations.

## Summary

PLIUS has been demonstrated in clinical studies and routine clinical practice to be a safe adjunctive therapy for the treatment of fractures including arthrodesis and osteotomy. Acceleration of fresh fracture healing has been shown in a number of studies subject to peer review either through the publication process or through regulatory body scrutiny, or in some cases through both. The literature indicates that PLIUS can have a positive impact in the prevention of complications, such as loss of reduction or slow healing, and that the prevention of nonunions is likely. The ability to resolve established nonunions that are not responding to conventional treatment, as well as delayed unions or slow healing fractures, is clearly evident. The data supports the efficacy of PLIUS in all bones excluding skull and vertebra (regardless of how superficial or deep the bone is), all types of fracture, and as an adjunctive treatment to primary fracture management, both surgical and conservative. Additionally, there is suggestive evidence to support the mitigation of risk factors such as smoking, disease state, or medication use, some of which may still need to be proved definitively. However, there may be cases in which PLIUS does not offer benefit, either fractures that are likely to heal optimally with no adjunctive treatments or those that are beyond help. In light of all this evidence, coupled with data from in vivo studies confirming that PLIUS accelerates the normal fracture healing process, PLIUS should be considered a safe, natural adjunct to appropriate fracture stabilization for acceleration and effective resolution of fractures.

## References

1. Busse JW, Bhandari M: Therapeutic ultrasound and fracture healing: A survey of beliefs and practices. *Arch Phys Med Rehabil* 2004;85:1653-1656.

2. Rubin C, Bolander M, Ryaby JP, Hadjiargyrou M: The use of low-intensity ultrasound to accelerate the healing of fractures. *J Bone Joint Surg Am* 2001;83:259-270.

3. Warden SJ, Bennell KL, McMeeken JM, Wark JD: Acceleration of fresh fracture repair using the sonic accelerated fracture healing system (SAFHS): A review. *Calcif Tissue Int* 2000;66:157-163.

4. Busse JW, Bhandari M, Kulkarni AV, Tunks E: The effect of low-intensity pulsed ultrasound therapy on time to fracture healing: A meta-analysis. *CMAJ* 2002;166:437-441.

5. Corradi C, Cozzolino A: The action of ultrasound on the evolution of an experimental fracture in rabbits. *Minerva Orthopedica* 1952;55:44-45.

6. Corradi C, Cozzolino A: Ultrasound and bone callus formation during a fracture. *Archivo di Orthopedia* 1953;66:44-45.

7. Reuter U, Strempel F, John F, Knoch HG: Modification of bone fracture healing by ultrasound in an animal experimental model. *Z Exp Chir Transplant Künstliche Organe* 1984;17:290-297.

8. Reuter U, Strempel F, John F, Durig E: Modification of bone fracture healing by ultrasonics in an animal model: Radiologic and histologic results. *Z Exp Chir Transplant Künstliche Organe* 1987;20:294-302.

9. Dyson M, Brookes M: Stimulation of bone repair by ultrasound. *Ultrasound Med Biol* 1983;2:61-66.

10. Klug W, Franke WG, Knoch HG: Scintigraphic control of bone fracture healing under ultrasonic stimulation: An animal experimental study. *Eur J Nucl Med* 1986;11:494-497.

11. Duarte LR: The stimulation of bone growth by ultrasound. *Arch Orthop Trauma Surg* 1983;101:153-159.

12. Pilla AA, Mont MA, Nasser PR, et al: Non-invasive low-intensity pulsed ultrasound accelerates bone healing in the rabbit. *J Orthop Trauma* 1990;4:246-253.

13. US Food and Drug Administration (FDA): *Sonic Accelerated Fracture Healing System (SAFHS), Model 2A: Summary of Safety and Effectiveness.* Premarket Approval P900009. Exogen, Inc, Rockville, MD, US Food and Drug Administration, October 5, 1994.

14. US Food and Drug Administration (FDA): *Exogen 2000, 3000, or Sonic Accelerated Fracture Healing System (SAFHS): Summary of Safety and Effectiveness.* Premarket Approval P900009/Supplement 6. Exogen, Inc, Rockville, MD, US Food and Drug Administration, February 22, 2000.

15. Heckman JD, Ryaby JP, McCabe J, Frey JJ, Kilcoyne RF: Acceleration of tibial fracture healing by non-invasive, low-intensity pulsed ultrasound. *J Bone Joint Surg Am* 1994;76:26-34.

16. Kristiansen TK, Ryaby JP, McCabe J, Frey JJ, Roe LR: Accelerated healing of distal radial fractures with the use of specific low-intensity ultrasound. *J Bone Joint Surg Am* 1997;79:961-973.

17. Cook SD, Ryaby JP, McCabe J, Frey JJ, Heckman JD, Kristiansen TK: Acceleration of tibia and distal radius fracture healing in patients who smoke. *Clin Orthop* 1997;337:198-207.

18. Wang SJ, Lewallen DG, Bolander ME, Chao EYS, Ilstrup DM, Greenleaf JF: Low-intensity ultrasound treatment increases strength in a rat femoral fracture model. *J Orthop Res* 1994;12:40-47.

19. Azuma Y, Ito M, Harada Y, Takagi H, Ohta T, Jingushi S: Low-intensity pulsed ultrasound accelerates rat femoral fracture healing by acting on the various cellular reactions in the fracture callus. *J Bone Miner Res* 2001;16:671-680.

20. Gebauer GP, Lin SS, Beam HA, Vieira P, Parsons JP: Low-intensity pulsed ultrasound increases the fracture callus strength in diabetic BB Wistar rats but does not affect cellular proliferation. *J Orthop Res* 2002;20:587-592.

21. Yang K-H, Parvizi J, Wang SJ, et al: Exposure to low-intensity ultrasound increases aggrecan gene expression in a rat femur fracture model. *J Orthop Res* 1996;14:802-809.

22. Spadaro JA, Albanese SA: Application of low-intensity ultrasound to growing bone in rats. *Ultrasound Med Biol* 1998;24:567-573.

23. Takikawa S, Matsui N, Kokubu T, et al: Low-intensity pulsed ultrasound initiates bone healing in rat nonunion fracture model. *J Ultrasound Med* 2001;20:197-205.

24. Emami A, Petren-Mallmin M, Larsson S: No effect of low-intensity ultrasound on healing time of intramedullary fixed tibial fractures. *J Orthop Trauma* 1999;13:252-257.

25. Leung KS, Lee WS, Tsui HF, Liu PPL, Cheung WH: Complex tibial fracture outcomes following treatment with low-intensity pulsed ultrasound. *Ultrasound Med Biol* 2004;30:389-395.

26. Mayr E, Rudzki MM, Borchardt B, Haüsser H, Rüter A: Does pulsed low intensity ultrasound accelerate healing of scaphoid fractures? *Handchir Mikrochir Plast Chir* 2000;32:115-122.

27. Strauss E, Ryaby JP, McCabe JM: Treatment of Jones' fractures of the foot with adjunctive use of low-intensity pulsed ultrasound stimulation. *J Orthop Trauma* 1999;13:310.

28. Rue JPH, Armstrong DW, Frassica FJ, Deafenbaugh M, Wilckens JH: The effect of pulsed ultrasound in the treatment of tibial stress fractures. *Orthopedics* 2004;27:1192-1195.

29. Frankel VH: Results of prescription use of pulse ultrasound therapy in fracture management. *Surg Technol Int* 1998;7:389-393.

30. Nolte PA, van der Krans A, Patka P, Janssen IMC, Ryaby JP, Albers GHR: Low-intensity pulsed ultrasound in the treatment of nonunions. *J Trauma* 2001;51:693-703.

31. Mayr E, Möckl C, Lenich A, Ecker M, Rüter A: Is low intensity ultrasound effective in treating disorders of fracture healing? *Unfallchirurg* 2002;105:108-115.

32. Frankel VH, Mizuno K: Management of non-union with pulsed, low-intensity ultrasound therapy: International results. *Surg Technol Int* 2001;10:1-6.

33. Romano C, Messina J, Meani M: Low-intensity ultrasound for the treatment of infected nonunions, in Agazzi M, Bergami PL, Cicero G, et al (eds): *Guarderni di infezione osteoarticolari.* Milan, Italy, Masson Periodical Division, 1999, pp 83-93.

34. Pigozzi F, Moneta MR, Giombini A, et al: Low intensity pulsed ultrasound in the conservative treatment of pseudoarthrosis. *J Sports Med Phys Fitness* 2004;44:173-178.

# Chapter 4
# Electric and Magnetic Stimulation of Bone Repair: Review of the European Experience

*Ruggero Cadossi, MD*
*Gian Carlo Traina, MD*
*Leo Massari, MD*

## Introduction

The employment of physical energy to modulate osteogenetic responses and ultimately to enhance fracture healing is a topic widely researched in Europe, where the relation between biologic systems and electric energy can be dated back as far as the studies by Galvani[1] and by Black[2] who, already in the 19th century, had identified the lesion currents and had perceived their role in repair processes. In the last century, studies performed by Fukada and Yasuda[3] and by Bassett and Becker[4] identified the relationship between mechanical loading and electric activity in bone. Since then it has become clear that bone generates two types of electric signals: one type in response to mechanical deformation (direct piezoelectric effect and electrokinetic phenomenon of the flow potential) and the other type in the absence of deformation (stationary bioelectric potential and stationary electric [ionic] current). The electric signals induced by mechanical deformation and those generated by unstressed bone have been interpreted as local control factors of bone remodeling and modeling and of reparative osteogenesis.

Several experimental studies have shown how and to what extent endogenous bone repair can be enhanced in various animal models and clinical conditions, particularly in situations where repair processes have remained incomplete.[2] It has indeed been possible to quantify the effect of electric stimulation on bone growth by calculating the mineral apposition rate, which has been shown to increase by 80%[5] (Fig. 1).

In humans, electric stimulation has been used to stimulate bone repair in nonunions as well as fresh fractures. These studies have enabled evaluation of (1) the relative effectiveness of methods of applying electric stimulation to the bone tissue, and (2) modalities, times, and doses needed to obtain a positive influence on osteogenesis. Devices have been approved for clinical use by the US Food and Drug Administration (FDA) and are employed in many countries to promote the formation of bone tissue. In Europe, research on the possible application of electric and magnetic energy to bone repair processes has been ongoing throughout the past century using electric current directly applied (faradic systems), capacitively coupled electric fields (capacitive systems), and pulsed electromagnetic fields (inductive systems).

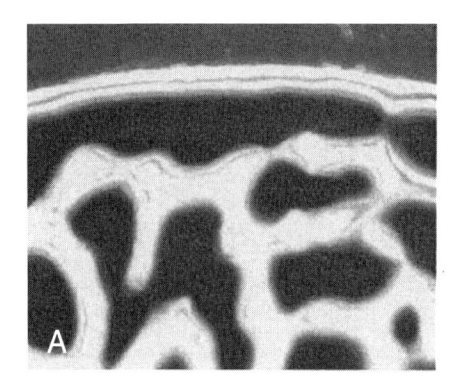

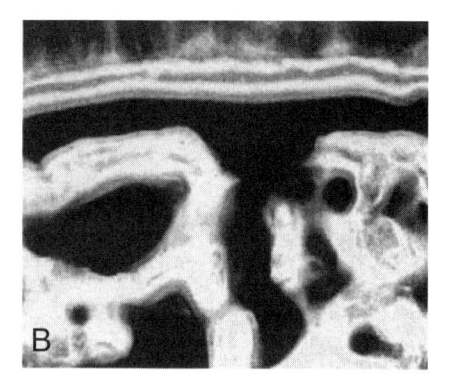

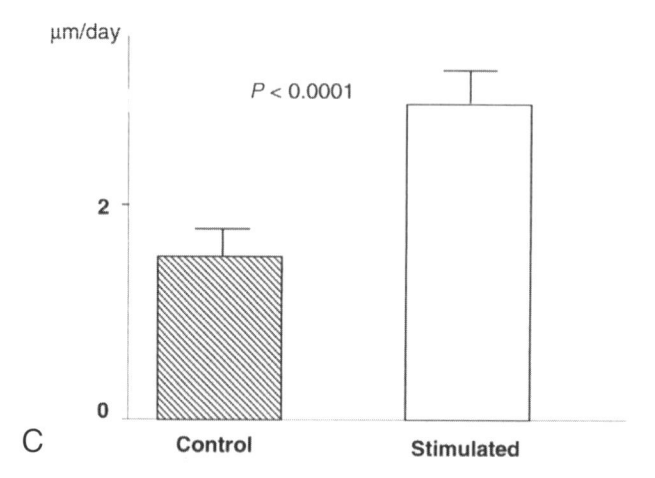

Section One    Biophysical Regulation of Clinical Bone Healing

**Figure 1** Mineral apposition rate of bone defects in the horse; tetracyclines were administered with an interval of 10 days. **A,** Labeling in control metacarpal bone. **B,** Labeling in stimulated metacarpal bone. **C,** Histogram shows the average mineral apposition rate in 12 controls (hatched bar) and in 12 stimulated (empty bar).[5]

## Directly Applied Electric Current: Faradic Systems

The effect of continuous electric current consists of both purely electric phenomena, which affect ions at the site of the fracture, and chemical-type phenomena, which lead to a reduction in the local tension of oxygen and a small increase in pH. With faradic systems, direct electric current is applied directly to the bone tissue. The therapeutic effectiveness of continuous electric current depends on its intensity. The cathode is supplied with an electric current ranging from 2 to 20 µA, a range considered optimal for stimulation of osteogenesis. The current is applied 24 hours per day; the negative pole must be positioned very precisely in the site of the fracture where stimulation of the osteogenic response is desired; the positive pole is placed in contact with the soft tissues, far from the site.[2]

In Europe, unlike in the United States, faradic techniques have never had much following, nor have they been applied beyond small series generally performed for purposes of research. Traina and Gulino[6] proposed using as a cathode an intramedullary nail covered with insulating material excluding the part near the fracture site, with the anode placed on the skin. The method was employed on a few patients, but further developments were limited, if not hindered, by technical problems connected with the difficulty of soldering the electric cable to the intramedullary nail. Jorgensen[7] suggested using the pins of the external fixation as electrodes, with the proximal and distal ones respectively nearer to the fracture site. Statistical analysis revealed a 30% acceleration in healing in the electrically treated group ($P < 0.001$). Zichner[8] developed an implanted stimulator (FKS), with the cathode in the fracture site and the anode in soft tissue or the medullary cavity. Fifty-three patients out of 57 with nonunion healed in 5.3 months on average.

## Capacitively Coupled Electric Fields: Capacitive Systems

With this noninvasive method, biologic effects are associated solely with a time-varying electric field. The method uses electrodes placed in contact with the skin by means of conductive gel. Optimal stimulation values are considered to be 60 kHz and an induced electric current density of 33 $\mu A/cm^2$.[2]

The European experience with the capacitive system for the stimulation of osteogenesis is extremely limited. The most relevant study was conducted by Scott and King.[9] In a prospective, randomized, double-blind study, 21 patients with established nonunion were treated with capacitive coupling (Orthopak, EBI, Parsippany, NJ). Results showed 60% healing in an active group, whereas none of the patients healed in the placebo group ($P = 0.004$) (Table 1). Zamora-Navas and associates[10] reported a success rate with capacitive coupling of 73% in an open series, including 22 patients with established nonunion. Positive results with capacitive coupling were also reported by Benazzo and associates,[11] who treated athletes with stress fractures. Recently, a success rate of 84% was achieved in a group of 30 patients with nonunion treated with pulsed capacitive coupling (A Mattei, unpublished data, 2003) (OsteoBit, IGEA, Carpi, Italy).

## Pulsed Electromagnetic Fields: Inductive Systems

Pulsed electromagnetic fields (PEMFs) are signals with complex waveforms, whose predominant frequency spectral content ranges from a few tenths to a few ten thousandths Hz. Application of an inductive technique to human bone was first described in 1972 by Kraus and Lechner.[2] They reported a success rate of 93% in patients with nonunion; however, the contribution of PEMF stimulation was difficult to quantify as these patients also underwent surgery. As a result of studies performed by Bassett and associates[12] in the United States, the 1980s witnessed widespread development throughout Europe of PEMF stimulation, resulting in broad clinical experience of scientific value.

**Table 1 Nonunion Studies: Summary of Results**

| Author | Study Design | Level of Evidence[35] | Number of Patients | Electric Stimulation Versus | Success Rate (Stimulation Versus Control) | Significance |
|---|---|---|---|---|---|---|
| Scott and King[9] | Double-blind | I | 23 | Casting | 55.5% vs 8.3% | $P = 0.004$ |
| Poli et al[14] | Controlled | II | 12 | Surgery | 100% vs 50% | $P < 0.001$ |
| Sharrard[15] | Double-blind | I | 45 | Casting | 50% vs 8% | $P < 0.002$ |
| Simonis et al[16] | Double-blind | I | 34 | Surgery | 89% vs 50% | $P = 0.02$ |
| Traina et al[17] | Controlled | II | 67 | Surgery | 88% vs 69% | $P < 0.05$ |

On the one hand, some clinicians have extended the US experience by developing a series of investigations using the US method. On the other hand, new and effective signals have been studied and clinically validated in Italy, the UK, and the Netherlands. As the clinical experience with PEMFs is extensive, we will review it according to the different pathologies treated.

## Stimulation of Reparative Osteogenesis in Congenital Pseudarthrosis

Congenital pseudarthrosis is a rare abnormality. The most common sequence of events leading to pseudarthrosis occurs in the tibia of an infant in whom there are either stigmata of neurofibromatosis—particularly café-au-lait spots—or a family history of neurofibromatosis. Either the tibia alone or the tibia and fibula may be affected; more rarely the condition may be located at the forearm.

An extensive review by Sharrard[13] of the treatment of congenital pseudarthrosis with PEMFs reported a success rate of 70%. The European clinical experience demonstrates the importance of combining orthopaedic procedures and electric stimulation. The treatment of congenital pseudarthrosis should aim not only at bone union but also at preventing refracture and protecting against the failure of the osteosynthesis devices used to maintain alignment. A prospective, controlled study of congenital pseudarthrosis has shown that employment of stimulation in support of surgical intervention with intramedullary devices is able to protect the patient from the risk of refracture. In a 4-year long-term follow-up, it was shown that failure of the nail and bone fracture occurred in 50% of the patients treated only with intramedullary nailing, but no refracture was observed in patients who underwent nailing accompanied by PEMF stimulation[14] ($P < 0.001$) (Table 1).

## Stimulation of Reparative Osteogenesis in Nonunion

Various studies refer to delayed union fractures as those that fail to consolidate in 6 to 9 months following trauma, whereas nonunion fractures are those that fail to consolidate after at least 9 months following trauma. It should, however, be emphasized that the distinction based on time alone is now believed to be insufficient and that the FDA has recently suggested that any fracture showing no progressive signs of healing be considered a nonunion. This definition will be used in this review regardless of time elapsed from trauma.

The efficacy of PEMF stimulation of bone healing has been tested in Europe both in prospective, randomized, double-blind studies as well as in large open series. The difficulties of conducting prospective, randomized, double-blind studies in patients with nonunion have always been acknowledged. Nevertheless, two double-blind studies yielding positive results have been performed in the UK (Table 1).

In 1990, Sharrard[15] demonstrated the efficacy of PEMF stimulation in a double-blind study involving 45 patients with nonunion of the tibia. Twenty patients were treated with active electromagnetic stimulation and 25 with inactive control units for 12 weeks; all nonunions were immobilized in a cast. The radiologist's assessment of union was positive in 50% of patients in the active group compared with 8% in the placebo group ($P < 0.002$). The author concluded that PEMFs significantly influence the healing of nonunion tibial fractures.

In 2003, Simonis and associates[16] reported the results of treatment of 34 consecutive patients with tibial nonunion followed over a period of 5 years. For each patient, the protocol consisted of fibular osteotomy followed by a unilateral external fixation. Half of the patients were treated with an inactive stimulator and half with an active stimulator for a maximum of 6 months. Sixteen out of 18 nonunions (89%) healed in the active group compared with 8 out of 16 (50%) in the inactive group. The authors found a statistically significant positive association between healing and electric stimulation: odds ratio 8, 95% CI: 1.5 to 41 ($P = 0.02$).

Traina and associates[17] observed that treatment of nonunions with PEMFs is particularly indicated when alignment, bone gap, and mobility at the fracture site are adequately controlled. Thus, they compared two contemporary groups of patients with nonunion—one treated with PEMFs, the other undergoing surgery. The success rate in the stimulated group was found to be higher than that in the operated group, 88% versus 69% ($P < 0.05$), and union was achieved more quickly with PEMFs (5.7 months) compared with surgery (7.8 months) ($P < 0.01$) (Table 1).

Large open series of nonunions treated with PEMFs have been reported. In 1985, Hinsenkamp and associates[18] reported the results of a European multicenter study using PEMFs with a success rate above 70%. Positive results were also described in France by Sedel and associates,[19] with a 83% success rate in the treatment of nonunions. In Italy, Marcer and associates[20] reported a success rate of 73% in a series of 147 patients treated with external fixation and PEMFs, the humerus being the least successful site. These studies were performed using the FDA-approved EBI signal. A different technology, no longer available, was developed in the UK by Dehaas and associates,[21] who reported positive results (80% success) in the treatment of nonunions.

In Italy, the technology developed by IGEA was used by Traina and associates,[22] who reported a success rate of 84% in a multicenter study involving

Table 2 Summary of European Nonunion Open Series: Level of Evidence IV[35]

| Author | Method | Number of Patients | Success Rate (%) |
|---|---|---|---|
| Hinsenkamp et al[18] | Inductive | 308 | 73 |
| Sedel et al[19] | Inductive | 35 | 83 |
| Traina et al[22] | Inductive | 248 | 84 |
| Vaquero[23] | Inductive | 137 | 74.5 |
| Fontijne and Konings[24] | Inductive | 139 | 85 |
| Marcer et al[20] | Inductive | 147 | 73 |
| Sharrard[15] | Inductive | 45 | 72 |
| Benazzo et al[11] | Capacitive | 21 | 88 |
| Zamora Navas et al[10] | Capacitive | 22 | 73 |

248 patients with nonunion. Average time to healing was 4.3 months; patients were followed for a minimum of 3 years to confirm the healing. The presence of infection did not influence the outcome of the treatments. The study identified some contraindications to the use of electric stimulation: (1) presence of bone gap larger than half the diameter of the long bone treated, (2) mobility at the fracture site, and (3) excessive angulation of the bone ends. The authors found that, among those patients who showed no radiographic progression toward healing after 3 months of stimulation (31 out of 248), the success rates at 6 and 12 months were respectively 5% and 20%. This observation suggests that, in the absence of radiographic progression, treatment should not be continued for longer than 3 months. Using the same technology, a multicenter study in Spain involving 1,710 patients with nonunion reported a success rate of 74% with an average treatment time of 4.8 months. The study showed the age of the patient ($P = 0.048$), the site of the fracture ($P < 0.001$), the presence of infection ($P = 0.01$), and the type of nonunion ($P = 0.02$) as factors influencing the results.[23]

Using high frequency electromagnetic fields, Fontijne and Konings[24] in the Netherlands reported a positive experience with a success rate of 85% in 139 patients (Table 2). In Europe, few devices are available besides those approved by the FDA; Figure 2 shows the characteristics of the signals used by those devices for which scientific and clinical documentation have been developed and reported above.

## Stimulation of Reparative Osteogenesis in Osteotomies and Fresh Fractures

*Osteotomies* The study of electromagnetic stimulation on osteotomies represents an original approach to quantifying the effects of PEMFs in clinical practice. Three prospective, randomized, double-blind studies have been performed on (1) human femoral intertrochanteric osteotomies,[25] (2) tibial valgus osteotomies,[26] and (3) osteotomies in patients undergoing massive bone graft[27] (Table 3). The studies on osteotomies of the femur and tibia showed that the application of electromagnetic stimulation results in enhanced bone healing. In the case of femoral osteotomies, 32 patients were investigated. PEMF-stimulated patients demonstrated an increased trabecular bridging on both femoral cortices. Digital analysis of the bone callus on the medial cor-

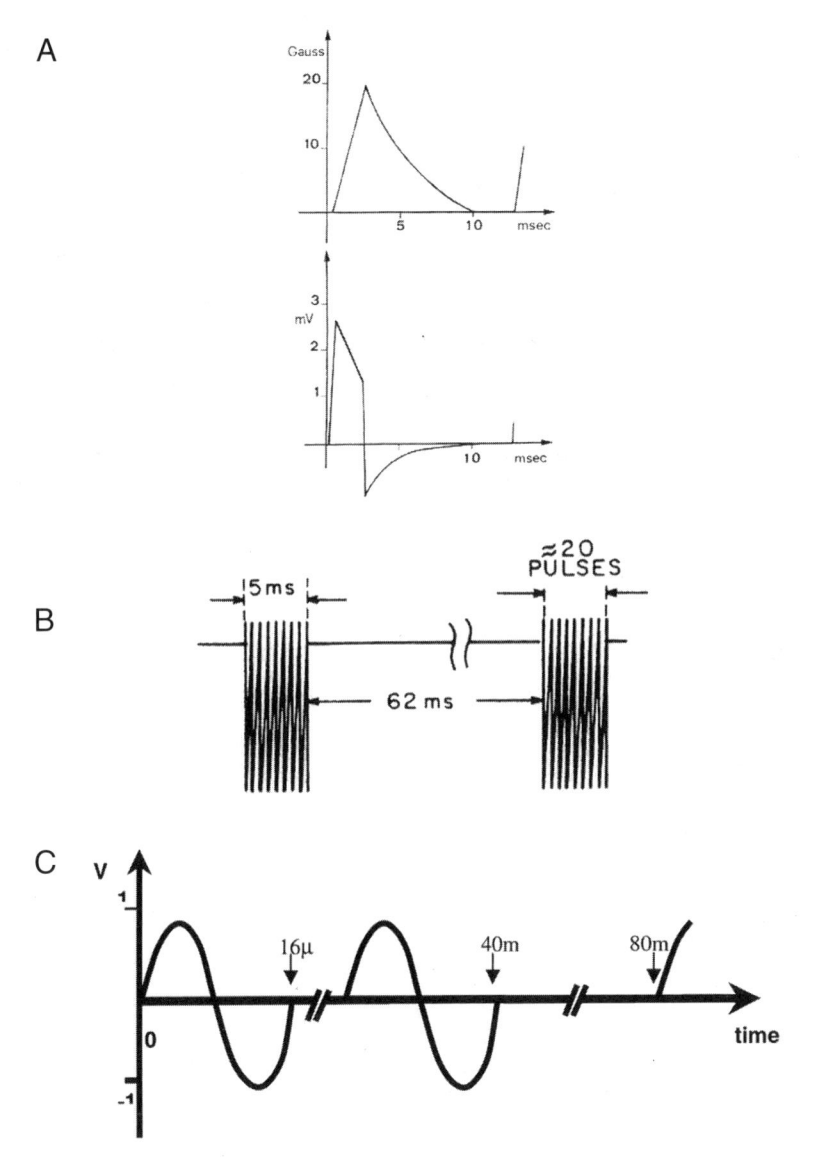

**Figure 2** Characteristics of the signal of devices used in clinical practice in Europe. **A,** Waveform of the magnetic field and induced electric field by Biostim (Italy). **B,** Waveform of asymmetrical PEMF used by OrthoPulse (Netherlands). **C,** Waveform of the electric field of the capacitive system by Osteobit (Italy).

tex indicated an increase in bone mineral content both at 40 and 90 days in the active group compared with the placebo group ($P < 0.05$).[25] In another study, 40 patients undergoing tibial osteotomies were evaluated, and bone healing was assessed at 60 days. The number of patients healed in the active group was 2.6 times that in the placebo group ($P < 0.04$).[26] In the third study,

**Table 3 Results of Pulsed Electromagnetic Fields Stimulation on the Healing of Osteotomies in Prospective, Randomized, Double-blind Studies (Level of Evidence I)[35]**

| Authors | Osteotomy | Active | Placebo | PEMF Outcome |
|---|---|---|---|---|
| Borsalino et al[25] | Femoral intertrochanteric | 15 | 16 | 68% enhanced healing ($P < 0.001$) and 54% increased bone callus mineral content ($P < 0.05$) |
| Mammi et al[26] | Tibial valgus | 18 | 19 | 43% X-ray enhanced healing ($P < 0.04$) |
| Capanna et al[27] | Osteotomy between massive allograft and host bone: 83 osteotomies in 46 patients | 40 | 43 | Shorter healing time (29%) in patients without chemotherapy ($P < 0.001$) |

the effect of PEMF stimulation on patients undergoing massive bone graft following tumor resection was studied. Forty-six patients were included in the study, with a total of 83 host graft junctions investigated. An analysis of variance of the different factors influencing healing with PEMF showed that the only significant association was with the use of chemotherapy ($F = 17.72$; $P = 0.0005$). Among patients who did not receive adjuvant chemotherapy, healing was achieved in 6.7 months on average in the active group and in 9.4 months in the placebo group ($P < 0.001$). No difference was observed between control and active groups in the survival number of patients and in the local or distal tumor recurrence.[27]

***Limb Lengthening*** Electromagnetic stimulation was also examined in two European studies in which the patients underwent limb lengthening following osteotomy. The first, performed in 1996 by Eyres and associates[28] in the UK, involved 13 patients randomly allocated to receive either an inactive placebo or an active PEMF coil; a total of 18 segments were investigated. The authors did not observe any difference in the rate or the amount of newly formed bone and the site of distraction between the two groups. However, DEXA investigation showed that bone loss in the segments of bone distal to the lengthening site was less when using active coils at both 2 and 12 months after surgery ($P < 0.0001$). In 30 patients undergoing bilateral limb lengthening, Luna and associates[29] demonstrated that it was possible to remove the external fixator on average 33 days earlier in stimulated limbs than in nonstimulated ones.

***Fresh Fractures*** Biophysical stimulation has been shown to accelerate healing of fresh fractures of the leg treated with casting. Fontanesi and associates[30] in 1986 investigated the effect of PEMFs in 40 consecutive patients,

20 of whom were treated with PEMFs. The average healing time was 109 days for patients treated with casting only compared with 85 days for patients in which PEMFs were added ($P < 0.005$). The authors pointed out that in no group did fractures heal before 70 days. Hinsenkamp and associates[31] described a positive effect of PEMF stimulation on fresh tibial fracture healing treated with external fixation. In a 1999 double-blind study involving 77 elderly patients with fracture of the femoral neck treated with three screws, Betti and associates[32] demonstrated a positive effect of PEMFs on the healing rate ($P < 0.05$). None of these authors suggested a generalized use of PEMF stimulation in fresh fractures; nevertheless, in those cases where the site, type of exposure, morphology of the fracture, or condition of the patient presage difficulties in the repair process, it was proposed to consider the use of PEMFs at an early stage to prevent nonunion. Stimulation should also be considered if radiographs show no bone callus 45 to 60 days from fracture.

## Rationale for Clinical Use of Biophysical Stimulation to Enhance Endogenous Bone Repair

Biophysical stimulation refers to the administration of electric, magnetic, or mechanical energy to bone tissue to enhance healing. The clinical use of biophysical stimulation as proposed by Bassett and associates[33] initially entailed immobilization of the bone in plaster and subsequent application of the stimulator until healing; some patients underwent treatment for 9 to 12 months or longer. In Europe, such lengthy stimulation was difficult for both the patients and the surgeons to accept. A rationale has been developed to guide the surgeon in choosing or rejecting biophysical stimulation as a means of treatment. It has been observed in particular that not all nonunions should be considered potentially eligible for stimulation. In addition, the time needed for healing should not be considered as a secondary factor, because healing time and consequently rehabilitation time are not negligible parameters in modern orthopaedics and traumatology. In Europe it has been considered necessary to pose the problem of the differential diagnosis, ie, to identify the causes underlying the nonunion.

Following the observations of Frost,[34] 50% of pseudarthrosis cases may be the result of a mechanical failure (ie, the conditions of stability, alignment, and contact of the stumps are not satisfied); 20% are the result of a biologic failure (ie, inadequate activation and conclusion of the reparative osteogenetic process); and in the remaining 30% of cases the failed union is accounted for by combined mechanical and biologic problems. Because biophysical stimulation aims to enhance endogenous bone repair, it is clear that only 50% of nonunions are potentially eligible for stimulation. Mechanical failure has been defined for many years; biologic failure can be described as inadequate activation and conclusion of the reparative osteogenetic process, often secondary to but not limited to infection, serious local osteoporosis, patient's age, or systemic diseases that inhibit the repair processes.

Based on both premise and clinical experience, a decision tree has been developed to guide the orthopaedic surgeon in identifying whether the

## Electromagnetic Stimulation of Bone Repair: Decision Tree

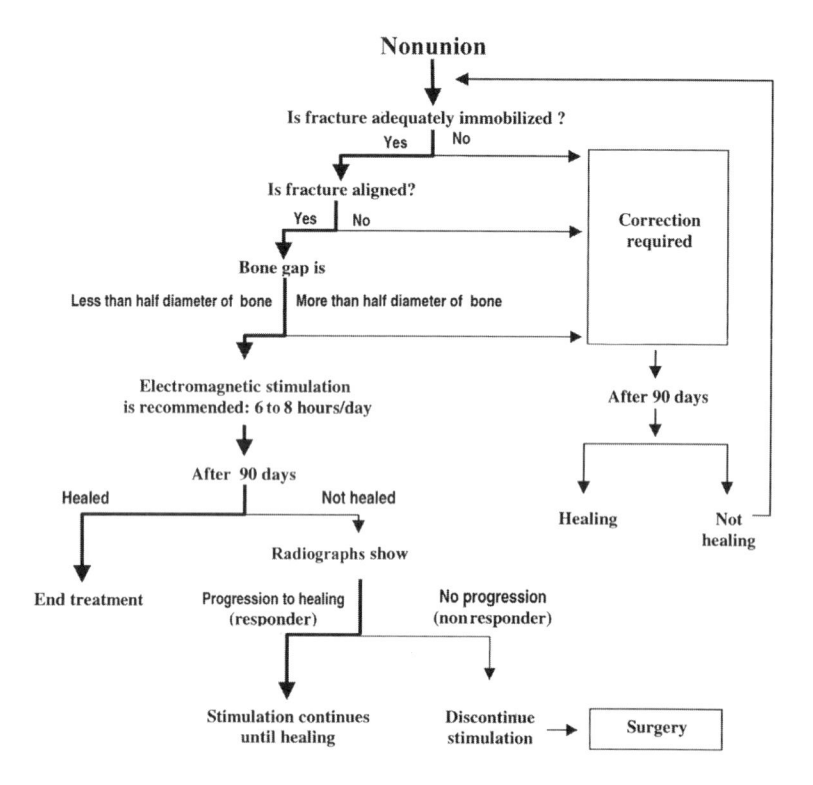

**Figure 3** Evaluation steps to identify patients with nonunion eligible for electric stimulation.

patient's nonunion is eligible for PEMF stimulation and when and how to evaluate stimulation results (Fig. 3).

## Conclusions

Overall, this review of the European experience is consistent with and complementary to the experience collected in the United States. The usefulness of electric stimulation in enhancing endogenous bone repair has been not only demonstrated in prospective, randomized, double-blind studies but also confirmed by extensive clinical experience, to the advantage of patients (avoidance of further surgical procedures) and the community (savings on health care costs).

Orthopaedic surgeons today have available various physical and chemical methods for the local enhancement of endogenous bone repair. The orthopaedic community has developed a sensitivity towards the biologic environment—particularly factors related to mechanical stability and local cellular activity—in which the repair of a fracture takes place. The availability of chemical and physical methods capable of maximizing the progression and conclusion of the endogenous osteogenic response represents opportunities for surgeons to reduce healing times and enable swifter functional and working recovery by the patient.

In Europe, the issue of prevention of nonunion has been addressed. Thus, fractures that do not show progression toward healing in 45 to 60 days from trauma or those located in bone areas that are known to be difficult to heal are considered eligible for early electric stimulation. The identification of biologic markers that will predict the failure of the healing process is fundamental for testing the hypothesis that the enhancement of endogenous osteogenic activity by bone growth stimulation is not only efficacious but also cost-effective.

The extensive European experience has undoubtedly been favored by the absence of legislation prescribing prior approval by EU authorities of these methods before their use on patients. Unlike the United States, where the entry of devices in the market is regulated by the FDA, there are no standards in Europe regarding the use of nonionizing radiation in humans. While this state of affairs has favored the development of new technologies and indications for use, it has also meant the proliferation of systems for treating patients with no scientific basis or studies demonstrating treatment effectiveness. This deficiency will certainly need to be remedied by the relevant authorities in the near future.

## References

1. Galvani L: *De Viribus Electricitatis in Motu Muscolari Commentarius.* Bologna, Italy, Accademia delle Scienze, 1791.

2. Black J: *Electric Stimulation: Its Role in Growth, Repair, and Remodeling of the Musculoskeletal System.* New York, NY, Praeger, 1987.

3. Fukada E, Yasuda I: On the piezoelectric effect of bone. *J Phys Soc Japan* 1957;12:121-128.

4. Bassett CAL, Becker RO: Generation of electric potentials in bone in response to mechanical stress. *Science* 1962;137:1063-1064.

5. Canè V, Botti P, Soana S: Pulsed magnetic fields improve osteoblast activity during the repair of an experimental osseous defect. *J Orthop Res* 1993;11:664-670.

6. Traina GC, Gulino G: Medullary rods as electrical conductors for osteogenic stimuli in human bone, in Brighton CT, Black J, Pollack S (eds): *Electrical Properties of Bone and Cartilage.* New York, NY, Grune and Stratton, 1979, pp 567-579.

7. Jorgensen TE: Electrical stimulation of human fracture healing by means of a slow pulsating asymmetrical direct current. *Clin Orthop* 1977;124:124-127.

8. Zichner L: Repair of nonunions by electrically pulsed current stimulation. *Clin Orthop* 1981;161:115-121.

9. Scott G, King JB: A prospective double blind trial of electric capacitive coupling in the treatment of non-union of long bones. *J Bone Joint Surg Am* 1994;76:820-826.

10. Zamora-Navas P, Borras Verdera A, Antelo Lorenzo R, Saras Ayuso JR, Pena Reina MC: Electric stimulation of bone non-union with the presence of a gap. *Acta Orthop Belg* 1995;61:169-176.

11. Benazzo F, Mosconi M, Beccarisi G, Galli U: Use of capacitive coupled electric fields in stress fractures in athletes. *Clin Orthop* 1995;310:145-149.

12. Bassett CAL, Mitchell SN, Sawnie RG: Pulsing electromagnetic field treatments in ununited fractures and failed arthrodeses. *JAMA* 1982;247:623-628.

13. Sharrard WJW: Treatment of congenital and infantile pseudarthrosis by pulsing electromagnetic fields. *Orthop Clin North Am* 1984;15:143-162.

14. Poli G, Dal Monte A, Cosco F: Treatment of congenital pseudarthrosis with endomedullary nail and low frequency pulsing electromagnetic fields: A controlled study. *J Bioelectr* 1985;4:195-209.

15. Sharrard WJW: A double-blind trial of pulsed electromagnetic field for delayed union of tibial fractures. *J Bone Joint Surg Br* 1990;72:347-355.

16. Simonis RB, Parnell EJ, Ray PS, Peacock JL: Electric treatment of tibial non-union: A prospective, randomised, double-blind trial. *Injury* 2003;34:357-362.

17. Traina GC, Fontanesi G, Costa P, et al: Effect of electromagnetic stimulation on patients suffering from non-union: A retrospective study with a control group. *J Bioelectr* 1991;10:101-117.

18. Hinsenkamp M, Ryaby J, Burny F: Treatment of non-union by pulsing electromagnetic field: European multicenter study of 308 cases. *Reconstr Surg Traumatol* 1985;19:147-151.

19. Sedel L, Christel P, Duriez J, et al: Resultats de la stimulation par champ electromagnetique de la consolidation des pseudarthroses. *Rev Chir Orthop Traum* 1981;67:11-23.

20. Marcer M, Musatti G, Bassett CA: Results of pulsed electromagnetic fields (PEMFs) in ununited fractures after external skeletal fixation. *Clin Orthop* 1984;190:260-265.

21. DeHaas WG, Watson J, Morrison DM: Non-invasive treatment of ununited fracture of the tibia using electrical stimulation. *J Bone Joint Surg Br* 1980;62:465-470.

22. Traina GC, Cadossi R, Ceccherelli G, et al: La modulazione elettrica della osteogenesi. *Giorn Ital Orthop* 1986;2:165-176.

23. Vaquero DH: Resultados y factores pronósticos de la electrostimulación en los trastornos de la consolidación ósea, in Vaquero H, Stern L (eds): *La Estimulación Electromagnetica en la Patologia Osea*. Madrid, Spain, San Martin IG, 1999, pp 171-188.

24. Fontijne WPJ, Konings PC: Botgroeistimulatie met PEMF bij gestoorde fractuurgenezing. *Ned Tijdschr Traum* 1998;5:114-119.

25. Borsalino G, Bagnacani M, Bettati E, et al: Electric stimulation of human femoral intertrochanteric osteotomies: Double blind study. *Clin Orthop* 1988;237: 256-263.

26. Mammi GI, Rocchi R, Cadossi R, Traina GC: Effect of PEMF on the healing of human tibial osteotomies: A double blind study. *Clin Orthop* 1993;288:246-253.

27. Capanna R, Donati D, Masetti C, et al: Effect of electromagnetic fields on patients undergoing massive bone graft following bone tumor resection: A double-blind study *Clin Orthop* 1994;306:213-221.

28. Eyres KS, Saleh M, Kanis JA: Effect of pulsed electromagnetic fields on bone formation and bone loss during limb lengthening. *Bone* 1996;18:505-509.

29. Luna GF, Arevalo RL, Labajos UV: La EEM en las elongaciones y transportes oseos, in Vaquero H, Stern L (eds): *La Estimulación Electromagnetica en la Patologia Osea.* Madrid, Spain, San Martin IG, 1999, pp 236-246.

30. Fontanesi G, Traina GC, Giancecchi F, et al: La lenta evoluzione del processo riparativo di una frattura puo essere prevenuta? *Giorn Ital Orthop Traumatol* 1986;12:389-404.

31. Hinsenkamp M, Bourgois R, Bassett C, Chiabrera A, Burny F, Ryaby J: Electromagnetic stimulation of fracture repair: Influence on healing of fresh fracture. *Acta Orthop Belg* 1978;44:671-698.

32. Betti E, Marchetti S, Cadossi R, Faldini C, Faldini A: Effect of stimulation by low-frequency pulsed electromagnetic fields in subjects with fracture of the femoral neck, in Bersani F (ed): *Electricity and Magnetism in Biology and Medicine.* New York, NY, Kluwer Academic/Plenum Publishers, 1999, pp 853-855.

33. Bassett CA, Pilla AA, Pawluk RJ: A non-operative salvage of surgically resistant pseudarthroses and non-unions by pulsing electromagnetic fields: A preliminary report. *Clin Orthop* 1977;124:128-143.

34. Frost HM: The biology of fracture healing: An overview for clinicians. Part I and II. *Clin Orthop* 1989;248:283-309.

35. Wright JG, Swiontkowski MF, Heckman JD: Introducing levels of evidence to the journal. *J Bone Joint Surg Am* 2003;85:1-3.

# Consensus Panel 1
# Evaluation of Biophysical Regulation of Clinical Bone Healing

**Dr. Roy Aaron:** The consensus panel is composed of people some of whom have an interest not only in physical stimulation but also in bone healing, bone grafting, and growth factors. I think it is great to be in a position to participate in a critical discussion of the state of the art. I also encourage anybody from the audience who wishes to ask a question or offer comment. I would like to develop some thoughts regarding what we do know and what we don't know, and some directions for proceeding in the future. So I would like to open the discussion with some general questions, as we often do in clinical medicine—where do we stand on this? What is known and accepted by good contemporary criteria of clinical trials? And what really represents a gap in our knowledge that might be considered critical to fill? Let me open broadly to any of the consensus people or anybody in the audience who wishes to address that or any other relevant question.

**Dr. Stephen Trippel:** I'm an orthopaedic surgeon, and I've had a long-standing interest in bone healing with emphasis not on the physical stimulation of bone healing but on growth factors. Several of the speakers alluded to the issue that for most fractures you don't really need adjunctive treatment, and that's probably true. What we need to decide is what patient should have this done, first those with fresh fractures and then those with nonunions. Probably every nonunion should be treated with adjunctive biophysical stimulation if they're going to be treated nonsurgically. And even if they are being treated surgically, the rate of success of surgical treatment is not 100%. Why not use this when it does clearly enhance bone healing? As far as the general group of patients who have fresh fractures is concerned, which fractures are at high risk for nonunion—smokers, people with diabetes, people with vascular problems, and the elderly?

**Dr. Joseph Lane:** I think there's no question that there is a biologic effect of biophysical techniques. I think there are excellent in vitro and in vivo data, and there is an impression from the clinical data that these techniques have an effect. So what are the problems out there? Problem number one is, you've got a bunch of cowboys who are the traumatologists, who think that they can solve everything with surgical instrumentation. Second, I think we have to identify the patients who are the candidates for adjunctive treatment in terms of their fracture location, the bone age, smoking, etc. We need a list of risk factors; we also need biologic markers to identify who is diverging from the normal pace of healing. There are clearly those fractures that heal rapidly, those that heal but more slowly, and those that don't heal. You have to be able to look at those biomarkers and pick out those that have stepped off the line, that are slower. I think that there's a world of new tools out there. Osteocalcin, bone alkaline phosphatase, N-telopeptides, and the collagen breakdown products are some. I think we need to characterize the biologic markers of fracture healing that will occur long before you're going to see it by radiographic changes. Then if one identifies those patients and their risk factors, one will feel very comfortable proceeding to add adjunctive biophysical stimulation. The third point is, does it make a difference? It has to make a difference in terms of some measurable outcome parameter, including the need for a secondary operation. This has to be determined. So what are the challenges? One, we have to define the risk factors, and two, we have to develop really acceptable clinical markers to indicate that a fracture stepped off the pace of normal healing. And I think we can do it. There are fabulous techniques, whether it's gene arrays or some biologic markers. I think these things are out there.

**Dr. Bruce Heppenstall:** One thing has to be done and that is to outline fractures at risk: the scaphoid fractures, distal tibia, comminuted fractures, etc. Those are the fractures in which biophysical techniques should be used. I think if one went from that standpoint forward, there would be more acceptance of these kinds of techniques, and I think it would be beneficial for the patients. Imagine an individual who is injured and needs to return to work. If you can decrease the healing time of his or her fracture by 30% or 40% as you heard this morning, that's a huge impact to that person and his or her family, and it's a huge impact to the employer.

**Dr. Deborah Ciombor:** One of the issues that seems to have come out of this discussion is the question of who should be treated and when. I'll ask Joe and the other members in a couple of seconds about the state of the art of biomarkers for fracture repair. But there are people here in the audience who have done work on the timing of the institution of physical regulation. Allen Goodship has done some work in mechanical stimulation of fractures—applying them late, and applying them early. The Germans have done some work as well. There are some data from our lab looking at the application of electric stimulation in early versus late endochondral bone formation. All of these studies with different techniques and different models have suggested that the earlier one applies the technique, the better the result—the better the endochondral bone formation, and in Allen's studies, the better the fracture healing. One wonders about the biologic potential of fractures to heal—when they begin to tail off and when they can be reactivated. Maybe you could tell us, Joe, about the state of the art of biomarkers.

**Dr. Joseph Lane:** We have an expert in our audience. Hari, you've looked at a lot of these markers in fracture healing. Do you think that there are markers that we could use very early on to pick up a delayed fracture healing?

**Dr. Hari Reddi:** We need to identify the earliest markers. Osteocalcin unfortunately is a very late marker. In fact, it's a marker that probably coincides with radiographic evidence of fracture healing. N- and C-telopeptides are definitely sensitive, but I'm not sure how sensitive they would be if you have a small fracture like scaphoid. Do you want to assay it in plasma or urine? The earliest marker would be alkaline phosphatase.

**Dr. Joseph Lane:** I know in animals things go up very quickly. But I have a feeling humans are a little bit slower, so this matter is going to require a very rigorous look at issues such as the volume of the bone involved and the location of the fracture. But I'm quite optimistic.

**Speaker:** Fractures heal with a cartilaginous intermediate, and the studies that have looked at diabetes and the effects of Adriamycin have all shown rather convincingly, I think, that when there is impaired healing, the effect is first seen on cartilage. That would seem to suggest that an earlier marker for a problem with healing than bone formation may indeed be cartilage formation. Therefore, a technique that would measure not bone markers but cartilage markers in serum would be particularly useful. I think a very intriguing possibility would be a technique that would image cartilage in the fracture callus. That would give you an early indication of whether the cartilage intermediate, which appears to be absolutely required for fracture healing, is indeed forming in a timely fashion.

**Speaker:** Those surgeons taking care of tumor patients today use a device called a PET scanner that looks at a biologic marker. The PET scan detects glucose metabolites. But there is excitement about using the fluoride 18 and others. And I think that combining a biologic marker with an imaging technique may be useful in measuring the potential of a fracture to heal.

**Speaker:** All these discussions are obviously germane not only to biophysical stimulation of fracture healing but also to growth factor applications as well as systemic agents. We're not working in a vacuum here. It's equally hard to justify using $5,000 worth of bone morphogenetic protein 2 (BMP-2) or osteogenic protein 1 (OP-1) as it is spending $2,000 for an Exogen device. We're obviously not going to use these expensive modalities for normal fresh fractures. We need to look at the local environment of problem fractures such as scaphoid, and then the nonunions. I think we should be concentrating our efforts on those fractures and on looking at biomarkers. I think the markers are important, but we still don't know what the right marker is, and it will be a ways down the line before we can use these markers to really understand the fracture healing process. The other thought I had in terms of getting acceptance of adjunctive modalities, and again it doesn't matter whether it's biophysical, growth factors, or systemic agents, is the mindset of the always operate (AO) group. They don't think about biology, although they think more about biology now than they used to, but they really have to be educated that this is an important adjuvant to their treatment. It's not a failure of their treatment but an adjuvant to their treatment. And until they get that in their mind, there's not going to be widespread acceptance regardless of the cost. Unless they really believe that the biophysical adjunctive makes a difference, they're not going to support its use. The question is, should we be using these techniques in fresh fractures at risk or all nonunions? That question needs to be answered.

**Dr. Joseph Lane:** I think part of the problem for clinical trials with biophysical stimulation is that they have not excluded the patients that are going to heal on time. It's just like giving iron for iron deficiency. Twenty-five percent of people are iron deficient; 75% are not. If you give iron to everybody, you're not going to see a benefit in changing the hemoglobin because the effect of treatment will be obscured by the 75% that are normal. So I think that when you do prospective, randomized, controlled studies, the exclusion criteria have to include the people who are going to heal on time. I think this is very important. One last thing I want to address is the issue about the analysis of the groups. Ruggero Cadossi emphasized that you cannot ask biophysical techniques to work if you don't have stable instrumentation or good alignment. So I think you're going to have to be a little bit more critical when deciding in which situations you will use biophysical techniques. The Italian algorithm would help in clinical decision making. This may mean a much more vigorous contribution by the companies that make these devices than traditionally has been the case.

**Speaker:** That algorithm is excellent, and it really should be part of the mainstay of educating the surgeon taking care of fractures. The only thing I would add to it would be that once one has a nonunion, I think the surgeon should strongly consider an adjuvant therapy to whatever the surgical treatment should be. I think there's strong enough evidence, and an economic argument could be made that you really have to be aggressive to get it to heal. I know the insurance companies don't like that, but I think it's reality.

**Speaker:** It's interesting when you talk about the fracture at risk versus treating all fresh fractures and the contamination of the data by fresh fractures. There's an implicit biologic assumption that you can't accelerate fresh fracture healing to the point where it has functional implications. Some of the people who are working on this clinically have different points of view. Is there something that is useful for treating fresh fractures or not?

**Speaker:** It's my understanding that the microanatomy of the nonunion is going to be critical. We heard from Allen Goodship that if there's motion, a fibrous nonunion generally forms, which means that now you have a new tissue interposed. And so it seems as if the second surgery is mandatory. I'm curious what your reaction to that is because I think the effort to go from 80% to 100% union rate is very likely to be jeopardized by application under circumstances where the tissue, the biology, is never being addressed.

**Speaker:** It's more complicated than that. We published a paper on the various types of nonunions. There is fibrous nonunion and there is also an entity that we described as synovial pseudarthrosis. Now, the AO group had a very difficult time accepting the synovial pseudarthrosis; however, I notice in all their communications they now refer to fibrous nonunion and synovial pseudarthrosis. The problem is that if you have a synovial joint between the bone ends, I don't care what technique you use, it's not going heal. If it's fibrous tissue in between, then I think you can possibly dedifferentiate cells and produce new bone. The exciting thing to me is all of these techniques appear to have some effect on bone. Several investigators demonstrated that when you use the ultrasound technique, you increase the blood flow 400%. Now that is a huge increase in blood flow, and we all know blood flow is very important for fracture healing. So I think there's something that turns on these cells and something that seems to be common to all of these various techniques, and to me the excitement is going to be finding that out.

**Dr. Barbara Boyan:** One of the things that jumps out to me in the talks that I saw this morning, from my perspective as a cell biologist, is that we're talking about what happens after the fact, we're not talking about the initiating events. Yet the pictures that Bruce Heppenstall and Ruggero Cadossi showed all start with the stem cell—the progenitor cell. We're trying to find a marker at some point down the line where there is a fault, but the fault is probably before we even know it, and I think that treating early is one of the values of these stimulation modalities, as we have seen with electric and mechanical stimulation. There's a sensitivity early, but I'm not sure that we're looking at the right point.

**Speaker:** I agree with you totally that the earlier you use biophysical stimulation, the biology would be advantageous. If you look at the data that were presented this morning, there is a clear cleavage of those who took it for 3 months and didn't take it for 3 months. So if you thought that the biology was receptive early, then just a short pulse at the beginning of fracture healing would have made the difference.

**Dr. Roy Aaron:** The comments from everybody are really coming together to me in an interesting way. There's an acceptance of the basic science underlying biophysical stimulation, that it is biologically effective. And the question of clinical efficacy is returning to biologic questions.

## Future Directions

- Identify fractures at risk for delayed or nonunion by both clinical and laboratory criteria. Target those fractures for clinical trials and treatment with biophysical techniques.
- Develop biochemical or imaging techniques to assist in both identifying fractures at risk and measuring the rate of fracture healing and outcomes after biophysical stimulation.
- Limit adjunctive biophysical techniques to at-risk fractures. Concentrate clinical research efforts on determining dosimetry and the appropriate timing of application of these techniques. Application of

biophysical techniques early in the healing process appears to be advantageous to at-risk fractures and has a good biologic rationale.

# Section Two
## Biophysical Regulation of Bone Healing in Animal Models

Chapter 5

# Bone's "Preferred Strain History" Provides Insight Into a Proposed Common Pathway for the Stimulation of Bone Formation by Distinct Biophysical Signals

*Clinton T. Rubin, PhD*
*Yi-Xian Qin, PhD*
*Michael Hadjiargyrou, PhD*
*Stefan Judex, PhD*

## Introduction

Bone is a tissue that is extremely sensitive to physical signals,[1] an attribute which can be harnessed to accelerate the healing of fractures, promote osseointegration, and augment bone quantity and quality as a nonpharmacologic strategy to combat osteoporosis. Physiologically-based physical signals play a central role in the proliferation of osteoblasts[2] and the inhibition of osteoclastogenesis,[3] thus representing a key regulatory factor in the preservation of balanced bone remodeling. It is now evident that physical signals are essential for even the viability of bone cells, because bone tissue devoid of stimulation may foster the apoptosis of osteocytes.[4] As we look toward new modalities to treat musculoskeletal injury and disease, bone's responsivity to mechanical, electric, and ultrasound signals represents a potent means to influence clinical outcomes. In this chapter, bone's "preferred strain history" is used as a road map to interpret how these distinct physical factors might use common parameters as strong anabolic signals to the skeleton.

Physical signals are endogenous to the skeleton, arising through load-bearing activities such as locomotion. In the clinical use of these signals to treat disease or injury, they can be introduced exogenously—and noninvasively—by a number of modalities, including applied mechanical loads, induced electric signals, and transcutaneous ultrasound. Although it may be difficult initially to recognize any commonality among a bout of exercise, a pulse of an electromagnetic field, and a burst of ultrasound, there are several common elements among these signals that may help identify the means by which physical stimuli are potent determinants of bone architecture and essential components of the healing process.

The sensitivity of bone tissue to alterations in its functional environment is evident in clinical studies that show the skeleton's graded response to levels of exercise[5] as well as the bone density lost due to reductions in gravitational force (space flight[6]) or bed rest.[7] As a result of functional load bearing, strain arises in the bone tissue,[8] whether it is the mandible during chewing,[9] the tibia during running,[10] or the humerus during flying.[11] Functional loading of the skeleton results in an extremely complex loading environment,[12] and investigation of the byproducts of bone strain, such as fluid flow and electric potentials, have led to several proposals as to the mechanisms responsible for controlling bone remodeling, including strain magnitude,[13] strain rate,[14] strain gradients,[15] electrokinetic currents,[16] piezoelectric currents,[17] fluid shear flow,[18] intramedullary pressure,[19] and strain energy density.[20]

Functional loading provides the physiologic foundations for essentially all exogenous modalities—such as modulating the pulse in a pulsed electromagnetic field—in which the time-varying component is designed to mimic the electric potentials that arise in the gait cycle.[17] An integral element of ultrasound, to name another example, is the goal of providing acoustic pressure waves to the site of a fresh fracture to ensure that the injured site retains an active mechanical milieu with all attendant physiologic benefits.[21] It is interesting to consider how small these exogenous signals are in comparison with endogenous ones. Strain equivalents of a 30 mW/cm² (milliwatts per square centimeter) acoustic pressure wave or a 100 µV/cm (100 microvolts per centimeter) electric field[22] are several orders of magnitude below the peak strain (2,000 to 3,000 µε, or 0.2% to 0.3% strain) signals that arise in bone tissue during locomotion.[23] In our laboratory, attempts to identify anabolic components within mechanical signals have led us to consider not the largest but the predominant component of the strain environment: extremely low-level, high-frequency mechanical signals.[24] The physiologic relevance and anabolic potential of extremely low-level mechanical signals is also used to demonstrate that there are common elements—and perhaps common pathways—between extreme exercise regimes to retain bone mass and extremely low-magnitude electric, acoustic, or mechanical interventions. As diverse as these signals may seem, they are all physical modalities, and all have elements—in their simplest form—of amplitude, frequency, and duration.

## The Physiologic Relevance of Low-level Mechanical Signals

In vivo recordings made from strain gages attached to the surfaces of bones allow a first order approximation of the range of physical signals to which the skeleton is ultimately subject, and permits some estimation of the conditions to be considered when designing signal paradigms intended to mimic or replace physical regulation of skeletal morphology. By examining strain data collected from a variety of animals over a range of activities[24] (including simple standing, invariably our predominant activity), a broad frequency range of bone strain is evident (Fig. 1). Spectral analysis of these data show that, while there are only a very few low-frequency, high-magnitude strain

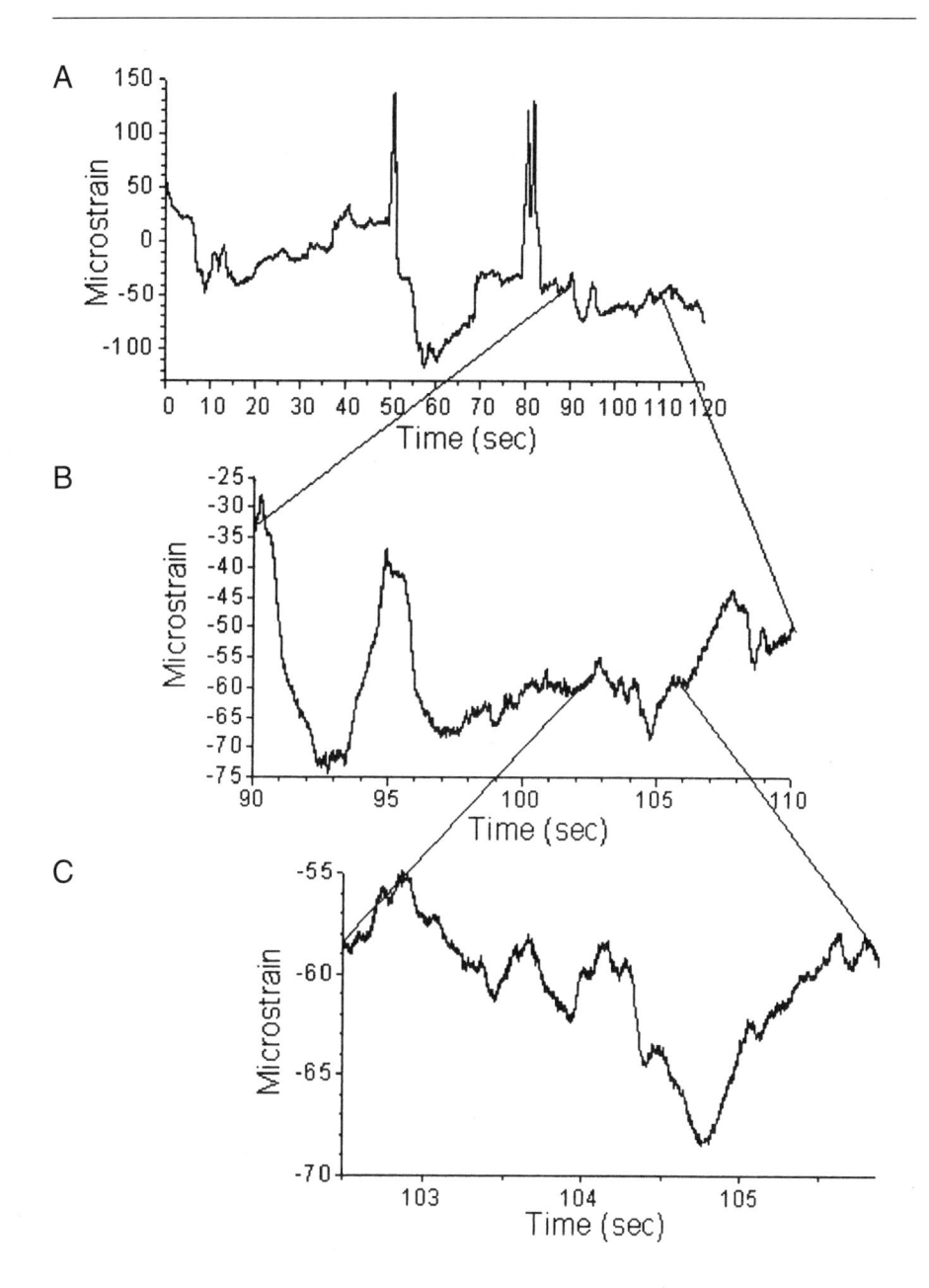

**Figure 1 A,** A 2-minute strain recording from the caudal longitudinal gage of the sheep tibia while the animal took a few steps with peak strains on the order of 200 µε. **B,** A 20-second portion of that strain record shows peak strain events as large as 40 µε. **C,** Further scaling down to a 3-second stretch of the strain recording illustrates events on the order of 5 µε. *(Adapted with permission from Fritton SP, McLeod KJ, Rubin CT: Quantifying the strain history of bone: Spatial uniformity and self-similarity of low-magnitude strains.* J Biomech *2000;33:317-325.)*

## Section Two  Biophysical Regulation of Bone Healing in Animal Models

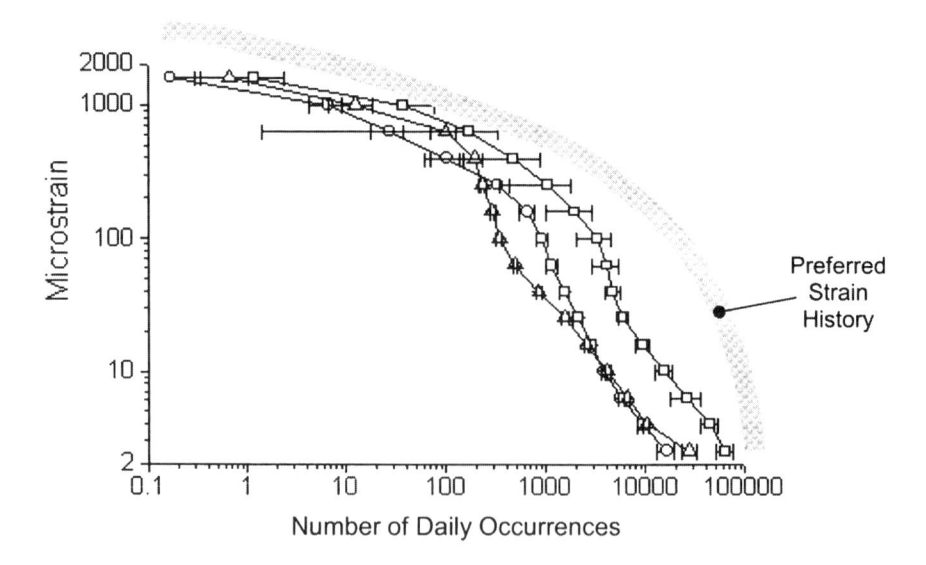

**Figure 2** When a bone's strain history is summed over a full 12-hour period, there are very few large strain events and tens of thousands of small strain events. This "preferred strain history" is illustrated by a curved line and represents a remarkable similarity in the 12-hour strain history of the tibia within a diverse range of animals, including dog (squares), sheep (circles), and turkey (triangles). *(Adapted with permission from Fritton SP, McLeod KJ, Rubin CT: Quantifying the strain history of bone: Spatial uniformity and self-similarity of low-magnitude strains.* J Biomech 2000;33:317-325.)

events (representing the peak strain magnitudes of vigorous activity), there is significant mechanical information extending out to even 50 cycles per second (Hz), and that these signals, summed over a period of 12 hours of standing, represent hundreds of thousands of extremely small strain events (Fig. 2). Thus, in addition to the peak strains of 2,000 µε that might sporadically occur, very small (< 5 µε) high-frequency strains are persistently bombarding the skeleton even during quiet standing (Fig. 1).

The frequency content of these signals indicates that they arise from the contractile activity of muscle spindles, and if these mechanical signals are important to the maintenance of the skeleton, the sarcopenia that occurs with aging or disuse ultimately will extinguish them.[25] From a stimulus standpoint, when these persistent, low-amplitude signals are summed, they may be at least as important in establishing skeletal morphology as the seldom-occurring and somewhat unpredictable strain events that arise from vigorous activity.[26] Of course, for mechanical signals below 5 µε to be pertinent to bone quantity and quality, it is essential to demonstrate that such signals can stimulate the formation of bone. Harnessing bone's sensitivity to physical signals can then be achieved without putting the skeleton at risk, as these low-level mechanical signals are several orders of magnitude below those strains known to cause damage to bone.[27]

# Bone Tissue's Responsivity to Low-level Mechanical Signals

The bone tissue modeling/remodeling response is sensitive only to dynamic (time-varying) strains; static strains are ignored as a source of osteogenic stimuli.[28] However, it is also clear that the osteogenic potential of mechanical signals is defined by a strong interdependence between cycle number, strain magnitude, and frequency. In cortical bone, 2,000 µε induced at 0.5 Hz (one cycle every 2 seconds) maintains bone mass with just four cycles of loading encompassing 8 seconds per day.[29] Reducing this strain to 1,000 µε at 1 Hz requires 100 cycles and 100 seconds to maintain bone mass.[30] If the loading frequency is raised to 3 Hz, bone mass can be retained with 1,800 cycles of only 800 µε,[31] whereas at 30 Hz the same 600 seconds require only 200 µε to maintain cortical bone, a protocol employing 18,000 cycles of loading. If the 30-Hz signal is increased to 1 hour per day (108,000 cycles), only 70 µε is necessary to inhibit bone loss. Plotted together, these data demonstrate that the sensitivity of cortical bone to mechanical loading goes up quickly with cycle number and that extremely low levels of strain will maintain bone mass if sufficient numbers are used (Fig. 3). Considered in the context of the interdependent relationship between the intensity of an electric field and bone strain, one microstrain per microvolt[32] indicates that induced fields on the order of tens of microvolts per centimeter, rather than thousands, would be sufficient to stimulate bone formation.[33]

Bone's sensitivity to high-frequency mechanical signals was used to determine if they could be used to promote bony ingrowth into porous-coated transcortical pins.[34] Over 28 days, disuse permitted an 8.3% (+ 5.5%) loss of bone area adjacent to the implant. One hundred seconds per day of a 1-Hz mechanical load sufficient to generate a peak strain of 150 µε at the pin-bone interface[35] stimulated the bone to grow into 28% (± 6.2%) of the implant area available for ingrowth. At 20 Hz, the amount of ingrowth increased to 69% (± 3.0%). These data indicate that at least some load bearing is ultimately beneficial to osseointegration but also suggest that the degree of bony ingrowth can be improved with a high-frequency signal.

# Noninvasive Introduction of Low-level Signals Into the Skeleton

The correlation between bone formation and exogenously applied physical signals indicates that bone mass can be retained with a very few number of large physical signals (which may also potentiate damage) or thousands—if not hundreds of thousands—of extremely low-level physical signals. The challenge then becomes identifying a means to get these signals to the skeleton noninvasively and in a trajectory relevant to weight bearing—something that can be achieved through foot-based whole body vibration,[36] which can efficiently transmit mechanical signals to the axial skeleton at least through 50 Hz.[37] DXA, peripheral quantitative computed tomography (pQCT), and histology (static and dynamic histomorphometry, µCT) were used to determine if daily 20-minute periods of vibration over an extended period of time

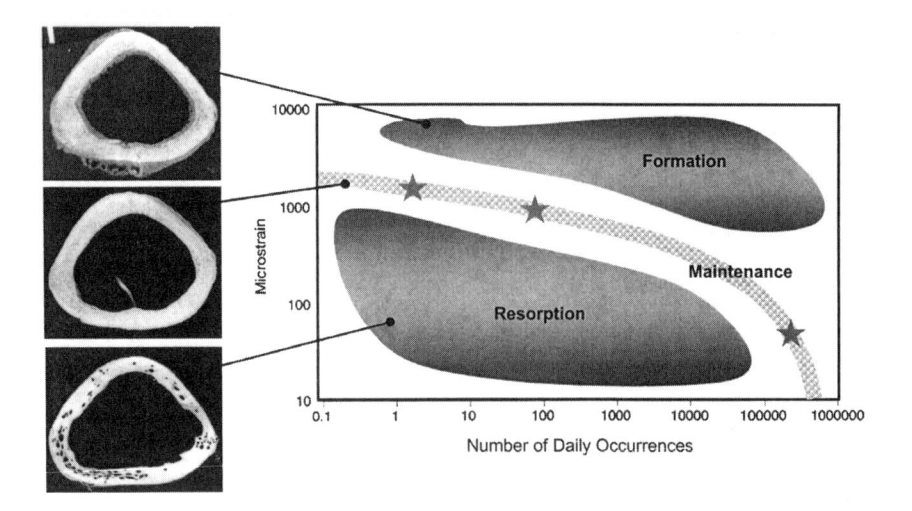

Section Two    Biophysical Regulation of Bone Healing in Animal Models

**Figure 3** The turkey ulna model is used here to determine the nonlinear interrelationship of cycle number and strain magnitude. It appears that bone mass can be retained through a number of distinct strategies (gray line); bone is preserved with either 4 cycles per day of 2,000 µɛ, 100 cycles per day of 1,000 µɛ, or tens of thousands of cycles of signals well below 100 µɛ (each represented as a star). It is proposed that falling below this "preferred strain history" would stimulate bone loss and that any combination exceeding this relationship would stimulate bone gain.

(12 months) could improve the structural status of the bone in adult sheep.[38] A vertical ground-based vibration oscillating at 30 Hz to create peak-peak accelerations of 0.3 g was used (1 g = earth's gravitational field, or 3.0 m/s$^2$); it induced peak strains on the order of 5 µɛ, or three orders of magnitude below that which generates damage in bone.

Compared with untreated controls, bone mineral density (BMD) of the proximal femur in stimulated animals was 5.4% greater, but this difference was not significant ($P < 0.1$). Although pQCT also failed to demonstrate a significant difference in the total density of the proximal femur (+ 6.5%; $P < 0.1$), a 34.2% increase in trabecular density was observed in mechanically stimulated sheep (Fig. 4; $P < 0.01$) when this assay was used to selectively evaluate cortical and cancellous bone at the lesser trochanter. Bone histomorphometry demonstrated substantial increases in trabecular bone volume and trabecular number and sharp decreases in trabecular spacing.[39]

To examine how these low-level signals would modulate the quality of the bone, high-resolution 3-dimensional (3-D) models were made of 1-cm cubes of trabecular bone harvested from the medial condyle of the femur.[40] Trabecular bone pattern factor, an index of connectivity, was decreased by 24.2% in the animals subject to the noninvasive stimulus ($P < 0.03$), reflecting a significant increase in connectivity and thus an improvement in the quality of bone. Stiffness in the longitudinal direction—at 410 MPa in the control animals—was 12.3% greater in the experimental animals (461 MPa;

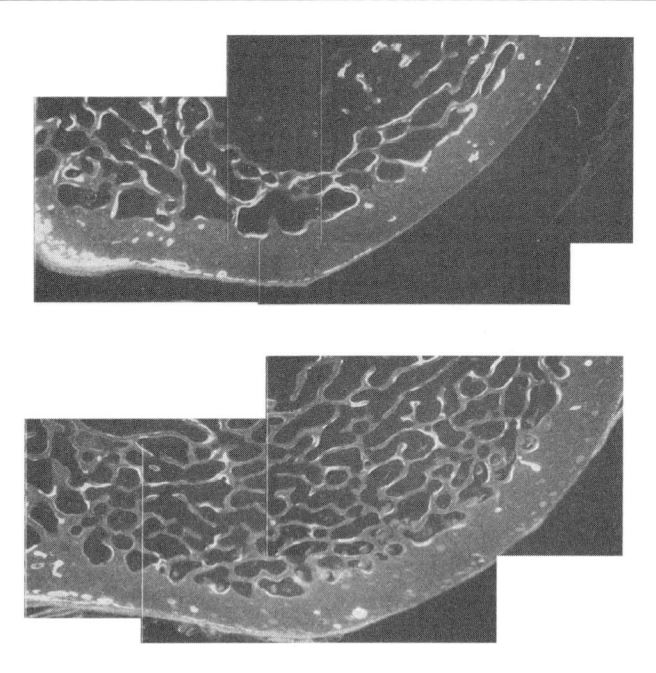

**Figure 4** Following 1 year of extremely low-level mechanical stimulation, parameters of both static and dynamic histomorphometry demonstrated a significant benefit to both the quantity and quality of bone from exposure to the biophysical stimulus. Shown here are fluorescent photomicrographs of a transverse section at the lesser trochanter of the femur, showing more trabeculae, which are thicker than control. *(Adapted with permission from Rubin C, Turner AS, Mallinckrodt C, Jerome C, McLeod K, Bain S: Mechanical strain, induced noninvasively in the high-frequency domain, is anabolic to cancellous bone, but not cortical bone.* Bone *2002;30:445-452.)*

$P < 0.04$). In the mediolateral direction there was a 6.1% increase, but it was not significant ($P = 0.22$), nor was a 2% drop in stiffness in the anteroposterior direction ($P = 0.39$). Strength to failure, measured only in the longitudinal direction, was 26.7% greater in the experimental animals ($P < 0.05$). These data indicate that the adaptive response of bone is preferential to the direction of weight bearing and results in an improvement in structural quality over controls.

## Inhibition of Disuse Osteopenia by Low-level Mechanical Signals

The above data demonstrate that these low-level mechanical stimuli are anabolic, yet it is unclear if they are effective in inhibiting the osteoporosis that parallels disuse. The rat-tail model of disuse osteoporosis as developed by Morey-Holton and Wronski[41] was used as a ground-based model to examine the impact of disuse and low-level mechanical signals on bone remodeling activity.[42] No significant changes in body mass were measured

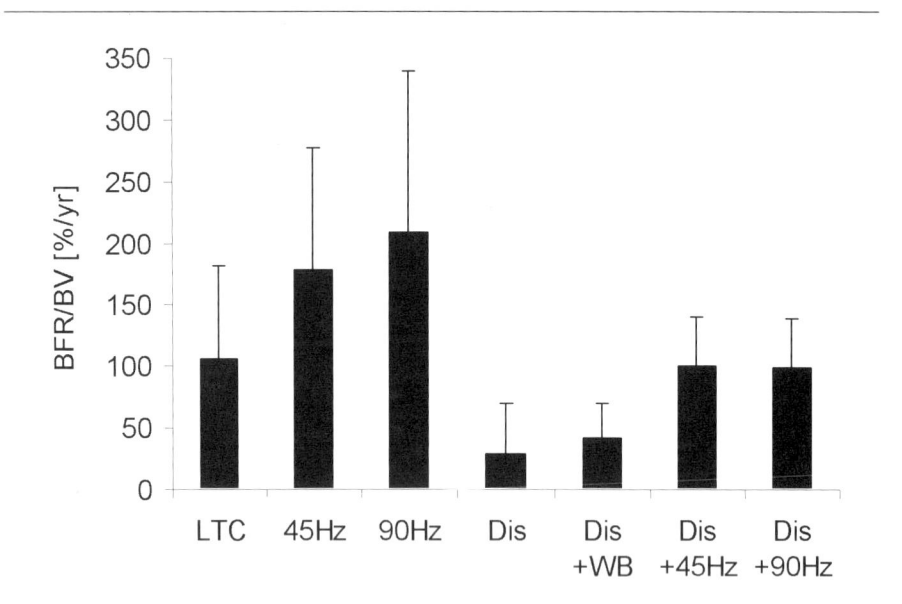

**Figure 5** Following 28 days of tail suspension (Dis) or disuse plus mechanical intervention, dynamic parameters of bone formation in the tibia were examined and compared with long-term control (LTC) as well as normal ambulation plus mechanical intervention (90 Hz, 45 Hz). Ten min/day$^{-1}$ negate the influence of disuse. A 10 min/day$^{-1}$ or 45 Hz (Dis + 45 Hz) restored bone parameters to those measured in LTC. Disuse was not significantly different from Dis + WB; both were significantly different from LTC, Dis + 90 Hz, and Dis + 45 Hz ($P < 0.05$). LTC was not significantly different from either Dis + 90 Hz or Dis + 45 Hz. Both 45 Hz and 90 Hz were significantly greater than LTC. N ≥ 12 for each group.

in any of the groups during the course of the 28-day study. Over the experimental period, 10 minutes per day of the 45 Hz or 90 Hz mechanical stimulation at 0.3 g significantly increased bone formation rate/bone volume (BFR/BV) by 67% or 97% compared with long-term controls (Fig. 5). In contrast, tail suspension suppressed BFR/BV by 72% ($P < 0.05$). Tail suspension interrupted each day by 10 minutes of normal weight bearing failed to reestablish the growth patterns suppressed by disuse; BFR dropped by 61% in this group ($P < 0.05$). In contrast, disuse interrupted each day by 10 minutes of either 45 Hz or 90 Hz loading maintained bone remodeling dynamics at control values; BFR/BV was 6% and 7% below control values respectively ($P > 0.05$).

In addition to the large strains typically associated with functional activity,[23] smaller magnitude strain signals are evident in bone.[24] These small strains persist over long durations, including in such passive actions as standing, and therefore represent a dominant component of the bone's functional strain history. The suspension of the rat hind limb from weight bearing removes this regulatory stimulus, uncoupling formation and resorption, and results in less bone than in control animals. The low-level, high-frequency mechanical signal effectively prevents osteoporosis from occurring, even when subject to 23 hours and 50 minutes of a strong stimulus for resorption, while 10 minutes per day of normal weight bearing fails to curb the loss. Given the anabolic potential of these thousands of extremely low-level mechanical signals, it is important to determine if they will be effective in all skeletons regardless of genetic makeup or if these epigenetic signals are ultimately dependent on a receptive genome.

## Bone's Sensitivity to Low-level Signals is Dependent on Genetic Variations

The great variability of bone loss in the aging and postmenopausal population[43] (a phenomenon also seen in the astronaut corps[44]) indicates that there is a genomic basis for vulnerability to osteoporosis.[45] Considering the link between bone morphology and mechanical function, this range of responses also indicates a varied sensitivity to altered mechanical environments. To address this issue, we used three distinct inbred mouse strains to determine if they were differentially sensitive to changes in their habitual mechanical environment.[46] Adult female B6, BALB, and C3H mice were subjected to 10 min/day of low-level mechanical signals (0.25 g at 45 Hz) or to disuse via hind limb tail suspension. Bone formation rates of B6 mice subjected to the low-level signal were 69% greater ($P < 0.04$) than those observed in intrastrain control mice. Despite the brief length of the low-level mechanical intervention, increased trabecular bone formation rates coincided with an 85% ($P < 0.01$) larger bone volume per total volume (BV/TV) and 50% larger trabecular thickness ($P < 0.009$) in vibrated mice. In contrast to the anabolic response to added mechanical signals, disuse failed to modulate histomorphometric indices in B6 mice.

In BALB mice, low-level mechanical signals increased bone formation rate per bone surface (BFR/BS) by 32% ($P < 0.04$) and BFR/BV by 34% ($P < 0.02$), but bone structural indices including BV/TV were unaffected. The increase in bone formation rates was primarily achieved by an increase in double-labeled surfaces (dLS/BS) (+ 56%, $P < 0.01$) rather than by increased mineral apposition rates (MAR). Disuse in BALB mice suppressed BFR/BS by 55% ($P < 0.02$), BFR/BV by 48% ($P < 0.002$), dLS/BS by 46% ($P < 0.04$), and MAR by 45% ($P < 0.001$), contributing to a 43% ($P < 0.007$) reduction in trabecular bone volume compared with controls. In contrast to the responsiveness of the B6 and BALB mice, no significant effects of mechanical stimulation or disuse were measured in tibial trabecular bone of C3H mice.

These data indicate a strong influence of genetic variability on the plasticity of trabecular bone to both anabolic and catabolic mechanical stimuli. Low-level mechanical signals superimposed on normal daily activities for 10 minutes per day were anabolic in the proximal tibia of both B6 and BALB mice, whereas no significant effect of this specific stimulus was detected in the high bone density C3H mice. The results of this study also suggest that some people who benefit from a genetically predetermined higher bone mass may ultimately be less sensitive to any form of physical intervention,[47] perhaps because the cells themselves are not responsive to the mechanical environment.

## Application of Low-level Mechanical Signals in the Clinic

The observations that high-frequency, low-magnitude mechanical stimuli can influence bone formation and resorption suggests that this signal can be used to inhibit or reverse osteoporosis. Certainly low-level mechanical signals are simpler and safer to impose into the skeletal system than large signals, and considering the inherent complications of pharmaceutical interventions to curb diseases such as osteoporosis, either in terms of their daily administration[48] or the potential consequences of extended use,[49] the development of a nonpharmacologic approach to the prevention of bone loss would clearly benefit treatment.[50]

Ultimately, our goal is to use low-level mechanical signals to inhibit or reverse osteoporosis in the human. Preliminary experiments demonstrate that mechanical signals induced for 20 min/day at 0.2 g and 30 Hz can prevent bone loss in women between 3 to 8 years past menopause.[51] Over the course of 2 years, 70 women were enrolled in our study, 50% in the active group and 50% in the placebo group. Using linear regression of the means normalized to body weight, BMD in the placebo group showed a 3.3% loss ($\pm$ 0.83%) in the lumbar spine and a 2.9% ($\pm$ 1.2%) loss in the trochanteric region of the femur. In the experimental group, loss of BMD in the spine was limited to $-0.8\%$ ($\pm$ 0.82%), a 2.5% benefit of treatment ($P < 0.04$). In the trochanter of the experimental group, a gain of 0.4% ($\pm$ 1.2%) was measured over the course of the year, a 3.5% benefit of treatment ($P < 0.02$). No differences were measured at the radius between the placebo and experimental groups. For lighter weight ($< 65$ kg) women who were compliant (compliance $\geq 60\%$), the benefits of therapy become significant ($P = 0.03$) with a 3% positive difference for the total spine and a $> 2\%$ positive difference at the femoral neck and trochanter (Fig. 6).

In young children with conditions such as cerebral palsy, osteoporosis is also a significant problem, caused at least in part by diminished locomotor function. To examine the ability of low-level mechanical signals to provide a surrogate for diminished muscular activity and thus restore bone loss in such children, a heterogeneous group of 20 prepubertal and postpubertal ambulant children with disabling conditions (14 boys, 6 girls; mean age 9.1 [$\pm$ 4.3], range 4 to 19 years) were randomized to stand on active (n = 10; 0.3 g at 90 Hz) or placebo (n = 10) devices for 10 min/day, 5 days/week for 6 months.[52] Pretrial and posttrial proximal tibial and spinal (L2) volumetric trabecular bone mineral density (vTBMD; in units of mg/mL) was measured by 3-D quantitative computer tomography (QCT). Over the 6-month trial, the mean proximal tibial vTBMD in children who stood on active devices increased by 6.27 mg/mL (+ 6.3%), whereas mean proximal tibial vTBMD in children who stood on placebo devices decreased by $-9.45$ mg/mL ($-11.9\%$). Thus the net benefit of treatment was +15.72 mg/mL (+ 17.7%)

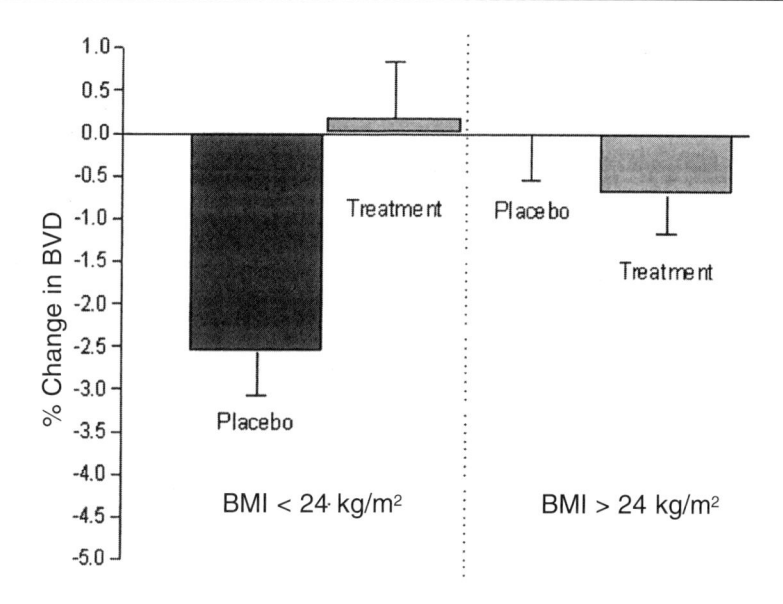

**Figure 6** Stratification based on body mass index (BMI) shows that the lighter women (BMI < 24) lost on the order of 2.5% bone from the spine over the course of the year. This loss was reduced ($P = 0.005$) when lighter women were exposed to low-level mechanical stimulation. Women with a BMI greater than 24 lost no bone over the course of the year; since no loss occurred, it was not possible to demonstrate the efficacy of treatment in these women ($P = 0.36$). *(Adapted with permission from Rubin C, Recker R, Cullen D, Ryaby J, McLeod K: Prevention of postmenopausal bone loss by a low magnitude, high frequency mechanical stimuli: A clinical trial assessing compliance, efficacy, and safety.* J Bone Miner Res *2004; 19:343-351.)*

(95% CI: 6.57, 24.87; $P = 0.0033$). At the spinal site, the net benefit of treatment as compared with placebo was +6.72 mg/mL, (95% CI: −2.60, 16.05; $P = 0.14$). This placebo-controlled, randomized, double-blind trial indicates that low-level mechanical signals are anabolic to trabecular bone in humans, perhaps by providing a surrogate for suppressed muscular activity in the disabled.[53] These preliminary results indicate the potential for a noninvasive, nonpharmacologic, and safe approach to improving trabecular vBMD in the limbs of children with disabling conditions.

## Summary

Extremely low-level physical stimuli in the form of mechanical, electric, or acoustic signals can represent strongly anabolic factors for bone. Several types of physical signals have great potential for direct clinical application in a number of situations, including osteoporosis, fracture healing,[21] or osseointegration.[34] Although Wolff's law is a well-accepted paradigm

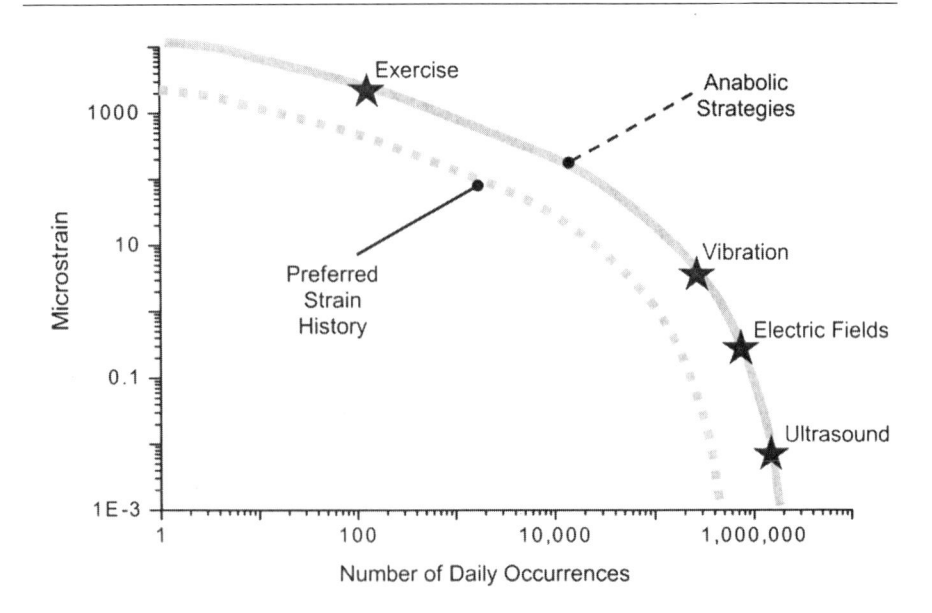

**Figure 7** This graph is intended to represent that there might be more than one way to harness bone sensitivity to physical signals. Considering the power:law relationship of cycle number and strain magnitude in defining the preferred strain history of bone (dashed line), this log-log plot proposes that stimulation of new bone formation in the healing callus using physical interventions can be achieved using a number of different strategies, as reflected by any modality that elevates the line at any given point (solid line; see also Figs. 1 and 2). With this in mind, bone formation could be stimulated by 36 cycles of 2,000 µε as generated by extreme exercise (star), tens of thousands of cycles of 2 µε as might be achieved by vibration, hundreds of thousands of cycles as might be achieved through a 0.2 µε equivalent of an induced electric field (eg, 1 µε = 1 µV), or millions of cycles of 0.02 µε as might be achieved using ultrasound. Exceeding this optimized line (perhaps by overloading a fracture) might cause hypertrophic nonunion, whereas not reaching even the "preferred strain history" would contribute to an atrophic nonunion.

emphasizing that bone responds to changes in its functional environment, it appears that bone's sensitivity to physical signals can be harnessed in a multitude of ways, whether with a few large events or a plethora of small ones (Fig. 7).

In contrast to systemic pharmaceutical interventions such as estrogens, parathyroid hormone (PTH), or bisphosphonates (and their attendant risks),[54-56] biophysical prophylaxes have numerous positive attributes: they are native to the bone tissue and safe at low intensities,[57] they incorporate all aspects of the remodeling cycle,[3] they will ultimately induce lamellar bone formation,[58] and the relative amplitude of the signal will subside as formation persists (self-regulating and self-targeting).[59] However, the widespread use of mechanical—or other physical—stimuli in the treatment of skeletal disorders and injuries will undoubtedly be delayed until a better understanding is achieved of the physical and biologic mechanisms by which they act.[60,61]

## Acknowledgments

This work has been kindly supported by grants from the National Institutes of Health; Juvent Inc; Exogen, Inc; the National Aeronautics and Space Administration; and the National Space Biomedical Research Institute. The authors would like to dedicate this chapter to Jack Ryaby, a pioneer in the science of physical signals in the treatment of musculoskeletal disorders.

## References

1. Wolff J: *The Law of Bone Remodeling*. Berlin and Heidelberg, Germany, Springer-Verlag, 1986.
2. Burger EH, Klein-Nulend J: Responses of bone cells to biomechanical forces in vitro. *Adv Dent Res* 1999;13:93-98.
3. Rubin J, Fan X, Biskobing DM, Taylor WR, Rubin CT: Osteoclastogenesis is repressed by mechanical strain in an in vitro model. *J Orthop Res* 1999;17:639-645.
4. Noble BS, Peet N, Stevens HY, et al: Mechanical loading: Biphasic osteocyte survival and targeting of osteoclasts for bone destruction in rat cortical bone. *Am J Physiol Cell Physiol* 2003;284:C934-C943.
5. Snow-Harter C, Bouxsein ML, Lewis BT, Carter DR, Marcus R: Effects of resistance and endurance exercise on bone mineral status of young women: A randomized exercise intervention trial. *J Bone Miner Res* 1992;7:761-769.
6. Vico L, Collet P, Guignandon A, et al: Effects of long-term microgravity exposure on cancellous and cortical weight-bearing bones of cosmonauts. *Lancet* 2000;355:1607-1611.
7. LeBlanc AD, Schneider VS, Evans HJ, Engelbretson DA, Krebs JM: Bone mineral loss and recovery after 17 weeks of bed rest. *J Bone Miner Res* 1990;5:843-850.
8. Fritton S, Rubin C: In vivo measurement of bone deformation using strain gages, in Cowin SC (ed): *Bone Mechanics Handbook*. Boca Raton, FL, CRC Press, 2001, pp 8.1-8.41
9. Hylander WL, Ravosa MJ, Ross CF, Johnson KR: Mandibular corpus strain in primates: Further evidence for a functional link between symphyseal fusion and jaw-adductor muscle force. *Am J Phys Anthropol* 1998;107:257-271.
10. Rubin CT, Lanyon LE: Limb mechanics as a function of speed and gait: A study of functional strains in the radius and tibia of horse and dog. *J Exp Biol* 1982;101:187-211.
11. Rubin CT: Skeletal strain and the functional significance of bone architecture. *Calcif Tissue Int* 1984;36:S11-S18.
12. Gross TS, McLeod KJ, Rubin CT: Characterizing bone strain distributions in vivo using three triple rosette strain gages. *J Biomech* 1992;25:1081-1087.
13. Rubin CT, Lanyon LE: Regulation of bone mass by mechanical strain magnitude. *Calcif Tissue Int* 1985;37:411-417.
14. O'Connor JA, Lanyon LE, MacFie H: The influence of strain rate on adaptive bone remodelling. *J Biomech* 1982;15:767-781.

Section Two    Biophysical Regulation of Bone Healing in Animal Models

15. Gross TS, Edwards JL, McLeod KJ, Rubin CT: Strain gradients correlate with sites of periosteal bone formation. *J Bone Miner Res* 1997;12:982-988.

16. Pollack SR, Salzstein R, Pienkowski D: Streaming potential in fluid filled bone. *Ferroelectrics* 1984;60:297-309.

17. Bassett CA: Biologic significance of piezoelectricity. *Calcif Tissue Res* 1968;1:252-272.

18. You L, Cowin SC, Schaffler MB, Weinbaum S: A model for strain amplification in the actin cytoskeleton of osteocytes due to fluid drag on pericellular matrix. *J Biomech* 2001;34:1375-1386.

19. Qin YX, Lin W, Rubin C: The pathway of bone fluid flow as defined by in vivo intramedullary pressure and streaming potential measurements. *Ann Biomed Eng* 2002;30: 693-702.

20. Carter DR, Fyhrie DP, Whalen RT: Trabecular bone density and loading history: Regulation of connective tissue biology by mechanical energy. *J Biomech* 1987;20: 785-794.

21. Rubin C, Bolander M, Ryaby JP, Hadjiargyrou M: The use of low-intensity ultrasound to accelerate the healing of fractures. *J Bone Joint Surg Am* 2001;83:259-270.

22. Rubin CT, Donahue HJ, Rubin JE, McLeod KJ: Optimization of electric field parameters for the control of bone remodeling: Exploitation of an indigenous mechanism for the prevention of osteopenia. *J Bone Miner Res* 1993;8:S573-S581.

23. Rubin CT, Lanyon LE: Dynamic strain similarity in vertebrates: An alternative to allometric limb bone scaling. *J Theor Biol* 1984;107:321-327.

24. Fritton SP, McLeod KJ, Rubin CT: Quantifying the strain history of bone: Spatial uniformity and self-similarity of low-magnitude strains. *J Biomech* 2000;33:317-325.

25. Huang RP, Rubin CT, McLeod KJ: Changes in postural muscle dynamics as a function of age. *J Gerontol A Biol Sci Med Sci* 1999;54:B352-B357.

26. Adams DJ, Spirt AA, Brown TD, Fritton SP, Rubin CT, Brand RA: Testing the daily stress stimulus theory of bone adaptation with natural and experimentally controlled strain histories. *J Biomech* 1997;30:671-678.

27. Burr DB, Martin RB, Schaffler MB, Radin EL: Bone remodeling in response to in vivo fatigue microdamage. *J Biomech* 1985;18:189-200.

28. Lanyon LE, Rubin CT: Static vs dynamic loads as an influence on bone remodelling. *J Biomech* 1984;17:897-905.

29. Rubin CT, Lanyon LE: Regulation of bone formation by applied dynamic loads. *J Bone Joint Surg Am* 1984;66:397-402.

30. Rubin CT, Lanyon LE: Osteoregulatory nature of mechanical stimuli: Function as a determinant for adaptive remodeling in bone. *J Orthop Res* 1987;5:300-310.

31. Qin YX, Rubin CT, McLeod KJ: Nonlinear dependence of loading intensity and cycle number in the maintenance of bone mass and morphology. *J Orthop Res* 1998;16:482-489.

32. Otter MW, Palmieri VR, Wu DD, Seiz KG, MacGinitie LA, Cochran GV: A comparative analysis of streaming potentials in vivo and in vitro. *J Orthop Res* 1992;10:710-719.

33. McLeod KJ, Rubin CT: The effect of low-frequency electrical fields on osteogenesis. *J Bone Joint Surg Am* 1992;74:920-929.

34. Rubin CT, McLeod KJ: Promotion of bony ingrowth by frequency-specific, low-amplitude mechanical strain. *Clin Orthop* 1994;298:165-174.

35. Qin YX, McLeod KJ, Guilak F, Chiang FP, Rubin CT: Correlation of bony ingrowth to the distribution of stress and strain parameters surrounding a porous-coated implant. *J Orthop Res* 1996;14:862-870.

36. Fritton JC, Rubin CT, Qin YX, McLeod KJ: Whole-body vibration in the skeleton: Development of a resonance-based testing device. *Ann Biomed Eng* 1997;25:831-839.

37. Rubin C, Pope M, Fritton J, Magnusson M, Hansson T, McLeod K: Transmissibility of 15-35 Hz vibrations to the human hip and lumbar spine: Determining the physiologic feasibility of delivering low-level, anabolic mechanical stimuli to skeletal regions at greatest risk of fracture due to osteoporosis. *Spine* 2003;28:2621-2627.

38. Rubin C, Turner AS, Bain S, Mallinckrodt C, McLeod K: Anabolism: Low mechanical signals strengthen long bones. *Nature* 2001;412:603-604.

39. Rubin C, Turner AS, Mallinckrodt C, Jerome C, McLeod K, Bain S: Mechanical strain, induced noninvasively in the high-frequency domain, is anabolic to cancellous bone, but not cortical bone. *Bone* 2002;30:445-452.

40. Rubin C, Turner AS, Muller R, et al: Quantity and quality of trabecular bone in the femur are enhanced by a strongly anabolic, noninvasive mechanical intervention. *J Bone Miner Res* 2002;17:349-357.

41. Morey-Holton E, Wronski TJ: Animal models for simulating weightlessness. *Physiologist* 1981;24:545-548.

42. Rubin C, Xu G, Judex S: The anabolic activity of bone tissue, suppressed by disuse, is normalized by brief exposure to extremely low-magnitude mechanical stimuli. *FASEB J* 2001;15:2225-2229.

43. NIH Consensus Development Conference: Osteoporosis prevention, diagnosis, and therapy. *NIH Consensus Statement* 2000;17:1-45.

44. Shackelford L, LeBlanc A, Feiveson A, Oganov V: Bone loss in space: Shuttle/Mir experience and bed rest countermeasure program. *1st Biennial Space Biomedical Investigators' Workshop* 1999;1:17.

45. Eisman JA: Genetics of osteoporosis. *Endocr Rev* 1999;20:788-804.

46. Judex S, Donahue LR, Rubin CT: Genetic predisposition to osteoporosis is paralleled by an enhanced sensitivity to signals anabolic to the skeleton. *FASEB J* 2002;16:1280-1282.

47. Torvinen S, Kannus P, Sievanen H, et al: Effect of 8-month vertical whole body vibration on bone, muscle performance, and body balance: A randomized controlled study. *J Bone Miner Res* 2003;18:876-884.

48. Neer RM, Arnaud CD, Zanchetta JR, et al: Effect of parathyroid hormone (1-34) on fractures and bone mineral density in postmenopausal women with osteoporosis. *N Engl J Med* 2001;344:1434-1441.

49. Enserink M: The vanishing promises of hormone replacement. *Science* 2002;297:325-326.

50. Eisman JA: Good, good, good... good vibrations: The best option for better bones? *Lancet* 2001;358:1924-1925.

51. Rubin C, Recker R, Cullen D, Ryaby J, McLeod K: Prevention of post-menopausal bone loss by a low magnitude, high frequency mechanical stimuli: A clinical trial assessing compliance, efficacy, and safety. *J Bone Miner Res* 2004;19:343-351.

52. Ward K, Alsop C, Brown S, Caulton J, Adams J, Mughal M: A randomized, placebo controlled pilot trial of low magnitude, high frequency loading treatment of children with disabling conditions who also have low bone mineral density. *J Bone Miner Res* 2001;16S:1148.

53. Ward K, Alsop C, Brown S, et al: Low magnitude, high frequency loading therapy increases volumetric tibial bone mineral density in children with disabling conditions. *J Bone Miner Res* 2004;19:360-369

54. Whyte MP, Wenkert D, Clements KL, McAlister WH, Mumm S: Bisphosphonate-induced osteopetrosis. *N Engl J Med* 2003;349:457-463.

55. Lacey JV Jr, Mink PJ, Lubin JH, et al: Menopausal hormone replacement therapy and risk of ovarian cancer. *JAMA* 2002;288:334-341.

56. Hirano T, Turner CH, Forwood MR, Johnston CC, Burr DB: Does suppression of bone turnover impair mechanical properties by allowing microdamage accumulation? *Bone* 2000;27:13-20.

57. Carter DR, Caler WE, Spengler DM, Frankel VH: Fatigue behavior of adult cortical bone: The influence of mean strain and strain range. *Acta Orthop Scand* 1981;52:481-490.

58. Rubin CT, Gross TS, McLeod KJ, Bain SD: Morphologic stages in lamellar bone formation stimulated by a potent mechanical stimulus. *J Bone Miner Res* 1995;10:488-495.

59. Judex S, Boyd SK, Qin YX, et al: Adaptations of trabecular bone to low magnitude vibrations result in more uniform stress and strain under load. *Ann Biomed Eng* 2003;31:12-20.

60. Rubin J, Rubin CT, McLeod KJ: Biophysical modulation of cell and tissue structure and function. *Crit Rev Eukaryot Gene Expr* 1995;5:177-191.

61. Hadjiargyrou M, Lombardo F, Zhao S, et al: Transcriptional profiling of bone regeneration: Insight into the molecular complexity of wound repair. *J Biol Chem* 2002;277:30177-30182.

# Chapter 6
# Mechanical Regulation of Bone Repair

*Lutz Claes, PhD*
*Peter Augat, PhD*

## Fracture Repair

Fractures heal by either osteonal healing (direct repair) or callus formation (indirect repair). Direct fracture repair occurs under extremely stable internal fixation and consists of simultaneous remodeling and formation of new bone at the fracture site without formation of periosteal callus tissue.[1] This type of healing occurs only under interfragmentary compression without significant mechanical regulation and is clinically seen very seldom in cases of internal fixation by compression plates.

Indirect repair of fractures is the more natural manner of fracture healing and is characterized by the formation of periosteal callus tissue. It is closely associated with flexible fixation of a fracture—for example, by external fixation or intramedullary nailing.[1] The fracture event induces a healing cascade that is categorized into the stages of inflammation, granulation, callus formation, and remodeling. All these stages occur with a significant degree of temporal and local overlap. Because of different mechanical situations at different sites, some of the healing stages occur simultaneously, whereas others may promote or retard each other. The inflammatory response causes hemorrhage, anoxia, cell death, and an aseptic inflammatory reaction. The fracture gap is initially filled with a hematoma and is gradually replaced by granulation tissue that contains fibroblasts, intercellular material, supporting cells, and numerous new vessels. Chondroblasts and osteoblasts recruited by cellular proliferation and differentiation form cartilage and directly deposit bone by intramembranous bone formation. In some distance from the actual line of fracture, periosteal callus formation commences by direct bony apposition of new bone. The development of the callus is associated with an increase in fracture stability. Further solidification is achieved by conversion of the cartilaginous callus into primary spongiosa or woven bone by endochondral ossification along with intramembranous bone formation. In the final stage of indirect repair, the woven bone is replaced by lamellar bone. Remodeling restores the bone's original shape.

Given sufficient vascularity, the whole course of bone healing seems to be largely influenced by the mechanical environment at the fracture site. The mechanical environment can mainly be characterized by the tissue strain in the fracture gap. The biomechanics of fracture healing, however, is a multifactorial process that includes fracture geometry (fracture type and gap size), amplitude and direction of interfragmentary movement and time-dependent

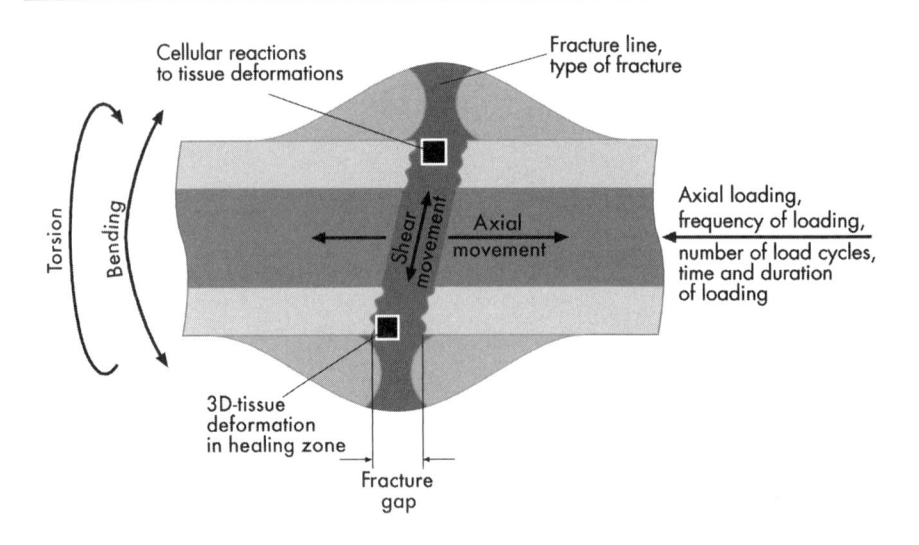

**Figure 1** Main mechanical factors influencing fracture repair.

loading, the number of loading cycles, and the speed of tissue deformation (Fig. 1).

## Axial Interfragmentary Movement and Fracture Gap Size

The biomechanical function of the callus is to reduce initial interfragmentary movement to the extent that the bone fragments can be united. This is achieved by enlarging the cross-sectional area of the bridging tissue (improving structural properties) and by tissue differentiation (improving material properties). A stiff fixation minimizes the amount of interfragmentary movement and results in limited stimulation of callus formation. A more flexible fixation is thought to enhance the callus formation and improve the healing process,[2,3] whereas an unstable fixation may lead to a nonunion.[1]

Another important mechanical factor is the quality of fragment reduction determined by the size of the fracture gap. Previous experimental studies from our group demonstrated that larger fracture gaps cause a delay in fracture healing.[4] Whereas small gap sizes are beneficial for a fast and successful healing process, larger gap sizes result in decreased callus formation and inferior mechanical stability (Fig. 2).

A theory that takes into account these two salient mechanical factors for fracture healing is the interfragmentary strain hypothesis,[5] which predicts that fracture healing will occur only if the local strain in the healing area is less than the rupture strain of bone. However, several studies in which interfragmentary movement and gap size were measured initially allowed much higher interfragmentary strain and yet had good results in terms of fracture

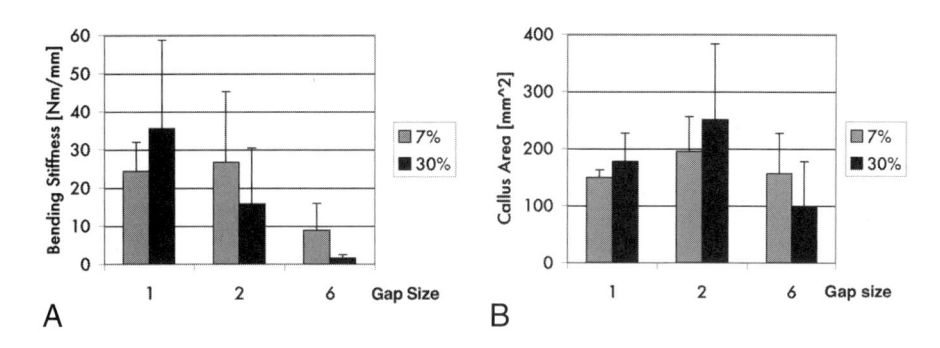

**Figure 2** Influence of gap size and interfragmentary strain (7%, 30%) on bending stiffness **(A)** and callus area **(B)**.

healing.[3] The interfragmentary strain hypothesis further predicts that, for a given interfragmentary movement, healing improves with increasing gap size. This concept disagrees with experimental and clinical experience.[4]

The idea of defining a global interfragmentary strain disregards the heterogeneity of the fracture callus. Although the mechanical situation of the whole bone may be well described by the gap size and the interfragmentary strain, the local tissue deformation that provides the actual stimulus is not exactly known. The structural and mechanical heterogeneity results in a complex distribution of stress and strain. These localized mechanical conditions guide the differentiation process of the various tissue types in the fracture.[6]

Pauwels[7] developed a theory on the differentiation of these tissues from mesenchymal cells depending on local mechanical stresses. He hypothesized that deviatoric stresses, which are always accompanied by strain in some direction, are a specific stimulus for the formation of fibrous connective tissue by fibroblasts. Hydrostatic stresses, on the other hand, are responsible for the formation of cartilaginous tissue by chondrocytes. No specific stimulus exists in this theory for the differentiation of bony tissue. However, as a secondary support tissue, bone is only formed on the basis of a rigid framework of connective tissue or cartilage under low hydrostatic pressure and tissue strain.

## Shear Movement

A controversial discussion persists over whether shear movement delays fracture healing more than axial movement of similar amplitude.[8-11] It is assumed that shear movements impede vascularization and promote fibrous tissue differentiation.[8] However, oblique tibial fractures treated with functional bracing show rapid natural healing[12] even though this type of fixation allows considerable shear movements of up to 4 mm.

The results of the experimental studies might be different because of varying experimental conditions. The studies compared various kinds of fracture models (oblique or transverse)[9] or showed various loading characteristics during the healing period.[10,11] A previous experiment by Augat and associates[11] compared the healing of a tibial osteotomy in sheep with a gap of 3 mm and an axial or plane shear movement of 1.5 mm. The results showed significantly more callus formation and larger flexural rigidity of the bones healed under axial movements in comparison with the bones healed under shear movements. A similar investigation, however, found better healing results for the shear movement.[10] In addition to differences in gap size (2.4 mm) and movement (0.6 mm), another major difference in these experiments was the timing of interfragmentary motion. The interfragmentary motion allowed in our experiment was not constant during the experiment. Because of postoperative pain, the interfragmentary motion was initially quite small and began to approach the full allowed magnitude only after several weeks of biofeedback regulation. In contrast, the motion in the other study was produced by a displacement-controlled hydraulic actuator with a force limitation that achieved interfragmentary motion independent of the biofeedback system of the animal in the early phase of healing.[10] Depending on the aim of the investigation, a study can be designed to answer a basic science question or to answer a clinically relevant question. From a clinical point of view, a study that allows the adaption of the loading by the biofeedback system seems to be more comparable with a clinical situation in a patient. This would explain why we found under our experimental conditions—as in clinical experience—a negative effect from shear movement.

## Time-dependent Changes in Loading and Interfragmentary Movements

Diaphyseal fractures of long bones are commonly treated by flexible fixation systems to allow interfragmentary movement, because motion at the fracture site stimulates the formation of periosteal callus and accelerates the process of endochondral ossification[3,12] if the fracture gap is not too large. By increasing loading or decreasing fixation rigidity (dynamization), investigators have applied specific micromotion at the fracture site to control and enhance this type of fracture healing. Dynamization of rigid external fixations has led to a more rapid consolidation,[13] an increased load-bearing capacity, and significantly more periosteal callus production in comparison with rigid control groups. Dynamization of less rigid external fixations has been effective only at distinct healing phases; very early or late application of micromotion had no beneficial effects on the mechanical properties of the healing fracture.[13] However, some of the positive effects on fracture healing seen under dynamization might simply be attributed to a reduction of the gap size. After dynamization, the fracture gap can be reduced by axial loading (if the implant allows this) and the bone ends remain in closer contact, enabling a more rapid bone formation and thus a faster healing response.[13,14]

A common way to apply micromotion to fractures treated with external fixators is through weight bearing. Retrospective clinical studies and experimental investigations have demonstrated the beneficial effects of weight bearing under flexible fixation of fractures.[3,14,15] Most of the widely used external fixation devices as well as intramedullary nailing systems are flexible enough to ensure enough interfragmentary motion and tissue strain at the fracture site during partial or full weight bearing. Experimental studies on the effect of weight bearing have generally focused on the temporal variation of stability and on the amount of micromotion of the fracture. These studies were based on the hypothesis that the optimal rigidity of fracture fixation may vary over time.

The results of a study by Augat[16] underline the importance of the early healing phase on the outcome of fracture healing. Prevention of early weight bearing under flexible fracture fixation resulted in a biomechanically more stable and histologically more differentiated tissue. Although early loading of a fresh fracture initiated an enormous amount of periosteal callus, the healing of the osteotomy was delayed and the quality of the newly formed tissue was reduced compared to fractures with a reduced loading situation. Instead of varying the onset of weight bearing, Egger[13] used a method of passive dynamization after various time periods to obtain different loading regimens. Early dynamization during the first 4 weeks of healing resulted in a decreased mechanical quality of the callus, although the amount of callus was increased significantly.

Fractures of the human tibial shaft are commonly treated with functional braces, external fixators, or intramedullary nails. All these devices provide a fixation system flexible enough to induce a natural healing pattern with abundant peripheral callus. They are therefore susceptible to stimulation of the healing process by active weight bearing. The amount of interfragmentary motion, which may be as high as several millimeters, is generally consistent with a successful healing process. The mechanical stimulus can be increased by increasing the load or decreasing the rigidity of the fracture fixation. Therefore, for the later healing phase, a flexible fixation that allows interfragmentary movement and encourages periosteal callus formation is the method of choice for fracture treatment. For the initial healing phase, however, the reduction of load transfer to the fracture site by delaying weight bearing or by using a more stable fixation is advantageous for fracture healing. An extremely rigid fixation or even immobilization of the fractured extremity should be avoided. Fractures in patients who may be able to bear weight should not be loaded extensively during the first few weeks after the occurrence of the fracture. However, small amounts of interfragmentary movement provided by partial weight bearing or muscle activity during the initial phase of fracture repair do induce the pathway of indirect healing without overburdening the elastic capacity of the callus tissue. The control of the amount of weight bearing is most efficiently performed by a biofeedback mechanism between the stability of the fracture and its sensibility to pain.[15] For those patients who are not able to bear weight within the first weeks of injury, dynamic interfragmentary motion may be initiated by physiotherapeutic activities. Active dorsiflexion and plantar flexion of the foot produces a spectrum of displacements similar to those seen with weight bearing.[17]

## External Mechanical Stimulation

Weight bearing in combination with flexible fracture fixation generates micromotion at the fracture site and stimulates the repair process. However, the amount of micromotion and hence the extent of the stimulus in weight bearing is not controlled and may vary considerably in individual patients and fractures. Inducing the micromovement by externally applying a known mechanical loading regimen enables the control of factors known to influence the healing response, such as number of loading cycles, amount of interfragmentary movement, or frequency. Controlled micromovement therefore provides an auspicious environment in which to study these factors in experimental and clinical trials. To establish the optimal environment for the enhancement of fracture healing, Goodship[2] compared a flexible fixation with externally induced micromovement to a rigid fixation in a sheep model of bone healing. The application of a controlled axial micromovement with an amplitude of 1 mm at a frequency of 0.5 Hz for 17 minutes daily was associated with an improvement in healing assessed biomechanically and radiographically. In further experiments, Goodship[2] demonstrated that micromovements with smaller amplitudes (0.5 mm) healed consistently better than larger displacements; however, the beneficial effects of controlled interfragmentary movement were always small compared with the rigidly fixed control group. In a group of mechanically stimulated osteotomies that was compared with a group of flexibly fixed osteotomies, differences in healing were no longer observed.[18]

In a comparison among stiff fixation, flexible fixation, and flexible fixation with external stimulation, no improvement of fracture healing was found for externally stimulated fractures under 1 Hz stimulation frequency and axial amplitude of 0.2 to 0.8 mm.[19] Callus formation, however, was significantly larger for fractures stimulated by 0.8 mm amplitude (1,200 load cycles per day) than for those with stiff fixation and was shown to increase with an increase in stimulation amplitude. The frequency of stimulation appears to have only minor effects on the bone healing process. In a sheep osteotomy healing study by Augat,[18] no differences were found in the flexural rigidity 9 weeks postoperatively when 0.2 and 0.8 mm axial amplitude with stimulation frequencies of 1, 5, and 10 Hz were compared.

The number of load cycles per day that are necessary to stimulate a callus formations appear to be very low. One load cycle per day with an amplitude of 1 mm stimulated larger callus formation in a rabbit osteotomy model (T Kato, MD, Tokyo, Japan, unpublished data presented at the International Society for Fracture Repair annual meeting, 1990). In other investigations,[2] 500 load cycles per day (0.5 Hz, 0.5 mm amplitude) led to a significant increase in torsional stiffness compared with a rigidly fixed group after 8 and 10 weeks of osteotomy healing in sheep.

When all data are compared, flexible fixation and weight bearing appear to be of similar stimulatory potency as a controlled externally applied loading regimen. External stimulation seems to have potential only in totally immobilized patients where even muscle activation with a small number of load cycles is impossible. Although the results provided by the research on fracture repair are abundant, it is still not possible to prescribe an optimal environment for efficient fracture treatment. This results only partly from the problem of general validity associated with the application of experimental results. It is the temporal variation of the mechanical environment and the structural heterogeneity of the newly formed tissue that impairs the exact specification of a mechanical environment that is most favorable for fracture repair. The pattern of fracture healing thus is largely a consequence of the progressively changing relationship between local displacement and histologic response.

## Summary

It is well accepted that mechanical factors regulate fracture repair when a sufficient blood supply is available. The major factors influencing the bridging of the fracture ends by callus formation seem to be interfragmentary movement and the fracture gap size, which together determine tissue deformation in the healing zone.

Adequate flexible fixation leads to interfragmentary motion and tissue deformation that stimulate callus formation and endochondral ossification. A stiff fracture fixation minimizes the amount of interfragmentary movement and results in a limited stimulation of callus, whereas an unstable fixation causes large movements and may lead to nonunions. Increased fracture gap delays bone healing because of the limited capacity for bone formation even under sufficient interfragmentary movement.

The time course of loading and interfragmentary movement can be modulated by changing the loading or the rigidity of the fixation device. Very early or late application of interfragmentary movements had no beneficial effects, whereas dynamization a few weeks postoperatively led to improved bone healing. The frequency and number of load cycles seem to have only a minor effect on the healing process. Few load cycles with small movement amplitudes (micromovements) may still stimulate bone formation.

## References

1. Schenk RK: Histophysiology of bone remodelling and bone repair, in Lin OC, Chao EYS (eds): *Perspectives on Biomaterials.* Amsterdam, Netherlands, Elsevier Science, 1986, pp 75-94.

2. Goodship AE: The influence of induced micromovement upon the healing of experimental tibial fractures. *J Bone Joint Surg Br* 1985;67:650-655.

3. Claes LE: Effect of dynamization on gap healing of diaphyseal fractures under external fixation. *Clin Biomech* 1995;10:227-234.

4. Claes L: Influence of size and stability of the osteotomy gap on the success of fracture healing. *J Orthop Res* 1997;15:577-584.

5. Perren SM: The concept of interfragmentary strain, in Uhthoff HK (ed): *Current Concepts of Internal Fixation of Fractures.* New York, NY, Springer-Verlag, 1980, pp 63-77.

6. Claes LE: Effects of mechanical factors on the fracture healing process. *Clin Orthop* 1998;355:S132-S147.

7. Pauwels F: Eine neue Theorie über den Einfluß mechanischer Reize auf die Differenzierung der Stützgewebe. *Z Anat Entwicklungsgeschichte* 1960;121:478-515.

8. Yamagishi M: The biomechanics of fracture healing. *J Bone Joint Surg Am* 1955;37:1035-1068.

9. Park SH: The influence of active shear or compressive motion on fracture-healing. *J Bone Joint Surg Am* 1998;80:868-878.

10. Bishop NE, Tami I, Van Rhijn M, Corveleijn R, Schneider E, Ito K: Effects of volumetric vs. shear deformation on tissue differentiation during secondary bone healing. *Trans Orthop Res Soc* 2003;28:114.

11. Augat P, Burger J, Schorlemmer S, Henke T, Claes L: Shear movement at the fracture site delays the healing of long bone fractures. *Trans Orthop Res Soc* 2003;28:113.

12. Sarmiento A: Tibial shaft fractures treated with functional braces: Experience with 780 fractures. *J Bone Joint Surg Br* 1989;71:602-609.

13. Egger EL: Effects of axial dynamization on bone healing. *J Trauma* 1993;34:185-192.

14. Aro HT: Biomechanics and biology of fracture repair under external fixation. *Hand Clin* 1993;9:531-542.

15. Goodship AE: The role of fixator frame stiffness in the control of fracture healing: An experimental study. *J Biomech* 1993;26:1027-1035.

16. Augat P: Early, full weightbearing with flexible fixation delays fracture healing. *Clin Orthop* 1996;328:194-202.

17. Goodship AE: Strain rate and timing of stimulation in mechanical modulation of fracture healing. *Clin Orthop* 1998;355:S105-S115.

18. Augat P: Mechanical stimulation by external application of cyclic tensile strains does not effectively enhance bone healing. *J Orthop Trauma* 2001;15:54-60.

19. Wolf S: The effects of external mechanical stimulation on the healing of diaphyseal osteotomies fixed by flexible external fixation. *Clin Biomech* 1998;13:359-364.

Chapter 7

# Pulsed Low-Intensity Ultrasound and Fracture Healing: A Proposed Mechanism of Action

*Javad Parvizi, MD*
*Sue J. Harris, PhD*
*Neill M. Pounder, PhD*

## Introduction

Pulsed low-intensity ultrasound (PLIUS) has been demonstrated to accelerate fracture healing by many clinical studies.[1-5] Over the last decade this treatment modality has become more widely accepted by the clinical community to accelerate healing of fresh fractures, to minimize delayed healing, and to stimulate healing of established nonunions. Although the use of PLIUS has increased, a lack of understanding remains as to how this therapy achieves its clinical effect. Rubin and associates[6] have published a comprehensive review of both the clinical and scientific evidence behind PLIUS. The aim of this chapter is to update one aspect of that review, focusing on the scientific data that contribute to understanding this therapy's mechanism of action.

## The Ultrasound Signal

The clinically effective ultrasound signal consists of 1.5 MHz ultrasound wave pulsed at 1 kHz with a 20% duty cycle at an intensity of 30 mW/cm$^2$ SATA (spatial average temporal average). Most of the research that has been carried out uses this signal, and the ultrasound signal will not therefore be specified when discussing experimental work unless it differs from the parameters outlined above.

## Physical Interaction With Biologic Material

The ultrasound signal is delivered via a transducer that is coupled to the skin (or experimental equipment) with water-based gel. The ultrasound waves are produced by vibrations in a piezoelectric material such as lead zirconate titante as a result of a high-frequency electric field set up across the material. Ultrasound may travel in a solid material in several different forms, the most common of which are longitudinal and shear waves. Longitudinal pressure waves are emitted by the transducer, and in the clinical scenario pass through the soft tissue to the bone. Mode conversion, or conversion from one wave type to another, occurs when a wave encounters an interface between

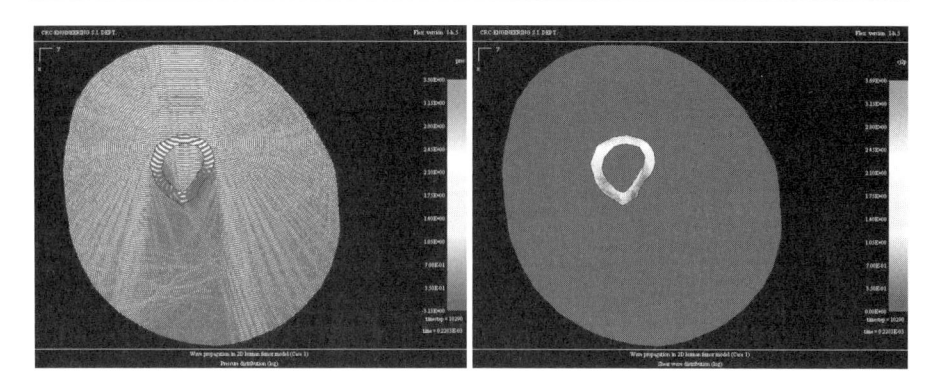

Section Two    Biophysical Regulation of Bone Healing in Animal Models

**Figure 1** Mathematical model of longitudinal and shear waves produced by low-intensity ultrasound incident on a tibia. *(N Fujimoto, MSc, Tokyo, Japan, personal communication, 2003.)*

materials of different acoustic impedance at an oblique angle of incidence. For example, when a longitudinal wave hits an interface (such as a bone) at an angle, some of the energy may cause particle movement in the transverse direction, resulting in a transverse, or shear, wave. Mathematical modeling has demonstrated that when the ultrasound signal reaches the bone surface, some longitudinal waves continue through the bone and some are reflected, converting into shear waves that pass around the bone (Fig. 1) (N Fujimoto, MSc, Tokyo, Japan, personal communication, 2003).

Leung and associates[5] reported the formation of fracture callus not only on the anteromedial surface of the tibia but also on the posterolateral surface, indicating that the stimulatory effect of ultrasound is not localized just to the area of direct stimulation. Such clinical observations alongside the physics of ultrasound transmission suggest that the combination of longitudinal and shear waves may be key to the clinical efficacy of this therapy.

As the ultrasound wave passes through the muscle and soft tissue to the bone, the amplitude of the signal attenuates, resulting in a loss of wave power (intensity). Attenuation coefficients are published for a range of biologic tissues and quoted in terms of dBcm$^{-1}$MHz$^{-1}$ (dB refers to decibels). Examples of intensity attenuation coefficients are given in Table 1.

Attenuation, expressed in decibels, is defined as $-10\log_{10}(I/I_0)$, in which $I_0$ is the incident ultrasound intensity and $I$ the attenuated intensity. Assuming that an ultrasound wave must pass through approximately 0.5 cm depth each of skin, fat, and tendon and 2 cm of muscle to reach a midshaft femur, then:

For 1.5 MHz ultrasound wave, total attenuation is:

$$1.5*[(0.5*0.6) + (0.5*0.6) + (2.0+1.5) + (0.5*1.2)] = 6.3$$

Therefore,

$$6.3 = -10\log_{10}\left(\frac{I}{I_0}\right)$$
$$\frac{I}{I_0} = 0.23$$

**Table 1 Attenuation Coefficients for Biologic Tissues**

| Material | Ultrasound Attenuation Coefficient (dBcm$^{-1}$MHz$^{-1}$) |
|---|---|
| Soft tissue (skin) | 0.6 (Wells[7]) |
| Fat | 0.6 (Wells[7]) |
| Muscle | 1.5 (Wells[7]) |
| Tendon | 1.2 (Goss et al[8]) |

**Table 2 Nonunion Success Rates for Different Fractures Treated With Ultrasound**

| Bone | Success Rate Quoted in Frankel[3] | Success Rate Quoted in Nolte et al[4] |
|---|---|---|
| Femur | 86% | 80% |
| Humerus | 70% | 100% |
| Tibia/Tibia-fibula | 83% | 100% |
| Scaphoid | 86% | 80% |
| Radius/Radius-ulna | 96% | 80% |
| Metatarsal | 81% | 100% |

Thus, for a 30 mW/cm² ultrasound signal at the skin surface, approximately 77% attenuation occurs, resulting in 7 mW/cm² reaching a damaged femur. For a superficial tibia, the approximate ultrasound power is 28 mW/cm². Frankel[3] and Nolte and associates[4] have both published fracture nonunion data for a range of different fracture sites. From these data (Table 2), the success rates for different fracture sites are seen to be independent of the depth of the fracture. Hence, although an ultrasound wave attenuates as it passes through soft tissue and bone, the clinical success rate appears to be independent of the ultrasound intensity reaching the fracture site.

As previously discussed, ultrasound is a high-frequency mechanical pressure wave. Absorption or reflection of this wave results in a steady radiation force that can generate a motion in the tissue. When the ultrasound is pulsed, the force would be expected to cycle on and off and lead to a vibration in the tissue at the pulse frequency. Greenleaf and associates (JF Greenleaf, PhD, Rochester, MN, unpublished data presented at the American Institute of Ultrasound in Medicine annual meeting, 2003) have reported the levels of motion generated by PLIUS in a cadaveric forearm model. A surgical opening was created in the cadaver to expose the distal radius. An osteotomy was then created in the radius. Ultrasound was applied to the underside of the arm and a laser interferometer targeted on the exposed radius to measure the motion of the distal and proximal edges of the bone fracture. The results showed that movement occurred at a frequency of 1 kHz, matching the pulse of the signal. At this frequency, the velocity of the bone ends and soft tissue ranges from 1 µms$^{-1}$ to 3.5 µms$^{-1}$, equating to 0.15 to 0.55 nm displacement respectively. These levels of motion are approximately 1,000 times less than micromotion,[9,10] in which accelerated fracture healing occurred with displacements between 0.5 and 2 mm. This work shows that PLIUS is providing motion on a nanometer scale, suggesting the mode of action is independent of fixation methods such as casting or external fixation where millimeter levels of motion can occur.[11] To understand how this treatment achieves a clinical effect, it is necessary to determine which of the many cell types and biologic processes involved in fracture healing are affected by the ultrasound signal.

## Biologic Response

Rubin and associates[6] reviewed the available scientific evidence and concluded that exposure of healing bone to ultrasound results in stronger and stiffer callus formation as demonstrated in a number of in vivo studies.[12,13] In vitro data showed that ultrasound accelerated the endochondral ossification process,[4] an observation supported by work in chondrocytes showing ultrasound-induced increases in proteoglycan synthesis.[14] Azuma and associates[15] have since shown that ultrasound benefits early, middle, and late phases of the fracture healing process. They also observed histologically that endochondral ossification was accelerated, thus validating the in vitro work of Nolte and associates.[4] Clearly endochondral ossification is crucial to the transition from soft to hard callus, but numerous other processes and cell types are involved that, according to Azuma and associates'[15] data, should also be positively affected by the ultrasound signal. In recent years, data on osteoblasts, marrow cells, and periosteal cells have been produced that provide mechanistic information to support the functional outcome of accelerated healing seen by Azuma and associates.[15] The remainder of this chapter will review this data and propose a basic mechanism of action by which PLIUS achieves its clinical effect.

### Effects on Chondrocytes

Parvizi and associates[14] demonstrated that rat chondrocytes responded to PLIUS (50 mW/cm$^2$ SATA, 1 MHz) with elevated levels of aggrecan mRNA and increased proteoglycan synthesis. Increased aggrecan mRNA in response to ultrasound had previously been demonstrated in a rat femoral fracture model[16] using a 50 mW/cm$^2$ SATA, 0.5 MHz signal. This study was followed up by work demonstrating that the chondrocytes responded immediately to ultrasound stimulation (50 mW/cm$^2$ SATA, 1 MHz) with rapid changes in intracellular calcium concentration[17] and that this calcium signaling was essential in mediating the ultrasound-induced increase in proteoglycan synthesis.

More recently, work on bovine chondrocytes shows increased proteoglycan synthesis (as measured by sulfate incorporation) in response to PLIUS. The latter occurred in 3-dimensional constructs seeded with chondrocytes, a culture system that provides a slightly more physiologic environment than the monolayer cultures. Interestingly, despite increased sulfate incorporation, the total sGAG content was not increased (Fig. 2) (NM Vaughan, BSc, London, England, unpublished data presented at the Orthopaedic Research Society annual meeting, 2005). This finding suggests that proteoglycan degradation is also increased, so ultrasound is accelerating proteoglycan

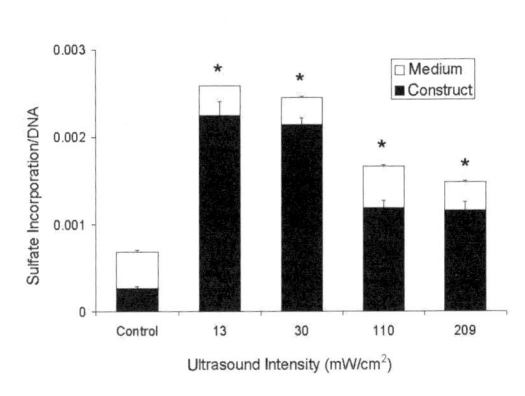

**Figure 2** Effect of pulsed ultrasound intensity applied every 24 hours on sGAG synthesis from day 8 to 9. Incorporation of $^{35}SO_4$ normalized to DNA levels in $\mu M^{35}SO_4/hr/\mu gDNA$. Error bars indicate SEM n = 7 (*$P < 0.001$). *(NM Vaughan, BSc, London, England, unpublished data presented at the Orthopaedic Research Society annual meeting, 2005.)*

turnover in chondrocyte cultures. An accelerated matrix turnover may facilitate faster remodeling at the fracture site as the callus transitions from fibrocartilage (soft callus) to mineralized tissue (hard callus). Understanding of the intracellular pathways mediating the ultrasound-induced proteoglycan synthesis is limited to the knowledge that intracellular calcium signaling increases aggrecan gene expression. Further discussion on signaling pathways is presented toward the end of this chapter.

## Response of Marrow Cells to Ultrasound

Bone marrow is an important source of undifferentiated cells during the fracture healing process,[18] contributing cells to the chondrocytic and osteoblastic lineages. ST2 cells, a bone marrow stromal cell line, have been shown to have a distinct temporal pattern of gene expression in response to daily PLIUS stimulation (J Ridgway, BSc, York, England, unpublished data presented at the International Society for Fracture Repair annual meeting, 2004). In vitro experiments were performed to investigate early gene transcription for up to 40 minutes following a single 20-minute dose of ultrasound and to study cell differentiation in response to daily ultrasound treatment over a 10-day period. The earliest response seen was increased expression of multiple genes belonging to the retinoic acid responsive signal transduction pathway. Genes such as cdx-1 and stra-8 showed a peak in transcription 20 minutes after ultrasound treatment (Fig. 3). Longer-term investigations showed retinoic acid–responsive genes such as MMP-13 to be upregulated after 48 hours (Fig. 4). Expression of this gene was not altered in the shorter timeframe (< 1 hour), suggesting that this upregulation is a downstream effect of the earlier response genes. Over a 10-day period in the presence of ascorbate, increased expression was seen for the osteogenic markers alkaline phosphatase and MMP-13 (J Ridgway, BSc, York, England, unpublished data presented at the International Society for Fracture Repair annual meeting, 2004).

These studies indicate that the transcriptional response to PLIUS in ST2 cells involves the early stimulation of the retinoic acid–responsive signal transduction pathway and subsequent upregulation of downstream genes in this

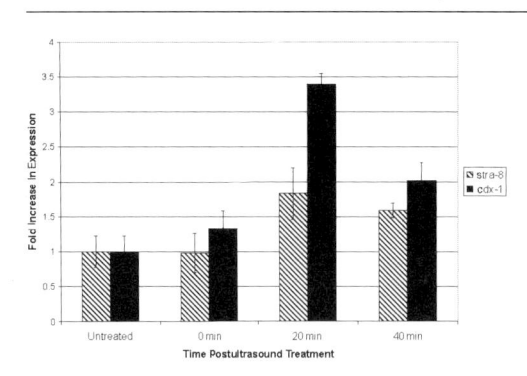

**Figure 3** Quantitative PCR data show increase in stra-8 and cdx-1 mRNA expression by ST2 cells 0, 20, and 40 minutes following a single 20-minute ultrasound stimulation. *(J Ridgway, BSc, York, England, unpublished data presented at the International Society for Fracture Repair annual meeting, 2004.)*

response pathway. This effect is followed by longer-term increases in the gene expression of osteogenic growth factors and markers of osteogenesis. This response suggests a mechanism by which ultrasound stimulates undifferentiated mesenchymal marrow cells in vivo to differentiate along osteogenic lineages, thus contributing to the formation of both soft and hard callus.[19-21]

## Periosteal Cell Response

Leung and associates[22] demonstrated PLIUS-stimulated human periosteal cell differentiation. The osteogenic markers osteocalcin and alkaline phosphatase were measured in the culture media after 2 and 4 days of ultrasound stimulation. After 20 minutes of stimulation per day for 4 days, osteocalcin, alkaline phosphatase, and vascular endothelial growth factor (VEGF) expression in the culture media was significantly increased compared with untreated control cultures. In addition, alizarin red staining showed significant increases in calcium nodule formation (representing mineralization) in cultures after 4 weeks of daily stimulation.

## Osteoblast Differentiation

Much of the in vivo data that has been published on PLIUS have shown significant enhancement of the mechanical properties of bone.[12,13,15] It has been suggested that this increase in strength is due to an acceleration of callus mineralization—that is, hard callus formation. In vitro studies now appear to support this hypothesis, including the study by Leung and associates[22] showing increased mineralization in periosteal cell cultures.

The MC3T3-E14 line is a murine preosteoblastic cell line that provides a model for studying osteoblastic differentiation in vitro. Two enzymes known to play important roles in the mineralization process are alkaline phosphatase and MMP-13. Unsworth and associates (J Unsworth, PhD, York, England, unpublished data presented at the Orthopaedic Research Society annual meeting, 2005) have shown that over a 10-day period the level of alkaline phosphatase in MC3T3 cultures increased but that this increase was significantly enhanced by daily stimulation with PLIUS. Significant differences ($P < 0.05$) were achieved on days 2, 4, 6, and 8 with the controls reaching the same levels by day 10. In addition to the acceleration in alkaline

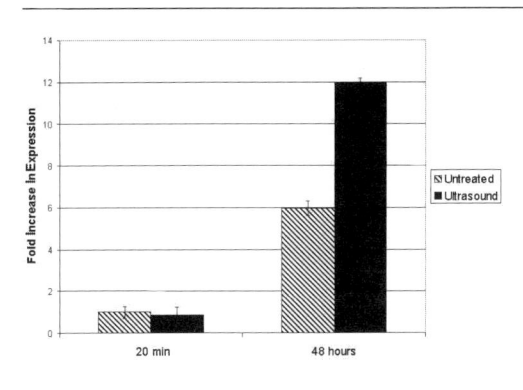

**Figure 4** Quantitative PCR data show increase in MMP-13 mRNA expression by ST2 cells following up to 2 days culture. *(J Ridgway, BSc, York, England, unpublished data presented at the International Society for Fracture Repair annual meeting, 2004.)*

phosphatase synthesis, MMP-13 mRNA levels in ultrasound-stimulated cultures followed the same temporal pattern that was seen in untreated controls but at a higher expression level. MC3T3 cultures stimulated for up to 25 days showed a significant increase in the degree of mineralization as determined by colorimetric analysis of alizarin red staining (J Unsworth, PhD, York, England, unpublished data presented at the Orthopaedic Research Society annual meeting, 2005).

Further evidence that ultrasound affects the mineralization process comes from Saito and associates,[23] who demonstrated accelerated calcium accumulation in MC3T3-E1 cultures. Significant increases (8.6-fold and 3.6-fold higher than untreated controls) were seen at day 25 and day 35 respectively. This study also showed that activity of enzymes involved in collagen cross-link formation was increased by a 30 mW/cm$^2$ ultrasound signal. These findings suggest that PLIUS accelerated calcium deposition and the formation of the collagen scaffold necessary for calcification of the bone matrix.

Collectively the findings of these studies demonstrate that, in a preosteoblastic culture system, PLIUS accelerates differentiation along the osteoblastic lineage, as shown by the rise in alkaline phosphatase synthesis and the raised level of MMP-13 expression (J Ridgway, BSc, York, England, unpublished data presented at the International Society for Fracture Repair annual meeting, 2004). These phenotypic changes facilitate an increased degree of mineralization, a process that includes accelerated calcium accumulation and collagen scaffold formation. Such effects in a fracture environment can benefit the formation of a mineralized callus, stabilizing the fracture and increasing the strength of the bone, as has been observed in animal studies.

## Transduction Processes

The beneficial effects of ultrasound demonstrated throughout the healing process cast doubt on the idea that a single transduction pathway converts the nanomotion reported by Greenleaf and associates (JF Greenleaf, PhD, Rochester, MN, unpublished data presented at the American Institute of

Ultrasound in Medicine annual meeting, 2003) to the biologic responses reviewed above. The following section of this chapter focuses on research into the transduction mechanism(s) and intracellular events that regulate these responses.

## Integrins Transduce the Ultrasound Signal

Research groups have used various models to understand the cellular pathways that regulate the cellular response to ultrasound. One group has used human dermal fibroblasts as its experimental model, having already shown that they proliferate in response to ultrasound.[24] This group investigated the integrin signaling pathway and clearly demonstrated the involvement of various downstream molecules in controlling the proliferative response.

Integrins are a family of transmembrane cell adhesion molecules that are known to respond to mechanical stimuli. One of their key characteristics is the capacity to switch between low- and high-affinity states. When in the high-affinity state and bound to their ligand (fibronectin or RGD peptide), the integrins cluster in the cell membrane, forming focal adhesions. Focal adhesion kinase (FAK) and paxillin are key proteins in the focal adhesion complex, and FAK binds directly to the integrin subunit molecules as well as to paxillin (an intracellular anchor protein), thereby providing the link between the integrin and the cytoskeleton.

As described above, a fundamental process in integrin signaling is the formation of focal adhesion complexes. Downstream of paxillin and FAK is MEK-1, an upstream regulator of ERK. Phosphorylation of ERK results in its translocation into the nucleus and therefore activation of transcription factors and gene transcription. Zhou and associates[24] showed that inhibiting MEK-1 using PD98059 prevented ultrasound-induced phosphorylation of ERK 1/2 (Fig. 5, *A*). The inhibition of ERK phosphorylation correlated with inhibition of DNA synthesis (Fig. 5, *B*), thereby demonstrating the involvement of the ERK cascade in ultrasound-induced cell proliferation. Having established that ERK 1/2 activation is affected by ultrasound, Zhou and associates[24] demonstrated that ERK activation is not required for focal adhesion formation and actin polymerization (ultrasound-induced focal adhesion formation still occurred in the presence of the MEK-1 inhibitor) (Fig. 6). In contrast, ERK phosphorylation does occur in response to TGF-α. The conclusions from these observations are that the proliferative effect of PLIUS in human dermal fibroblasts is mediated through integrins and paxillin upstream of MEK-1-regulated ERK 1/2 phosphorylation. Supporting this concept are data showing the ultrasound-induced DNA synthesis to be abolished in the presence of β1-integrin-blocking antibody or RGD peptide. Experiments using integrin-blocking antibodies have been performed on human dermal fibroblasts[24] and rat chondrocytes (ME Bolander, MD, Rochester, MN, personal communication, 2002). These experiments support the involvement of integrins in mediating cellular response to PLIUS.

The data obtained in fibroblasts are strong evidence that integrins are involved in the transduction of PLIUS, converting the signal from a mechanical stimulus to a cellular signaling cascade. Further observations regarding the intracellular effects of ultrasound on cell types directly involved in frac-

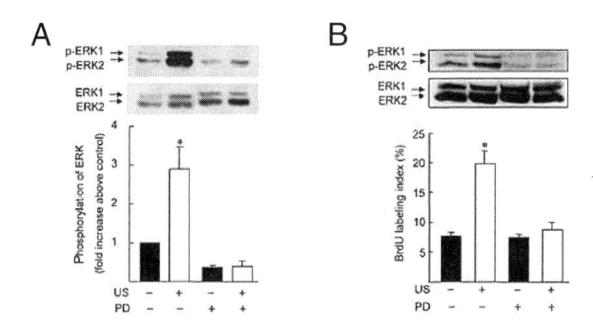

**Figure 5** Ultrasound-induced activation of ERK 1/2 is regulated by MEK-1 and required for ultrasound-induced BrdU incorporation. Quiescent skin fibroblasts were incubated with 20 mM PD98059 (PD) for 1 hour followed by 11 minutes of ultrasound stimulation. Phosphorylation of ERK 1/2 was analyzed by Western blotting with antibody to threonine and tyrosine dual phosphorylated ERK 1/2. **A,** Quantitation of phosphorylation was performed by scanning densitometry from three separate experiments, presented as the increase in phosphorylation of ERK1/2 above control unstimulated level. **B,** BrdU incorporation data represent the mean ± SE percentage of BrdU-positive nuclei in three independent wells per condition. *$P < 0.05$ compared with control cells. (Zhou et al[24])

ture healing provide insights into additional signaling pathways that contribute to the clinical efficacy of PLIUS.

## Transduction Pathways in Osteoblastic Cells

As discussed previously, work on ST2 cells has indicated that retinoic acid–responsive genes are immediately upregulated by PLIUS with subsequent increases in alkaline phosphatase and MMP-13 expression (J Ridgway, BSc, York, England, unpublished data presented at the International Society for Fracture Repair annual meeting, 2004). Other published work using the same ST2 cell line has demonstrated an increase in cyclooxygenase-2 (COX-2) mRNA in response to PLIUS, with a corresponding increase in prostaglandin synthesis ($PGE_2$).[25] The pathway involved in this response was delineated by the addition of an inhibitor of MEK-1 and -2 phosphorylation (PD98059), an inhibitor of PI3K (LY294002), and an inhibitor of p38 MAPK (SB203580). These experiments demonstrated that the increased COX-2 expression was downstream of the p38 MAPK and PI3K pathways but not dependent on ERK 1/2 phosphorylation. This state of affairs contrasts with the ERK-dependent proliferative response of human dermal fibroblasts[24] referred to earlier.

Studies of a number of preosteoblastic cell lines indicate that other cell-signaling pathways are also affected by PLIUS. Chen and associates[26] used a human fetal preosteoblast line and observed gene upregulation of the transcription factor Cbfa1/Runx2 and a downstream osteogenic marker, osteocalcin. The upregulation of both these genes was dependent on phosphory-

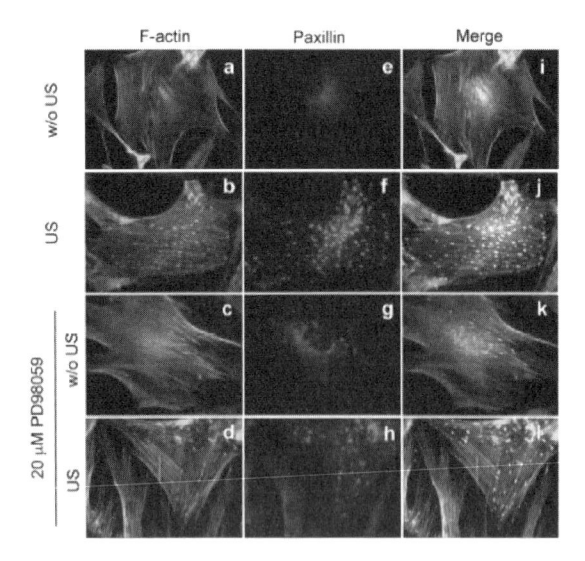

**Figure 6** Ultrasound-induced focal adhesion formation occurs in the presence of PD98059. Quiescent fibroblasts grown on glass coverslips were stimulated with ultrasound for 11 minutes in the absence **(A, B, E, F, I, J)**, or presence **(C, D, G, H, K, L)** of 20 mM PD98059. The cultures were fixed 45 minutes after stimulation with 4% paraformaldehyde in PBS. F-actin filaments were visualized by Alexa-phalloidin **(A, B, C, D)**; paxillin was determined by indirect immunofluoresence and visualized with Texas Red conjugate **(E, F, G, H)**; nuclei were visualized with Hoechst 33258. Photos **I, J, K,** and **L** are merged pictures of F-actin, paxillin, and nucleus. (Zhou et al[24])

lation of ERK, which in turn was found to be downstream of Gαi protein. The involvement of a G protein indicates that another transmembrane receptor or ion channel outside the integrin family can transduce the ultrasound signal.

Another intracellular response to ultrasound was identified by Wang and associates[27] using MG63, SaOS2, and hFOB 1.19 cells (human preosteoblast line). Ultrasound stimulation induced an increase in VEGF-A levels (mRNA and protein) in all three cell lines (VEGF expression is also increased in human periosteal cells; see Leung and associates[22]). Upstream regulators of this response were identified as nitric oxide (NO) (regulated by iNOS) and cGMP, inducing the transcription factor HIF-1α. NO donors alone induced the increase in VEGF but failed to replicate the ultrasound-induced proliferation and alkaline phosphatase activity. This finding indicates that both cGMP and NO are necessary to result in the proliferative and alkaline phosphatase activity and that, although VEGF contributes to these functional responses (as shown by antibody-blocking experiments), it acts in concert with other proteins not identified by this study.

In summary, a number of pathways respond to PLIUS. Integrins transduce the signal in human dermal fibroblasts and are implicated in chondrocytes. A marrow cell line responds by upregulation of retinoic acid–responsive genes. Preosteoblastic lines have been shown to respond through Gαi proteins or cGMP- and NO-regulated pathways.

## Conclusions

Given our knowledge that PLIUS has a positive impact throughout the fracture healing process,[17] it is to be expected that numerous cell types and biologic processes show measurable responses to this mechanical stimulus. Within this chapter a number of signaling pathways have been discussed, and in certain instances the findings of some studies may appear to contradict one another (eg, ERK activation in preosteoblastic cells[26] but not in ST2 cells[25]). When considering such data, the differences in cell type and stage of cell differentiation (often dependent on small variables in culture conditions) must be remembered. When all available evidence is considered as a whole, it is clear that, as might be expected, ultrasound affects a number of intracellular pathways. Understanding the interactions of those pathways with one another, the involvement of different pathways at various stages of osteoblast differentiation, and the impact of downstream events on other cell populations in a fracture environment are all challenges that remain for those seeking to understand ultrasound as a bone-healing therapy.

## References

1. Heckman JD, Ryaby JP, McCabe J, Frey JJ, Kilcoyne RF: Acceleration of tibial fracture healing by non-invasive, low-intensity pulsed ultrasound. *J Bone Joint Surg Am* 1994;76:26-34.
2. Kristiansen TK, Ryaby JP, McCabe J, Frey JJ, Roe LR: Accelerated healing of distal radial fractures with the use of specific, low-intensity ultrasound. *J Bone Joint Surg Am* 1997;79:961-973.
3. Frankel VH: Results of prescription use of pulse ultrasound therapy in fracture management, in Szabo Z, Lewis JE, Fantini GA, Savalgi RS (eds): *Surgical Technology International, VII.* San Francisco, CA, University Medical Press, 1998, pp 389-393.
4. Nolte PA, van der Krans A, Patka P, Janssen IMC, Ryaby JP, Albers GHR: Low-intensity pulsed ultrasound in the treatment of nonunions. *J Trauma* 2001;51:693-703.
5. Leung KS, Lee WS, Tsui HF, Liu PPL, Cheung WH: Complex tibial fracture outcomes following treatment with low-intensity pulsed ultrasound. *Ultrasound Med Biol* 2004;30:389-395.
6. Rubin C, Bolander M, Ryaby JP, Hadjiargyrou M: The use of low-intensity ultrasound to accelerate the healing of fractures. *J Bone Joint Surg Am* 2001;83:259-270.
7. Wells PNT: Ultrasonic imaging of the human body. *Rep Prog Phys* 1999;62:671-722.
8. Goss SA, Frizzell LA, Dunn F: Ultrasonic absorption and attenuation in mammalian tissues. *Ultrasound Med Biol* 1979;5:181-186.
9. Kenwright J, Goodship AE: Controlled mechanical stimulation in the treatment of tibial fractures. *Clin Orthop* 1989;241:36-47.
10. Kenwright J, Richardson JB, Cunningham JL, et al: Axial movement and tibial fractures. *J Bone Joint Surg Br* 1991;73:654-659.

11. Kenwright J, Gardner T: Mechanical influences on tibial fracture healing. *Clin Orthop* 1998;355:S179-S190.

12. Pilla AA, Mont AA, Nasser PR, et al: Non-invasive low-intensity pulsed ultrasound accelerates bone healing in the rabbit. *J Orthop Trauma* 1990;4:246-253.

13. Wang SJ, Lewallen DG, Bolander ME, Chao EYS, Ilstrup DM, Greenleaf JF: Low-intensity ultrasound treatment increases strength in a rat femoral fracture model. *J Orthop Res* 1994;12:40-47.

14. Parvizi J, Wu CC, Lewallen DG, Greenleaf JF, Bolander ME: Low intensity ultrasound stimulates proteoglycan synthesis in rat chondrocytes by increasing aggrecan gene expression. *J Orthop Res* 1999;17:488-494.

15. Azuma Y, Ito M, Harada Y, Takagi H, Ohta T, Jingushi S: Low-intensity pulsed ultrasound accelerates rat femoral fracture healing by acting on the various cellular reactions in the fracture callus. *J Bone Miner Res* 2001;16:671-680.

16. Yang KH, Parvizi J, Wang SJ, et al: Exposure to low-intensity ultrasound increases aggrecan gene expression in a rat femur fracture model. *J Orthop Res* 1996;14:802-809.

17. Parvizi J, Parpura V, Greenleaf JF, Bolander ME: Calcium signaling is required for ultrasound-stimulated aggrecan synthesis by rat chondrocytes. *J Orthop Res* 2002;20: 51-57.

18. Friedenstein AJ, Piatetzky-Shapiro II, Petrakova KV: Osteogenesis in transplants of bone marrow cells. *J Embryol Exp Morphol* 1966;16:381-390.

19. Weston AD, Rosen V, Chandraratna RAS, Underhill TM: Regulation of skeletal progenitor differentiation by the BMP and retinoid signaling pathways. *J Cell Biol* 2000; 148:679-690.

20. Li X, Schwarz EM, Zuscik MJ, et al: Retinoic acid stimulates chondrocyte differentiation and enhances bone morphogenetic protein effects through induction of Smad1 and Smad5. *Endocrinology* 2003;144:2514-2523.

21. Skillington J, Choy L, Derynck R: Bone morphogenetic protein and retinoic acid signaling cooperate to induce osteoblast differentiation of preadipocytes. *J Cell Biol* 2002; 159:135-146.

22. Leung KS, Cheung WH, Zhang C, Lee KM, Lo HK: Low intensity pulsed ultrasound stimulates osteogenic activity of human periosteal cells. *Clin Orthop* 2004;418:253-259.

23. Saito M, Soshi S, Tanaka T, Fujii K: Intensity-related differences in collagen post-translational modification in MC3T3-E1 osteoblasts after exposure to low- and high-intensity pulsed ultrasound. *Bone* 2004;35:644-655.

24. Zhou S, Schmelz A, Seufferlein T, Li Y, Zhao J, Bachem MG: Molecular mechanisms of low intensity pulsed ultrasound on human skin fibroblasts. *J Biol Chem* 2004;279: 54463-54469.

25. Naruse K, Miyauchi A, Itoman M, Mikuni-Takagaki Y: Distinct anabolic response of osteoblast to low-intensity pulsed ultrasound. *J Bone Miner Res* 2003;18:360-369.

26. Chen YJ, Wang CJ, Yang KD, et al: Pertussis toxin-sensitive Gαi protein and ERK-dependent pathways mediate ultrasound promotion of osteogenic transcription in human osteoblasts. *FEBS Letters* 2003;554:154-158.

27. Wang FS, Kuo YR, Wang CJ, et al: Nitric oxide mediates ultrasound-induced hypoxia-inducible factor-1α activation and vascular endothelial growth factor-A expression in human osteoblasts. *Bone* 2004;35:114-123.

Chapter 8
# Pulsed Electromagnetic Fields on Osteotomy Healing and Normal Bone Turnover

*Edmund Chao, PhD*
*Isao Ohnishi, MD*
*Bahman Rafiee, MD*
*Rainer Meffert, MD*
*Teresa Wu, MD*
*Dennis Cullinane, PhD*
*Bruce Simon, PhD*
*Nozomu Inoue, MD, PhD*

## Introduction

Pulsed electromagnetic field (PEMF) stimulation has been in clinical use for over 25 years, and has been shown to be effective in a multitude of clinical case reports.[1-3] Double-blind studies have confirmed the clinical effectiveness of PEMF stimulation on osteotomy healing[4,5] and delayed union fractures.[6] A substantial number of in vitro studies have shown positive effects of electromagnetic fields on the proliferation and activity of osteoblasts.[7-9] Although PEMF treatment has long been in clinical use, additional in vitro and animal studies are still being conducted to clearly understand the functional mechanism and dose effects of PEMF at the cellular and tissue levels. Small animal models, such as rabbit and rat, have been used to test the various PEMF signals for bone healing.[10,11] Large animal models are necessary to develop clinical application protocols and to validate the benefit of PEMF treatment for functional outcomes.

Despite the well-established positive effect of PEMF on osteogenic activities,[10-13] the results obtained using large animal models, such as horses, canines, and sheep, are still controversial. Positive effects of PEMF on new bone formation have been shown in a bone defect model using the metacarpal bones of the horse.[14,15] Conversely, no benefit of PEMF treatment was found in a dog nonunion model and a sheep osteotomy model.[16,17] The effect of PEMF treatment on delayed osteotomy gap healing in a canine model[18] would be clinically relevant because the study results may provide the needed assurance of successful bony union in cases where the clinical and radiographic signs of fracture healing are not well demonstrated. However, this study did not report the measured dose effect or the influence of PEMF on normal bone turnover at sites away from the osteotomy and on the contralateral intact bone exposed to the same but weaker electromagnetic field for an extensive period of time.

We have established a highly standardized delayed union model using a canine midtibial transverse osteotomy fixed with a rigid external fixator.[19-22] Delayed union in this model was defined by a significant reduction in bone strength and limb load-bearing function when compared with the osteotomized bone that was dynamized by allowing the gap to close under the same rigid fixation.[19-21] This model was also used to test the effectiveness of fixed doses of PEMF stimulation on bone osteotomy healing under external fixation.[18] Our working hypothesis was that PEMF effects on callus formation and osteotomy healing would be dose dependent and that such stimulation may also influence normal bone turnover. The objective of this study was to compare the dose effect of the same PEMF signal using two stimulation time periods on the osteotomy gap model in canine midtibia stabilized under a rigid external fixator. Normal bone turnover in the cortex adjacent to the osteotomy site and the intact contralateral tibia exposed to the same but weaker PEMF field was also investigated.

## Methods

### Animal Model

Eighteen adult male mixed-breed dogs were divided into three experimental groups: the 1-hour PEMF group, the 4-hour PEMF group, and the control group without PEMF stimulation. Standardized transverse middiaphyseal tibial osteotomies were performed unilaterally. The osteotomies were stabilized with a 2-mm gap using a rigid custom-made unilateral 6-halfpin external fixator. The external fixator had no adjustable joint except a telescoping mechanism with a lock bolt to permit fine adjustment of gap distance. The telescoping mechanism was fixed with polymethylmethacrylate postoperatively to avoid any subsequent movement. This external fixation system provided a rigid fixation at the osteotomy in order to create the delayed union environment. Immediate weight bearing and mobilization were allowed postoperatively as tolerated by the animal. PEMF treatment started 4 weeks after surgery and was continued for 8 weeks until sacrifice at 12 weeks. The experimental protocol was approved by the Institutional Animal Care and Use Committee.

### Surgical Procedure

Six 4-mm stainless steel tapered fixation pins were inserted perpendicular to the tibia in a craniolateral position (30° cranial to the lateral plane) after predrilling with a 3.2-mm drill before the application of the unilateral fixator. A 5-cm longitudinal medial skin incision was made, followed by subperiosteal elevation to expose the midtibia. A transverse tibial osteotomy was performed with saline irrigation at the midpoint between the proximal and distal fixation pins using a Stryker saw (Model 1370; Stryker Corp, Kalamazoo, MI). The pin brackets of the fixator were separated by 75 mm over the osteotomy, and the fixator body was positioned 50 mm away from the centerline of the midtibia. The 2-mm gap was achieved using a thickness gauge as a spacer between the bone ends during adjustment. The telescoping mechanism built into the fixator body was immediately locked and reinforced with bone cement to maintain a constant osteotomy gap distance.

## PEMF Stimulation

A PEMF stimulation signal waveform (EBI, LP, Parsippany, NJ) was used with 30 millisecond bursts of asymmetric pulses repeated at 1.5 Hz. During each pulse, the magnetic field rose from 0 gauss to approximately 2 gauss in 230 μs and then returned to 0 gauss in 30 μs.[10] The dogs were treated daily starting at 4 weeks after surgery and lasting for a total of 8 weeks. The coil and signal generator were designed to deliver peak magnetic fields between 1.0 and 2.4 gauss within the bone at the osteotomy site. The animals were divided into PEMF-stimulated for 1 hour (PEMF 1 hour, n = 6), stimulated for 4 hours (PEMF 4 hour, n = 6), and nonstimulated control (n = 6) groups. In all groups, the daily treatment regimen lasted for 4 hours with the animals lightly sedated using acepromazine maleate (5 mg, intramuscularly) in separate cages. The 4-hour treatment program was selected to subject all animals to an identical management protocol to investigate the dose effect. In the PEMF-stimulated groups, the signal generator was activated for 1 hour and 4 hours per treatment period, whereas no signal was generated in the nonstimulated control group. All dogs remained in a resting position in small cages throughout the treatment period with the contralateral intact limb placed within the proximity of the PEMF coil (Fig. 1, *A*). Using a magnetic field intensity calculation formula based on the coil geometry and an experimental measuring technique, we estimated the average PEMF intensity for the intact tibia at a distance of 5 cm to 20 cm from the center of the coil to be 64% to 28% of the peak strength at the osteotomy site (Fig. 1, *B*).

## Load Bearing

Load bearing was measured before surgery and at 4-, 8-, and 12-week time points postoperatively. Each dog was led by a leash over a dynamic force plate (Model OR-6-6, Advanced Mechanical Technologies, Inc, Nugent,

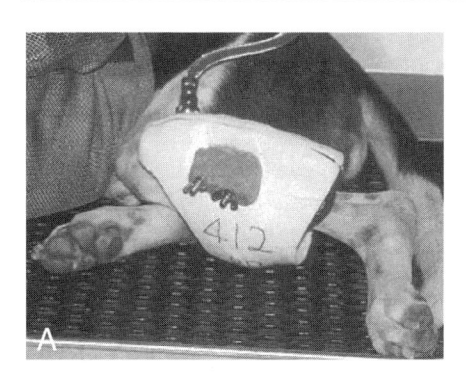

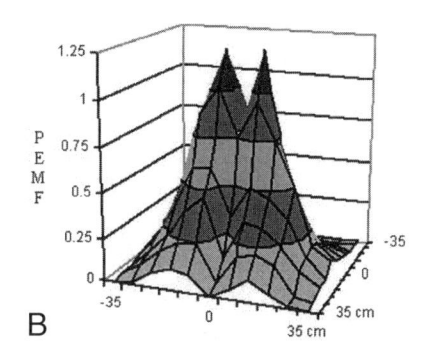

**Figure 1 A,** Position of the contralateral hind limb during PEMF stimulation. **B,** External field intensity normalized by surface values versus distance from coil center.

MA), with an approach distance of 4 meters to reach a steady-state running cadence before dynamic measurement. An observer recorded each successful foot-strike, which was defined by complete contact of either the left or right hind limb within the margins of the force plate surface. At least 6 valid maximum vertical ground reaction force measurements for each hind limb were recorded, and the mean of hind limb dynamic weight bearing was calculated at each preoperative or postoperative time point.[20,21]

## Radiographic Analysis

Craniocaudal and mediolateral radiographs were taken before surgery to exclude abnormal radiographic findings and to ascertain closure of the distal femoral epiphyseal plate. Radiographs were also taken immediately after surgery and at 2, 4, 6, 8, 10, and 12 weeks postoperatively under sedation with ketamine (8 mg/kg intramuscularly) and xylazine (0.8 mg/kg intramuscularly). Because the external fixator was placed 30° cranial to the lateral plane, the external fixator did not overlap with the periosteal callus in the mediolateral or craniocaudal radiographs. Periosteal callus size was measured directly on craniocaudal and mediolateral radiographs using an image analysis software package (Bioquant System IV, R & M Biometrics, Inc, Nashville, TN) and a sonic digitizer (Summa Sketch II Plus, Summagraphics, Seymour, CT).

## Biomechanic Testing

After euthanasia at 12 weeks postoperatively, the tibiae including the intact side from all animals were harvested for biomechanic and histologic evaluations. An axial torsion test at a low strain rate (15°/min) in external rotation was performed on the osteotomized tibiae and the contralateral intact tibia using an MTS mechanical testing machine (MTS Bionix 858, MTS Systems, Eden Prairie, MN). The slope of the initial linear portion of the curve was measured as torsional stiffness. Ultimate strength was defined as the maximum torque applied until fracture failure. Maximum torque and torsional stiffness of the osteotomized tibiae were normalized against the respective values of the contralateral tibiae or the body weight of each animal.

## Histologic and Histomorphometric Analyses

After mechanical testing, specimens were repositioned and prepared for undecalcified histologic study. The specimens were fixed in 70% ethanol, dehydrated in increasing concentrations of ethanol, defatted in acetone, and embedded in methylmethacrylate (Technovit 9100, Kulzer GmbH, Wehrheim, Germany). Midlongitudinal and transverse sections were cut to a thickness of approximately 200 μm and ground to a thickness of 100 μm. After taking contact microradiographs, toluidine blue-stained slides were analyzed on the midlongitudinal plane. New bone, cartilage, and fibrous tissue areas were measured using a digital image analysis system (Bioquant System IV, R & M Biometrics, Inc, Nashville, TN). Mineral apposition rate of the cortical bone adjacent to the osteotomy site was measured using a bone labeling technique. Animals were given the following bone labels biweekly postoperatively: xylenol orange (90 mg/kg intravenously), calcein blue (30 mg/kg intravenously), alizarin complexone (30 mg/kg intravenously), and oxytetracycline (30 mg/kg intramuscularly). Unstained transverse sections at 1, 3, 5, and 10 mm away from the osteotomy edge were analyzed under ultraviolet light using the same bone histomorphometric analysis system. The intact tibia specimens were studied in a similar manner at the diaphyseal region corresponding to the osteotomy on the operated tibiae.

Contact microradiographs were made using a high-resolution film (Industrex SR, Kodak-Industrie, Chalon sur Saône, France) exposed at 35 kV and 20 mA for 45 seconds in a self-contained x-ray cabinet (Faxitron X-ray Corp., Buffalo Grove, IL). A target-to-specimen distance of 20 cm was used to obtain the microradiographs. The films were developed for 3 minutes in a Kodak film developer (D-19 developer, Eastman Kodak, Rochester, NY). The contact microradiographs of the transverse sections were used for porosity measurement using light microscopy. The contact microradiographs were digitized using a charged coupled device camera (DXC-151, Sony, Tokyo, Japan) attached to the microscope. Digitized image data were transferred to a SiliconGraphics Workstation (Iris Indigo Elan; SiliconGraphics, Mountain View, CA), and bone area was measured using a threshold optimization procedure.[23] Porosity of the cortex was expressed as a percentage of the bone area not occupied by mineralized tissue.

## Statistical Analysis

Data from the three groups were compared using an unpaired Student's $t$ test. Time-sequential changes in periosteal callus area and load bearing and the porosity and mineral apposition rate in the different sites were compared using analysis of variance with Tukey's post hoc test. A difference was considered significant when $P$ values were less than 0.05. The results are reported as the mean and standard deviation.

# Results

## Load Bearing

All animals were able to stand unassisted on the day after surgery and thereafter. In both PEMF-stimulated groups, load bearing on the operated limb decreased at 4 weeks after surgery ($P < 0.05$) but increased during the PEMF treatment period between 4 and 8 weeks ($P < 0.05$) and returned to the preoperative level at 12 weeks. In the control group, load bearing decreased at 4 weeks after surgery ($P < 0.05$), but the improvement from 4 weeks to 8 weeks was not significant (Fig. 2). A significant increase in the control group occurred only from 8 to 12 weeks ($P < 0.05$), with recovery to the preoperative level at 12 weeks. Load bearing in the PEMF groups at 8 weeks was significantly higher than that in the control group ($P < 0.02$). There was no difference between the PEMF 1-hour and PEMF 4-hour groups.

## Radiographic Analysis

There was a significant increase in the periosteal callus area after 4 weeks in both of the PEMF-stimulated groups but not in the control group (Fig. 3). At 12 weeks, only the periosteal callus of the PEMF 4-hour group was signifi-

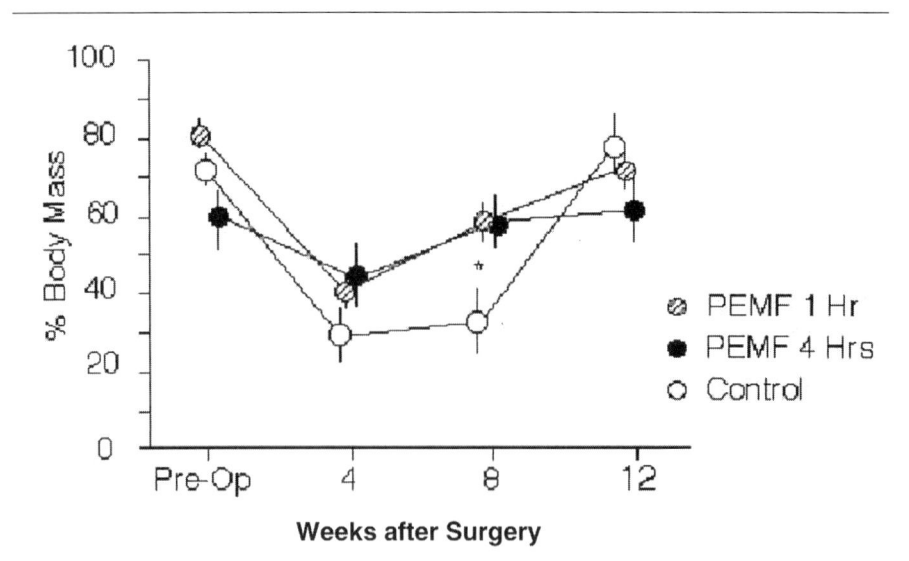

Section Two    Biophysical Regulation of Bone Healing in Animal Models

**Figure 2** Results of the operated limb weight bearing during gait (*$P < 0.05$ compared with the control group, mean ± SEM).

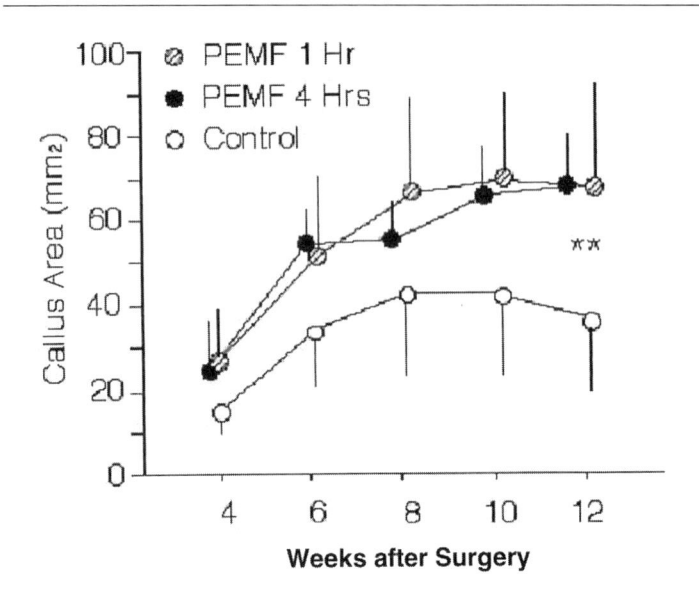

**Figure 3** Radiographic results of periosteal callus measured in two orthogonal projections (**$P < 0.05$ between the 4-hour PEMF and the control group, mean ± SEM).

cantly greater than that of the control ($P < 0.05$). However, there was no significant difference between the PEMF 1-hour and 4-hour groups. The increase of callus following surgery at 6 weeks and thereafter was significant ($P < 0.01$) and the same occurred from 2 to 8, 10, and 12 weeks ($P < 0.01$) in the stimulated groups. In the control group, significant increase of periosteal callus was observed only at 8 and 10 weeks after surgery ($P < 0.05$). No significant difference between the mean values for periosteal callus area in the PEMF and control groups could be detected at any time during the study.

## Biomechanic Testing

The maximum torques to failure for the PEMF 1-hour and 4-hour groups and the control group were $21.4 \pm 6.6$, $22.4 \pm 3.4$, and $18.6 \pm 6.4$ Nm (mean ± SD) respectively. The corresponding torsional stiffness values were $132 \pm 20.5$, $138 \pm 25.6$, and $89.8 \pm 29.6$ Nm/rad. There was a strong trend toward higher maximum torque in the stimulated groups ($P = 0.06$ and $P = 0.08$ for the 1-hour and 4-hour groups when compared with the control). A significant increase in torsional stiffness was found in both the PEMF-stimulated groups compared with the control. There was no significant difference between the PEMF 1-hour and 4-hour groups. When the maximum torques were normalized against the contralateral intact tibia, those of the 1-hour stimulated group were significantly greater than those of the control ($P < 0.04$). However, normalizing the biomechanic data against the contralateral tibia was considered inappropriate due to the possible PEMF spill-off effects on the intact tibiae exposed to the magnetic field without adequate shielding.

The torsional stiffness of the contralateral intact tibia normalized against the animal's body weight was significantly higher for the 4-hour stimulated group ($P < 0.05$) and with a strong trend of higher value for the 1-hour group ($P < 0.08$) when compared with the controls (Fig. 4). The maximum torque of the intact tibiae normalized against the body weight was significantly greater in the PEMF 4-hour group ($P < 0.004$) but only with a strong trend toward greater value in the 1-hour group ($P < 0.08$) as compared with the control.

## Histologic and Histomorphometric Analyses

The percent area of new bone in the gap region was significantly greater in the PEMF groups ($P < 0.05$). Total new bone area within the periosteal, gap, and endosteal areas was also significantly greater in the PEMF groups than in the controls ($P < 0.05$). Cartilage made up less than 1% of the total area in both the PEMF and control groups. The mineral apposition rate was significantly higher in the PEMF 1-hour group than in the control group in the cortex 3 and 5 mm away from the osteotomy line (Fig. 5). In the PEMF group, the mineral apposition rate of the experimental side at every level in the cortex was higher than that in the contralateral intact side ($P < 0.05$). The cortical bone porosity in both PEMF groups was significantly decreased compared with the control group in the cortex 1, 3, 5, and 10 mm away from the osteotomy line. At 3 mm away, the porosity in the PEMF 4-hour group

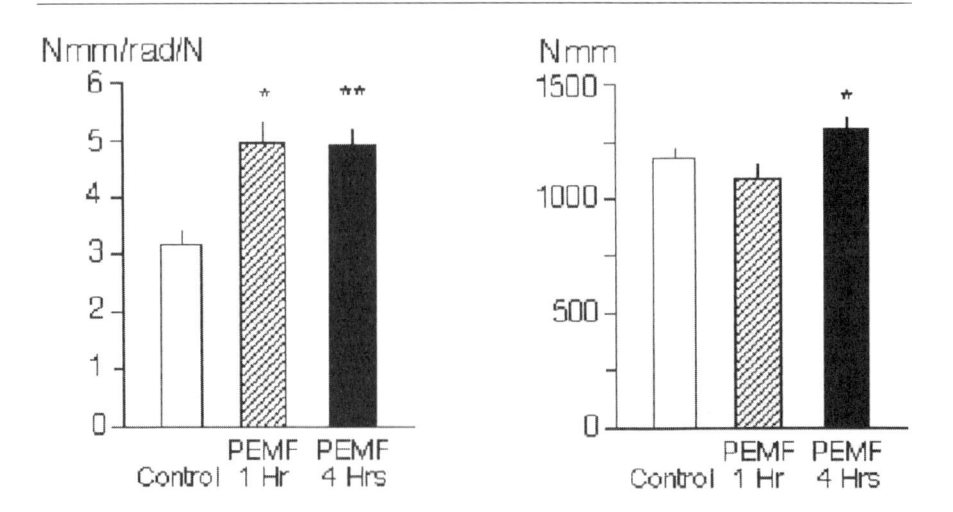

**Figure 4** Torsional stiffness, left (*$P < 0.08$ and **$P < 0.05$ compared with control), and maximum torque, right (*$P < 0.004$ for the 4-hour group when compared with the control, mean ± SEM), of the contralateral untreated intact tibiae. The values showed here were normalized against the animals' body weight.

was significantly decreased when compared with that in the PEMF 1-hour group (Fig. 6).

In the contralateral intact tibiae, the mineral apposition rates in the midshaft corresponding to location of the osteotomy for the PEMF 1-hour, 4-hour, and control groups were 0.99 ± 0.13, 1.03 ± 0.12, and 1.47 ± 0.48 mm/day (mean ± SD) respectively. The mineral apposition rate was significantly higher in the 4-hour stimulated group versus the control group ($P < 0.03$) and when compared with the 1-hour stimulated group ($P < 0.02$) (Fig. 7). There was no difference between the 1-hour PEMF group and the control group. There was no significant difference in cortical porosity in the intact tibiae among the three groups.

## Discussion

This study showed that PEMF stimulation provided faster recovery of dynamic load bearing, a significant increase in new bone formation, and higher mechanical strength of a healing midtibial osteotomy using the canine osteotomy gap delayed healing model. The similar results from two animal groups in the dose effect study also served as a strong added validation of the positive effect of PEMF on osteotomy gap healing enhancement. More interesting was the fact that a significant side effect was discovered on the contralateral intact tibiae due to the PEMF signal spread from the intended treatment area.

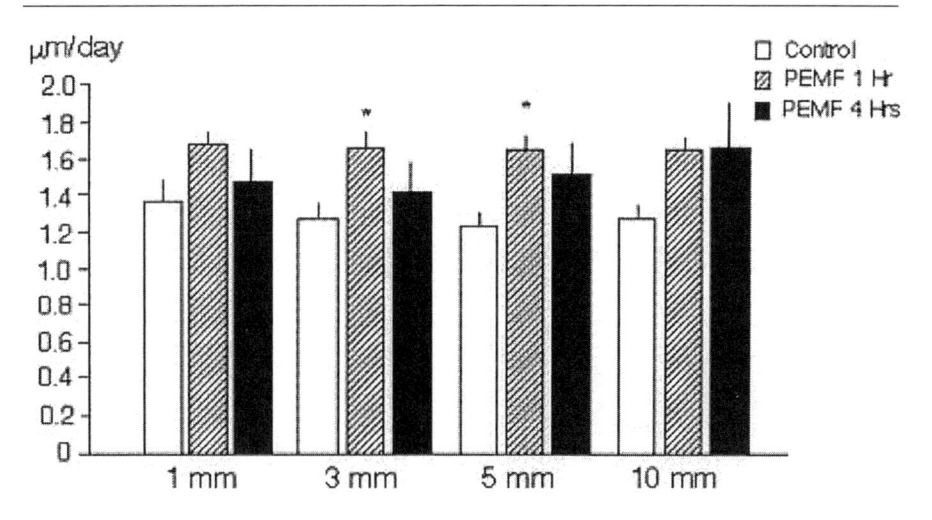

**Figure 5** Cortical bone mineral apposition rate for the 1-hour PEMF group at the transverse sections at 1, 3, 5, and 10 mm away from the osteotomy line and inside the innermost pins of the fixator (*$P < 0.05$ compared with the control group, mean ± SEM).

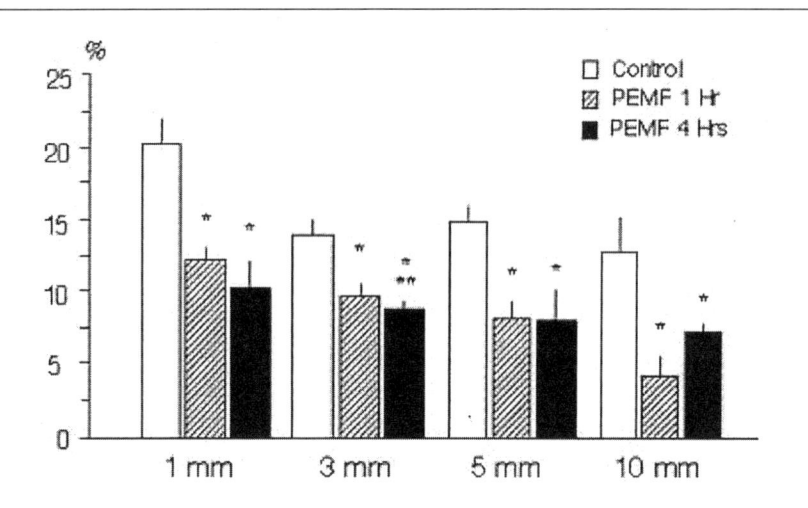

**Figure 6** Cortical bone porosity analyses using transverse sections at 1, 3, 5, and 10 mm away from the osteotomy line and inside the inner pins of the fixator (*$P < 0.05$ compared with the control group, **$P < 0.05$ compared between the 1-hour and 4-hour PEMF groups, mean ± SEM).

The current animal model possessed unique features that made it particularly useful for investigating the effects of any form of biophysical stimulation on the late phase of osteotomy healing: stable and rigid external fixation of the osteotomized long bone, a transverse middiaphyseal osteotomy with a 2-mm gap, and the stimulation implemented 4 weeks after surgery.

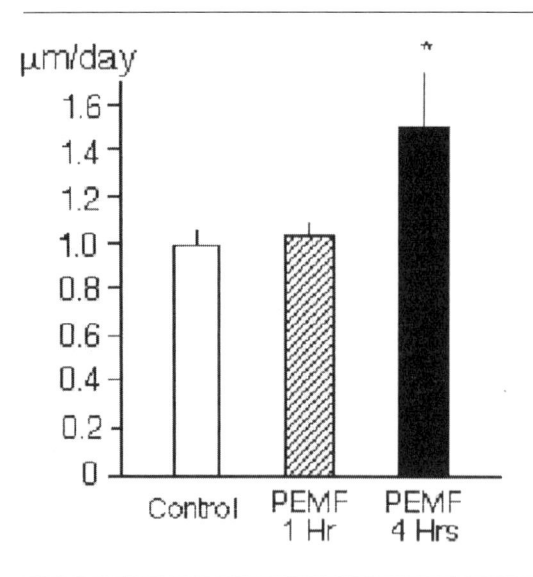

Section Two   Biophysical Regulation of Bone Healing in Animal Models

**Figure 7** Mineral apposition rate (*$P < 0.03$ between the control and the 4-hour PEMF-treated group and $P < 0.02$ between the 1-hour and the 4-hour PEMF-treated groups, mean ± SEM) in the contralateral untreated intact tibiae.

Stability and rigidity of the bone defect fixation and size of the osteotomy gap have been found to be critical factors in achieving consistent osteotomy gap healing and in the determination of the mechanical properties of the healed osteotomy.

The timing of the initiation of biophysical stimulation is considered to be an important factor because it may cause different biologic responses during bone healing phases. PEMF stimulation was introduced 4 weeks after surgery to investigate its effect after the initial phase of osteotomy healing. Gene expression of bone morphogenetic proteins and other growth factors that induce new bone formation during fracture repair typically decreases by 4 weeks after fracture.[24,25] The genetic expression of different collagen fiber types also was found to decrease at the same time period after surgery. Therefore, the initiation of PEMF stimulation 4 weeks after surgery was selected to study its effects on the late phase of bone healing, which may have significant implication on the appropriate management of delayed union fracture.

Increased new bone formation in the osteotomy gap area under PEMF stimulation was shown in the present study. Grace and associates[26] studied the effect of PEMF on early chondrogenesis during fresh osteochondral repair in the rat and found that a prolonged use of such stimulation may have a deleterious effect, ie, enhancing chondrogenesis beyond a point observed in normal repair could delay normal subsurface trabeculation. In the present study, however, increased chondrogenesis was not observed at 12 weeks after surgery, and the deleterious effect of PEMF described in the previous study was not found in our model under two different stimulation doses. Previous studies using a similar canine osteotomy healing model with rigid external fixation and a 2-mm midtibial transverse osteotomy showed a small amount of chondrogenesis during bone healing.[20-22] The mode of bone healing in a stable mechanical environment, such as cortical bone defect healing[18,27] (N Inoue, MD, PhD, Baltimore, MD, unpublished data presented at the Orthopaedic Research Society annual meeting, 2003) and osteotomy healing under rigid fixation, was primarily an intramembranous ossification process. In addition to the differences in the animal model and type of the signal, this finding may explain the lack of remarkable cartilage formation in the gap area under PEMF stimulation in the present study.

The animal's load bearing and the torsional properties of the tibial specimen evaluated in the present study reflect not only the strength of the healing tissue but also that of the adjacent cortical tissue. In the adjacent cortical bone, the porosity was lower and the mineral apposition rate was higher in the PEMF-stimulated tibiae. Therefore, the higher torsional stiffness and strength in the PEMF-stimulated tibiae might be caused by new bone formation or by decreased porosity in the adjacent cortical bone or by a combination of both factors that could not be identified using the testing method in the present study. To evaluate the mechanical properties of the new bone formed in the gap area alone, a standard material indentation test of the gap tissue will be required.[22] However, the significance of the weakening of the cortical bone adjacent to the osteotomy site after long-term rigid external fixation has been reported.[28] The structural testing used in the present study evaluated the strength of the entire midtibial segment including the healing osteotomy, which would reflect the functional requirement of the entire long bone. The effect of PEMF on the maintenance of bone density in the adjacent cortex during limb lengthening was recognized clinically.[2] This finding, together with the results in the present study, suggests an additional benefit of PEMF stimulation for prolonged fracture treatments such as delayed fracture union and nonunion cases in order to avoid osteopenia of the treated bone and provide better structural strength.

The PEMF signal used in the present study has proved to have enhancing effects on osteotomy healing in both rabbit and canine models.[10,18] However, other PEMF signals have demonstrated varying effects with different stimulation timing and periods described earlier.[16,17] The rabbit study also demonstrated that 1-hour stimulation had a better effect on bone healing compared with 30-minute stimulation. Hence, dose effect in different stimulation signal and bone fracture environment must be carefully investigated to optimize clinical efficacy.

There was no additional gain in osteotomy healing augmentation by increasing the stimulation time from 1 hour to 4 hours, even though several bone histomorphometric parameters showed benefits with a longer stimulation time period. Fredericks and associates[10] studied the effects of the same PEMF signal in a rabbit tibia osteotomy model and found that 1 hour of stimulation was more efficacious than 30 minutes of stimulation. In a rat endochondral bone induction model using the same signal, the investigators demonstrated that a 1-hour daily stimulation dose was significantly more effective than 8 hours per day in a histomorphometric study (RK Aaron, MD, Providence, Rhode Island, personal communication, 2003).

The distribution of electromagnetic fields varies within the bone at the osteotomy site and in the adjacent bone and soft tissues. The present study used a flexible elliptical PEMF coil that was placed between the external fixator and the skin and positioned between the two inner pins of the fixator. Peak magnetic field strengths at the osteotomy site within the coil were between 1.0 and 2.4 gauss. Magnetic fields decrease significantly in soft tissues adjacent to the PEMF coil, with peak strengths of 0.35 gauss at a position 1 cm distal to the coil and 0.1 gauss at a position 4 cm distal to the coil, for example.

Tabrah and associates[29] demonstrated an increased bone mineral density (BMD) in distal radii of osteoporotic women treated with 10 hours of PEMF stimulation per day for 12 weeks using a different signal. An increase in BMD in the opposite, untreated arm was also observed; investigators suggested that this increase was the effect of a weak field outside of the primary treatment area. During the daily treatment intervals in the present study, the nontreated legs were noted to be within 5 cm to 20 cm of the PEMF coil. At such distances, the field intensity of the PEMF was estimated to be 64% to 28% of that at the coil surface. This finding suggested a crossover effect by the stimulation signal spill-off that should be carefully considered both in animal experiment design when the unshielded contralateral limb is used as the control, and in clinical application when the use of biophysical stimulation may lead to unexpected or unwanted bone and organ change at a site distant from the intended treatment area.

Current PEMF stimulation is primarily used clinically to treat delayed fracture unions and nonunions. In the present study, this mode of biophysical stimulation increased new bone formation when it was applied in the late phase of bone osteotomy healing. Together with the results from the previous studies, it is reasonable to conclude that a stable fixation is required to optimize the effects of PEMF on fracture healing. The present study also helped to establish the efficacy of the lower energy PEMF signal, which has been previously demonstrated in a rabbit model. Although the optimal dose has not been established, longer daily treatment time did not show any added benefit. The reduced stimulation time is not only convenient to the patient, but it may also minimize any stimulation side effects on normal tissue adjacent to the intended area of treatment.

## Acknowledgment

This study was supported in part by a gift from EBI, LP.

## References

1. Bassett CAL: Fundamental and practical aspects of therapeutic uses of pulsed electromagnetic fields (PEMFs). *Crit Rev Biomed Eng* 1989;17:451-529.
2. Eyres KS, Saleh M, Kanis JA: Effect of pulsed electromagnetic fields on bone formation and bone loss during limb lengthening. *Bone* 1996;18:505-509.
3. Ryaby JT: Clinical effects of electromagnetic and electric fields on fracture healing. *Clin Orthop* 1998;355:S205-S215.
4. Borsalino G, Bagnacani M, Bettati E, et al: Electrical stimulation of human femoral intertrochanteric osteotomies. *Clin Orthop* 1988;237:256-263.

5. Mammi GI, Rocchi R, Cadossi R, Massari L, Traina GC: The electrical stimulation of tibial osteotomies. *Clin Orthop* 1993;288:246-253.

6. Sharrard WJW: A double-blind trial of pulsed electromagnetic fields for delayed union of tibial fractures. *J Bone Joint Surg Br* 1990;72:347-355.

7. Bodamyali T, Bhatt B, Hughes FJ, et al: Pulsed electromagnetic fields simultaneously induce osteogenesis and upregulate transcription of bone morphogenetic proteins 2 and 4 in rat osteoblasts in vitro. *Biochem Biophys Res Comm* 1998;50:458-461.

8. Fitzsimmons RJ, Farley JR, Adey WR, Baylink DJ: Frequency dependence of increased cell proliferation, in vitro, in exposures to a low-amplitude, low-frequency electric field: Evidence for dependence on increased mitogen activity released into culture medium. *J Cell Physiol* 1989;139:586-591.

9. Fitzsimmons RJ, Ryaby JT, Mohan S, Magee FP, Baylink DJ: Combined magnetic fields increase insulin-like growth factor-II in TE-85 human osteosarcoma bone cell cultures. *Endocrinology* 1995;136:3100-3106.

10. Fredericks DC, Nepola JV, Baker JT, Abbott J, Simon B: Effects of pulsed electromagnetic fields on bone healing in a rabbit tibial osteotomy model. *J Orthop Trauma* 2000;14:93-100.

11. Pienkowski D, Pollack SR, Brighton CT, Griffith NJ: Low-power electromagnetic stimulation of osteotomized rabbit fibulae: A randomized, blinded study *J Bone Joint Surg Am* 1994;76:489-501.

12. McLeod KJ, Rubin CT: The effect of low-frequency electrical fields on osteogenesis. *J Bone Joint Surg Am* 1992;74:920-929.

13. Moore DC, Chapman MW, Manske D: The evaluation of a biphasic calcium phosphate ceramic for use in grafting long-bone diaphyseal defects. *J Orthop Res* 1987;5:356-365.

14. Canè V, Botti P, Farneti D, Soana S: Electromagnetic stimulation of bone repair: A histomorphometric study. *J Orthop Res* 1991;9:908-917.

15. Canè V, Botti P, Soana S: Pulsed magnetic fields improve osteoblast activity during the repair of an experimental osseous defect. *J Orthop Res* 1993;11:664-670.

16. Enzler MA, Sumner-Smith G, Waelchli-Suter C, Perren SM: Treatment of nonuniting osteotomies with pulsating electromagnetic fields: A controlled animal experiment. *Clin Orthop* 1984;187:272-276.

17. Law HT, Annan I, McCarthy ID, et al: The effect of induced electric currents on bone after experimental osteotomy in sheep. *J Bone Joint Surg Br* 1985;67:463-469.

18. Inoue N, Ohnishi I, Chen DA, Deitz LW, Schwardt JD, Chao EYS: Effect of pulsed electromagnetic fields on osteotomy gap healing in a canine tibial model. *J Orthop Res* 2002;20:957-966.

19. Aro HT, Kelly PJ, Lewallen DG, Chao EYS: The effects of physiologic dynamic compression on bone healing under external fixation. *Clin Orthop* 1990;256:260-273.

20. Egger EL, Gottsauner-Wolf F, Palmer J, Aro HT, Chao EYS: Effects of axial dynamization on bone healing. *J Trauma* 1993;34:185-192.

21. Larsson S, Kim W, Caja VC, Egger EL, Inoue N, Chao EYS: Effect of early axial dynamization on tibial bone healing: A study in dogs. *Clin Orthop* 2001;388:240-251.

22. Markel MD, Wikenheiser MA, Chao EYS: Formation of bone in tibial defects in a canine model: Histomorphometric and biomechanical studies. *J Bone Joint Surg Am* 1991;73:914-923.

23. Keller TS, Moeljanto E, Main JA, Spengler DM: Distribution and orientation of the human lumbar vertebral centrum. *J Spinal Disord* 1992;5:60-74.

24. Aro HT, Eerola E, Aho AJ: Determination of callus quantity in 4-week-old fractures of the rat tibia. *J Orthop Res* 1985;3:101-108.

25. Sandberg MM, Aro HT, Vuorio EI: Gene expression during bone repair. *Clin Orthop* 1993;289:292-312.

26. Grace KLR, Revell WJ, Brookes M: The effects of pulsed electromagnetism on fresh fracture healing: Osteochondral repair in the rat femoral groove. *Orthopedics* 1998; 21:297-302.

27. Shapiro F: Cortical bone repair: The relationship of the lacunar-canalicular system and intercellular gap junctions to the repair process. *J Bone Joint Surg Am* 1988;1970:1067-1081.

28. Simpson AH, Kenwright J: Fracture after distraction osteogenesis. *J Bone Joint Surg Br* 2000;82:659-665.

29. Tabrah F, Hoffmeier M, Gilbert F: Bone density changes in osteoporosis-prone women exposed to pulsed electromagnetic field (PEMFs). *J Bone Miner Res* 1990; 5:437-442.

# Consensus Panel 2

# Evaluation of Biophysical Regulation of Bone Healing in Animal Models

**Dr. Roy Aaron:** I am interested in the issue of dosimetry because it's the way we think about developing clinical signals. It's interesting because we know that the Goodship-Kenwright group has shown acceleration of fracture repair with mechanical stimulation. Other groups, particularly in Germany, have not shown that effect, but they've shown differences in the healing rates with the timing of the application. Certainly electromagnetic fields (EMF) have a variety of dosimetric relationships. And ultrasound, by the strength of the signal and by dosimetric relationships, can be thermal or nonthermal, or it can even break things pretty nicely, including methylmethacrylate. So the amplitude, the frequency, the duration of application, and the way these signals are applied really are critical if we are going to develop clinically relevant signals. The other thing I found particularly interesting was this idea of responders versus nonresponders, whether they are heavy women or bone morphogenetic protein (BMP)-deficient mice. This is an analogy to the at-risk fracture that we heard about this morning; and then the specificity of targeting of signals, particularly to the aggrecan promoter. This was interesting because fracture healing is really a developmental sequence and targets may change over time. To optimize the way physical stimulation works, we may need to target chondrocyte behavior at one time and bone cell behavior at another time. So I'd be interested to hear what the consensus panel thought about these issues, and then perhaps questions and conversation from the floor.

**Speaker:** You asked me earlier, Roy, what my thoughts were regarding dosimetry. We know, for example, from the BMP literature that as we go up in animal species, the dose that is required to have a substantial biologic affect has increased from the microgram to the milligram range. And these are really super-therapeutic doses. I'm curious (almost as a lay audience here looking at the specifics of the doses applied): is the dose different in these different species and different animal models? I think the dose to the tissue or the specific cell that you're targeting varies a lot depending on the depth of the tissue. Should we just be applying the same ultrasound dose to a skinny person as an obese person? Similarly, what tissues are being stimulated? Cartilage is only evident in fracture healing during a certain period. Perhaps intramembranous ossification in the bridging part of the callus is affected by biophysical stimulation. I think we probably need more basic science about how biophysical stimuli works, because just as it doesn't make sense to throw in 5 mg of BMP-2, I don't think it makes sense to throw the same electric or other biophysical stimuli to the callus for the duration of healing. I think we need to tailor the application: make it the right dose, the right magnitude, the right amount of energy. And that may be different as the fracture heals.

**Dr. Joseph Lane:** These are difficult questions concerning the design of physical signals, including duration, pulse shape, and so forth. Number one, I believe strongly in the hierarchical concept developed for demineralized bone matrix (DBM). This starts off with an in vitro test for efficacy of DBM and then moves to the mouse and the rat, then to the rabbit, then to the dog and the primate, and finally to the human. Number two, we are going to have to find an in vitro cell system for signal screening. Once this is done, I think you probably should consider the advantage of the mouse because you can then explore prospective mechanisms with all the transgenic mice. Once the cellular target is identified, you can then move up more selectively. You're not going to do a dose curve on a dog. So I move toward mechanisms of action and screening techniques to help the choice of signal profiles. I'm totally convinced that biophysical stimuli work now that I look at the literature and listen to the presentations. But I think there are big opportunities in this area.

**Dr. Bruce Simon:** One problem with pulsed fields is that the metric is an induced electric field, and the magnitude of the induced electric field depends on the target of the tissue. So if you take a particular signal and treat a rat, and if you take the same signal and treat a human tibia—which is 20 to 30 times the size of a rat's—the induced field is going to be 20 to 30 times as large. And it gets worse if you do tissue culture. You have induced fields that you know very well with tissue culture. You then treat human tissue and the induced electric field is very complicated. Is it the periosteum, the cortical bone, where's the target? The induced field is very different in different tissues in the body.

**Dr. Roy Aaron:** These are testable hypotheses that you've outlined. And in fact there has been some work done in small and larger animals looking at dosimetry and scaling. Do you want to comment on that?

**Dr. Bruce Simon:** Many animal studies have been performed, several in Roy's lab and the lab at the University of Iowa. We observed 50% acceleration in fracture healing in the rabbit model and enhanced ossicle formation. But the induced electric field in these animal models was much smaller than the induced electric field in humans. And data presented today indicate that there are amplitude windows as well. So we went back to the ossicle model to screen signals and did a dose response and in fact found that smaller amplitude gave a much larger result. This is consistent with what Ed Chao presented. So it's quite difficult to go from a cell model where you can very accurately calculate the induced electric field to a full animal model where you cannot.

**Dr. Ruggero Cadossi:** I would also like to stress the point that we know a lot of things—there are reliable models that have been developed, and there are clinical results from many researchers, and we know something about mechanisms. We know that we can interfere with the reaction between the ligand and the receptor. And we can stimulate the synthesis of growth factors locally. There are studies from our own lab on cytokine expression in human lymphocytes. And we have several animal models: the fibular osteotomy in the rat, the osteotomy in the rabbit, and our model in the horse. These have been used with different signals.

**Dr. Deborah Ciombor:** One problem in particular with the electric and magnetic field work is that we don't have a recognition site at the cell. We don't know whether the biologic effects are due to the magnetic field, the induced electric field, or some combination thereof. The DC and even capacitively coupled fields are a little bit clearer, but the inductively coupled fields give a lot of headaches to a lot of people. We need to get a recognition site at the membrane that is amplifying the signal in some fashion because the fields are so low that they are orders of magnitude below the transmembrane potential. There's obviously a recognition site on the cell, but we don't know what it is, and we don't know if it's the same from a muscle cell, a chondrocyte, or a bone cell. And because the cell lends specificity, it's very important. So it's going to be very hard to come down to a single screening method.

**Dr. Solomon Pollack:** I would like to elaborate a little bit more on what Mikki was just talking about. We talk at this conference about biophysical signals as if they were all alike, and yet they are so different. And it's very important to understand the difference. Just take the difference between a pulsed EMF and a capacitively coupled signal. A capacitively coupled signal we calculate and measure at the tissue level, not at the cell level. We haven't solved that problem ourselves. The target tissue level is about 20 mV/cm. Now that's about two volts per meter, and that's a pretty large field. That field is actually capable of perturbing a calcium channel. In the case of pulsed EMFs, the electric component of it is proportional to the magnitude of the magnetic field times how rapidly it changes—the frequency or the derivative of it with respect to time. If it's changing very rapidly, the electric field component will be larger. If it's changing very slowly, the electric field component will be small. That electric field is two orders of magnitude smaller, and it is not readily obvious that it can perturb a calcium channel. So it isn't clear that the site at which transduction occurs and the mechanism that is involved is even the same. There's no question that it works, but it's not necessarily the same. And with each of these two, there are clear dose response relationships in terms of the amplitudes of those fields.

Another matter deals with the geometry of the tissue when you apply these fields. Just to give you an example that Bruce probably knows better than I do: if you were applying a pulsed EMF to a fracture callus of a long bone and you ask, what are the fields in the fracture callus? Well, that's not a simple question. But if you model it and you say, let's assume that the fracture callus has some average electric and magnetic properties, then you can calculate an average value of that field. The value for that field will depend on the ratio of its height to its distance. So if it's small, you will get a different value for that electric field component even though the magnetic field value will be the same. If you put the coils so that they line up along where the axis of the coils are parallel to the axis of the long bone, then the electric field in that callus is very dependent on the radius from the centerline of that coil; therefore, it's a high nonuniform electric field. And so to say that we used PEMF is like saying I used a drug and then I show you all my data, but I don't tell you the milligrams per kilogram of body weight. Underlying all of these studies is a confounder that makes it impossible to extract the key information on dosing. It's not good enough to say I used capacitive coupling, I have to say I used capacitive coupling with a value of the applied fields on a surface of this for which the electric field and the tissue compartment that was the target is so many volts per centimeter. The situation is similar in pulsed EMFs. And if I change it from the rapid pulse rate for so many seconds and then off, and I change it to the kind that you saw presented a little earlier, it's a very different magnetic field and a very different electric field because the time rate of change is different for the two different pulsed EMFs.

The mechanical problem also is not simple because the application of a mechanical force on a tissue produces the following things: it produces deformation of the matrix and any cell that is attached to it, and it can produce pressure oscillation depending on the time variation of the force. But pressure changes in fluid. It could cause fluid motion, which in itself could result in electric fields and streaming potentials. Pressure changes could result in shear stresses, which could cause conformational variations at the membranes of cells. You apply a simple force, but depending on the targeted tissue, many phenomena take place that ultimately have to be quantified if you're going to compare one experiment to another and if you're going to start looking in detail at dose-related mechanisms. And so there probably isn't a single cell that you're going to use as a model. There probably isn't a single mechanism because, although the word *biophysical* is a single word, underlying it are a lot of physical phenomena that can cause and alter cellular behavior. These are complex elements of the physicochemical environment of the cell. The underlying assumption is that there are some biophysical forces of the types I just described that are somehow causing the cell to alter its behavior. There's some transduction of that signal, some nuclear response, some synthesis, and some expression.

**Dr. Stephen Trippel:** I have a sense that there's an intrinsic assumption that these effects are occurring through local stimulation, and I don't want to suggest that that assumption isn't right, but it might be worthwhile to look at this issue in a little bit of a different way. We heard some very interesting data from Ed Chao that when he applied a field to a fractured limb, he saw an effect on the contralateral limb. Now that may be because the one-tenth field strength at the other side was biologically effective locally, but it raises the possibility that there is a systemic effect being produced by this signal. And work from Mikki and Roy's group has very elegantly shown that there are data to support that possibility. TGF-β, for example, might be a mediator for some of these biologic effects.

**Dr. Hari Reddi:** If you take a defect, like let's say a gap model in a dog, 2 mm. There is not one cell but rather a cellular population that is responding to this physical signal. There are stem cells in the marrow, there are periosteal cells, there are endosteal cells, and there are regional differences in the periosteum. And there are differences in the response of osteoprogenitor cells and osteoclasts. Has there been work looking at formation and resorption? This is a very important issue because, first of all, we haven't defined the physical signal, and secondly, we haven't defined the responding cells. We then have the complication that Sol introduced, that in fact these cells are surrounded by an ocean of extracellular matrix. There are, in fact, observations that it's not osteoprogenitors that are responding to mechanical signals but rather an osteocyte network. I haven't yet heard anybody talk about osteocytes, yet we have discussed the aforementioned issues. So please enlighten me, because I would like to be enlightened.

**Dr. Mone Zaidi:** I'm an endocrinologist and I understand very little about either biomechanics or indeed orthopaedic surgery, but let's look at some of the more mechanistic paradigms. In response to your question, Bruce Simon and I did some work many years ago that had actually showed that pulsed EMFs could affect osteoclast function. We couldn't understand the mechanism at that time, but now there are two ways in which one could look at the mechanism. One of them is to use a microarray approach in which you apply fields to in vitro cells, then you look at a host of genes that might go up and down. Then you can actually select patterns of genes that turn off and on with these fields, which might lend some mechanistic information as to the specific cell types that are being targeted as well as the specific molecules. Another more interesting way to do this would be to use knockout mice and see if fractures do heal in an accelerated fashion using a knockout model. Bruce Simon tells me that 20 or so papers are now available showing that TGF-β and BMP are upregulated. Why not use either a tissue-specific knockout mouse or indeed a noggin-overexpressing mouse that overexpresses this BMP inhibitor in bone cells—particularly in osteoblast but also in osteoprogenitor cells—and look at whether these pulsed EMFs have anything to do with that. And I would imagine a BMP is one of the signals, for that matter, that should shift the response curve if you overexpress the inhibitor. So these kinds of elegant molecular approaches can now be used to look at more mechanistic aspects of how pulsed EMFs or, for example, mechanical fields and activation could affect remodeling and fracture healing.

**Dr. Roy Aaron:** Mone just put his finger right on the target. Sol, I think you've done an elegant characterization. Do you think, Sol, that you could establish criteria for a minimal amount of information you would need to see in an article that would allow you to compare it with somebody else's article?

**Dr. Solomon Pollack:** There are enough standardized animal models out there that one can do a side-by-side comparison of stimulation techniques. There are gap models and there are closed fracture models out there, and mouse or rat models can be used as screen tools. The dose can be recalculated too so that each company can have what they think is the optimal dose delivered to that animal model. We should do the side-by-side comparison, and then do the more elegant molecular biologic approaches.

**Dr. Roy Aaron:** We're talking about two related things—mechanism and efficacy. Mechanism is something we're going to talk more about in the next couple of days. Today's discussion about animal models is largely related to efficacy. I brought up the issue of dosing because dosing and scaling from one size animal to another is probably one of the most limiting features of this entire field. And it's important to realize that until this year—which is probably 20 years or 25 years after this all got started—the issue of dosimetry in EMF was not even considered. We haven't done a clinical trial or a large animal trial to demonstrate that the dosimetry shown in small animals holds up as you scale up. So that's really the state of the art.

**Dr. Edmund Chao:** The prediction of local intensity of any physical stimulation method or signal is something that we can do very well actually. But we really never tried that. If you look at the radiation therapy field, they are using very accurate numerical simulation techniques. So I think that it's essential, if the industry and academic field wish to do it. That is a problem that we certainly can solve.

## Future Directions

- Dosimetric relationships of applied biophysical stimulation need further study, including scaling to experimental animal size, human body proportion, and specific tissues as fractures heal.
- There is a need to develop rapid screening techniques to identify optimum signal parameters and then scale results to the human.
- Mouse models allow an approach to mechanism in the whole animal by using selective knockouts and molecular techniques.
- Direct comparison of biophysical techniques could be done using a standardized model. We need to identify signal parameters that should be reported to facilitate comparisons.
- The target cells and tissues that respond to biophysical stimulation need to be identified. Some stimulation may be systemic and not just local.

# Section Three
## Biophysical Regulation of Skeletal Cells and Tissues

# Chapter 9
# Biophysical Regulation of Cell and Tissue Function

*Alan J. Grodzinsky, ScD*
*Jon Szafranski, MS*
*Michael DiMicco, PhD*
*Nora Szasz, PhD*

## Introduction

Musculoskeletal tissues are subjected to a wide range of loading forces associated with ambulation and joint motion. Mechanical loading forces can in turn induce a variety of endogenous mechanical and electrical fields, forces, and flows within tissues and cells. Stimulation via exogenous mechanical and electrical signals has also been used clinically to induce repair and in studies to understand basic cell signal transduction mechanisms. To understand tissue repair mechanisms that may be regulated by electrical, mechanical, or ultrasound stimulation of cells, investigators have performed studies in vivo and in vitro to address several fundamental questions: What are the endogenous physical signals in the environment of the cell? What are the cellular responses to tissue-level endogenous physical signals in vitro and in vivo? What are the transduction mechanisms by which cells can respond to these physical signals? Can exogenous physical signals be optimized to harness these same physical transduction mechanisms and thereby initiate repair responses in vivo?

A major challenge in the study of bone and dense connective tissues has been to integrate the results of studies in vitro at the cellular and tissue levels with the results of animal and human studies. While isolation of cells can technically facilitate the study of biological signaling mechanisms, the response of isolated cells to physical stimuli may be very different than that of cells in their native dense extracellular matrix (ECM) environment. Recent studies suggest that there are multiple regulatory pathways by which connective tissue cells sense and respond to mechanical stimuli. These pathways include upstream signaling and changes at the level of gene transcription, protein translation, and posttranslational modifications of newly synthesized macromolecules. Experiments have focused on a range of upstream and downstream intracellular processes. Although the details of many of these pathways remain to be elucidated, significant advances have been made.

This chapter first focuses on the magnitude and frequency of physiologic levels of endogenous physical forces at the tissue, cellular, and molecular levels. It then highlights selected in vitro model systems that have been developed to quantify cellular responses to mechanical and electrical stimuli. In particular, the focus is on the effects of physiologic levels of mechanical compression and tissue shear applied to intact cartilage explants, as well as electric currents applied to chondrocytes in agarose gel disks. Distinct patterns of chondrocyte biosynthesis and gene expression in response to these physical signals have emerged; these patterns provide significant clues regarding the mechanisms by which cells respond to physical signals. Methodologies and approaches used to identify electromechanical signal transduction mechanisms are described.

## Physical Signals in the Environment of the Cell

In articular cartilage, the biophysical signals of interest at the cellular level are directly related to the static and dynamic compressive and shear mechanical loads on the tissue that are produced by joint articulation (Fig. 1). Many physical forces and flows that occur in cartilage during loading in vivo have been identified and quantified in vitro. Dynamic compression of cartilage results in deformation of cells and extracellular matrix,[1,2] hydrostatic pressurization of the tissue fluid, pressure gradients and the accompanying flow of fluid within the tissue, and streaming potentials and currents induced by tissue fluid flow[1-3] (Fig. 1). These latter electromechanical phenomena are examples of classic electrokinetic effects that are inherent to mechanical deformation-induced fluid flows with respect to the ECM that occur in any charged, hydrated, porous medium.[4] In contrast, the components of tissue loading that result in pure tissue shear deformation of the ECM cause a concomitant local cell-level deformation of ECM and cells but little or no associated intratissue fluid flow. Such tissue shear deformations, therefore, are not accompanied by local pressure gradients and streaming potentials (Fig. 1).

In addition, the local changes in tissue volume caused by static compression lead to physiochemical changes within the ECM, including alterations in matrix water content, fixed charge density, mobile ion concentrations, and osmotic pressure.[5-7] Any of these mechanical, chemical, or electrical phenomena in the environment of connective tissue cells may signal the cell and thereby affect cellular metabolism. An understanding of the tissue-level spatial distribution of these forces and flows within cartilage during compression has been aided by the development of theoretical models for the mechanical, physicochemical, and electromechanical behavior of cartilage.[3,8,9] Recent studies of cell and matrix nanoindentation using atomic force microscopy or other specialized instruments has further extended our understanding of local physical stimuli in the environment of the cell.

## Biosynthetic Response of Chondrocytes to Mechanical Compression and Shear

### Compression
Studies using animal and human cartilage explants have shown that static compression of up to 50% can cause a dose-dependent decrease in the biosynthesis of proteoglycans, collagens, and other ECM proteins as rapidly as 1 hour after the onset of compression.[10] Cell-level quantitative autora-

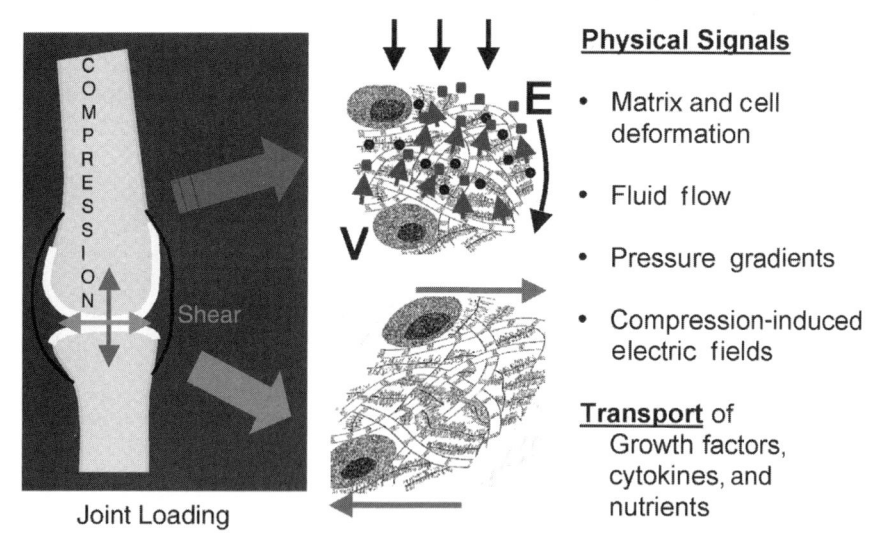

**Figure 1** Joint loading, left, leads to a complex combination of compression and shear deformation of cartilage, center, which produces multiple fields, forces, and flows that can act as signals to the chondrocytes and can also affect transport of soluble factors, nutrients, and waste products.

diography has been used to visualize the distribution of newly synthesized matrix molecules around individual cells in response to compression.[11] It was thus discovered that static compression could stimulate directional deposition of secreted proteoglycans around chondrocytes superimposed on an inhibition of synthesis. Dynamic compression in the 0.01 to 1 Hz frequency range (Fig. 1) can markedly stimulate the production of ECM molecules by chondrocytes in cartilage and in alginate and agarose gel culture systems in a manner dependent on amplitude and location within the tissue.[10,12-14] Quantitative autoradiography showed increased proteoglycan and protein deposition in regions of the tissue where relatively higher levels of fluid flow and cell deformation would occur, further suggesting the importance of these physical stimuli.[11,15] Recent studies by Bonassar and associates[16] showed that application of dynamic compression and simultaneous addition of insulin-like growth factor-1 (IGF-1) to the medium enhanced proteoglycan and protein in bovine explants almost twofold to threefold more than that achieved by either stimulus alone. Although cyclic compression also accelerated the transport of IGF-1 into the explants, the increase in biosynthesis caused by the combined effects of compression and IGF-1 was not simply due to mechanical augmentation of transport but rather to the combined but separately acting biological and mechanical cytokines.

## Dynamic Tissue Shear

Dynamic tissue shear (Fig. 1) can also stimulate cartilage biosynthesis over a range of strain amplitudes (1% to 3%) and frequencies (0.01 to 1 Hz) relevant to normal joint loading.[17] At 0.1 Hz, this stimulation of biosynthesis increased in a dose-dependent fashion with shear strain amplitude (1% to 6% strain). Quantitative autoradiography[17] showed that the increase in synthesis caused by tissue shear was spatially uniform within the explants, a finding consistent with the more uniform matrix deformation and the absence of localized fluid flow compared with that induced by dynamic compression. Dynamic tissue shear also failed to produce an increase in the transport of soluble factors such as IGF-1, again consistent with the notion that local tissue shear does not induce fluid flow with respect to the ECM. In contrast to dynamic compression, dynamic shear increased collagen synthesis significantly more than proteoglycan synthesis (in the presence of serum).[17] It is possible that this difference is related to the importance of collagen fibrils in providing resistance to shear loading in cartilage, suggesting that chondrocytes may recognize specific patterns of mechanical loading.

## Effects of Physical Forces on Chondrocyte Gene Expression

Recent advances in real-time polymerase chain reaction (PCR), the methodologies for extraction of RNA from intact cartilage tissue, and the use of clustering analysis to examine the trends in expression of multiple genes have allowed quantitative approaches in the study of the effects of physical forces on chondrocyte gene expression. A recent study by Fitzgerald and associates,[18] using real-time PCR, characterized the response of 28 genes after application of ramp-and-hold compressive strains to bovine cartilage explants for periods between 1 and 24 hours. Compression time courses were performed in the presence of an intracellular calcium chelator or an inhibitor of cyclic AMP-activated protein kinase A to address questions regarding mechanotransduction mechanisms. We found that both anabolic and catabolic genes were induced by static compression, but they exhibited contrasting expression patterns. Intracellular calcium and cAMP were found to play a fundamental role in the mechanical regulation of gene transcription.

### Direct Mechanical Compression

An example of the mechanical stimulus is shown in Figure 2, *A*: explants were slowly compressed over a ~3-minute period to 25% or 50% strain (based on cut thickness) and maintained at these static strain levels for 1, 2, 4, 8, or 24 hours, with disks kept in free-swelling conditions as controls. During joint loading in vivo, cartilage experiences a complex mixture of compressive and shear deformation having both static and dynamic components. For example, in vivo joint loading can result in high peak mechanical stresses (15 to 20 MPa)[19] that occur over very short durations (< 1 second) causing cartilage compressive strains of only 1% to 3%. In contrast, sustained (static) physiologic stresses applied to knee joints for 5 to 30 minutes can result in compressive strains in certain knee cartilages as high as 40% to 45%.[20] Application of a slow compression such as that seen in Figure 2, *A* causes an initial transient intratissue pressurization and fluid flow within the matrix immediately following compression and during a 15- to 30-minute

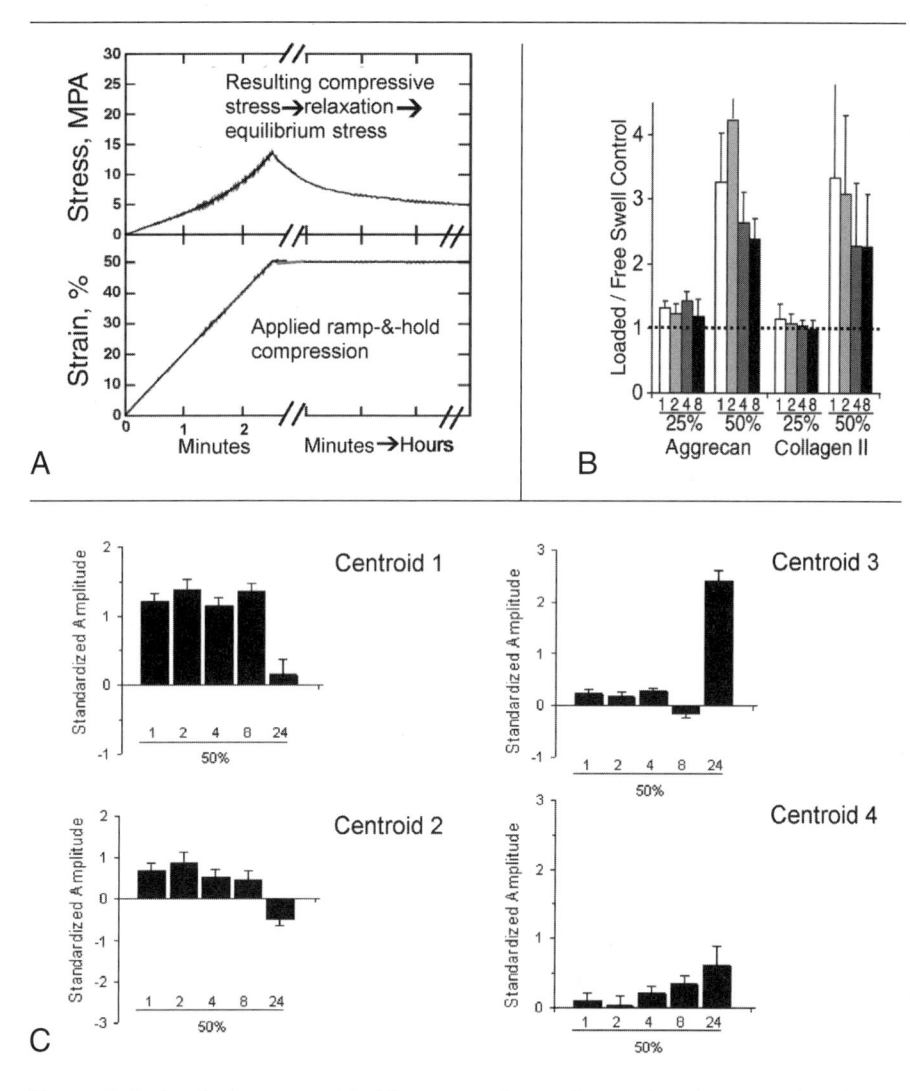

**Figure 2 A,** Applied ramp-and-hold compression and associated stress relaxation waveforms. **B,** Changes in mRNA levels of aggrecan and collagen II relative to free swelling controls. *(Data adapted with permission from Fitzgerald JB, Jin M, Dean D, Wood DJ, Zheng MH, Grodzinsky AJ: Mechanical compression of cartilage explants induces multiple time-dependent gene expression patterns and involves intracellular calcium and cyclic AMP. J Biol Chem 2004;279:19502-19511.)* **C,** Four main expression trends induced by 1 to 24 hours of 50% static compression of cartilage explants. Centroid vectors were calculated from the average projection coordinates of genes within each group; optimal groups were found using k-means clustering. Group 1: aggrecan, collagen II, c-fos, c-jun; Group 2: link protein, MMP-1, TIMP-2, sox-9, fibromodulin, MAPK1; Group 3: MMP-3, MMP-9, MMP-13, TIMP-1, ribosomal 6P, collagen 1; Group 4: ADAMTS-4, ADAMTS-5, TIMP-3, fibronectin, HSP-70, TGF-β, COX-2. *(Data adapted with permission from Hodge WA, Fijan RS, Carlson KL, et al: Contact pressures in the human hip joint measured in vivo. Proc Natl Acad Sci USA 1986;83:2879-2883.)*

period of stress relaxation. After stress relaxation has ended, fluid flow ceases and intratissue pressure returns to zero (ie, that of the medium) as the new equilibrium compressed state of the tissue is reached. Thus, the initial compression transient has certain physical attributes of slow dynamic compression, whereas the final compressed state mimics the static component of in vivo compression. Therefore, the objective of this study was to explore the kinetics of changes in gene expression to both the initial transient loading and final static loading phases.

Static compression has been shown to decrease proteoglycan and type II collagen synthesis within 1 to 2 hours.[10] However, transcription levels for aggrecan and type II collagen were upregulated approximately twofold to threefold during the first 8 hours of 50% compression (consistent with previous studies that used Northern analyses)[21] and subsequently downregulated to levels below that of free-swelling controls by 24 hours (Fig. 2, B). Thus, the temporal kinetics of transcriptional and biosynthetic responses to compression loading appeared considerably different, though they converge by 24 hours after application of static compression. The transcription of aggrecan and type II collagen genes may be more sensitive to the dynamic components of compression. Recent experiments have shown that ERK 1/2 and p38 phosphorylation levels peak within 10 minutes of static compression.[22] It has been suggested that such an initial transient response is due to the dynamic components of static compression, which may similarly explain the transient transcriptional upregulation of matrix proteins observed here. In addition, loading may affect the apparatus for transcription and translation differently. Studies have shown that high pressure can cause changes in cell morphology and disorganization of the Golgi and microtubules in chondrocytes.[23] Compression of cartilage explants also reduces cell volume and the volumes of several intracellular organelles; however, the volume of the Golgi appears to remain unaffected by static compression of up to 50% strain.[24] Thus, the synthesis of proteins that require significant posttranslation modification may be affected by compression differently than transcription is.

Transcription levels of matrix metalloproteinases-3, -9, -13, aggrecanase-1, and the matrix protease regulator cyclooxygenase-2 increased with the duration of 50% compression 2- to 16-fold up to 24 hours.[18] Thus, transcription of proteins involved in matrix remodeling and catabolism dominated over anabolic matrix proteins as the duration of static compression increased. Immediate early genes c-fos and c-jun were dramatically upregulated 6- to 30-fold respectively during the first 8 hours of 50% compression and remained upregulated after 24 hours.[18]

Clustering analysis[25,26] and principal component analysis[27,28] were used to elucidate the main expression trends and to highlight genes that appeared to be coregulated by mechanical compression. These computational techniques help to classify groups of genes with common upstream signaling pathways and may help to predict certain cell behavior. Cluster analysis of the data revealed four main expression patterns (Fig. 2, C): two groups containing either transiently upregulated or duration-enhanced expression profiles could each be subdivided into genes that did or did not require intracellular calcium release and cyclic AMP-activated protein kinase A for their mechanoregulation.[18] We found that the presence of BAPTA-AM during mechanical loading suppressed the upregulation of many genes, including aggrecan, type II collagen, link protein, c-jun, and many MMPs.[18] The selective suppression by BAPTA-AM supports the idea that intracellular calcium is a common but not complete upstream signaling event controlling the mechanoregulation of anabolic, catabolic, and anticatabolic genes. Interestingly, expression of stress protein HSP70 during compression was significantly greater in the presence of BAPTA-AM.[18] Hence, intracellular calcium release may also be required to elicit the stress-protective response seen in chondrocytes during loading.[29]

**Hydrostatic and Osmotic Pressure**
Extensive research studies have also focused on the effects of medium osmolarity, pH, and applied hydrostatic pressure on chondrocyte biosynthesis, gene expression, and ion channel transport. The primary focus here is on the effects of direct mechanical deformation; however, there are several excellent reviews on this subject.[7,30,31] The study of mechanisms in such cases has often necessitated the use of isolated chondrocyte culture systems. Such isolated cell systems are extremely important models for investigating chondrocyte mechanotransduction; however, the relevance to cellular mechanisms in native tissue must be confirmed independently due to the complex interactions that exist between the chondrocyte and the ECM in vivo.

## Cell Environment and Morphology

Loading of cartilage produces deformations at the tissue, cellular, and molecular length scales. Confocal microscopy[32] and quantitative stereology[2] have demonstrated that compression of cartilage tissue results in similar magnitude reductions in cell height and cell volume. Deformations within the pericellular matrix also affect the physicochemical microenvironment of the chondrocyte[1,11] and may in turn signal the cell to modulate its biosynthetic response. Cell-surface connections to the ECM, including integrin receptors, enable pericellular deformations to be transmitted through the cell membrane to intracellular organelles via cytoskeletal elements such as actin microfilaments, microtubules, and intermediate filaments.[32-34] Compression may also affect the morphology of other intracellular organelles related to matrix metabolism, such as the rough endoplasmic reticulum (rER) and the Golgi apparatus. Since the rER and Golgi are sites of posttranslational modifications of ECM macromolecules (eg, glycosylation and sulfation of aggrecan),[35] changes in Golgi morphology and function with compression may play a critical role in the known changes in glycosaminoglycan (GAG) chain length and sulfation caused by static compression.[36] There is also increasing evidence that cell-membrane-ECM connections play a role in mechanotransduction signaling events. Integrins can convert extracellular mechanical stimuli into intracellular signals in a variety of cell types.[37] Several recent studies have also demonstrated a role for mitogen-activated protein kinases (MAPKs) in alteration of matrix gene expression and changes in matrix production by chondrocytes within cartilage under load. This family of ubiquitous signaling molecules includes extracellular-signal regulated protein kinases (ERK 1/2), c-Jun N-terminal kinase, and p38. Several groups have discovered the activation of MAPKs in chondrocytes within bovine cartilage explants subjected to static and dynamic compression. Isolated bovine chondrocytes exposed to fluid shear have also been shown to have increased levels of activated ERK 1/2.[38]

## Electric Stimulation Affects Chondrocyte Biosynthesis and Gene Expression

The regulation of cellular behavior by endogenous electric currents has been investigated for many physiologic processes, including embryonic development,[39] wound healing,[40,41] and neural action potential propagation.[42] Interactions between exogenous electric currents and chondrocytes have been demonstrated in several previous studies showing that externally applied electric and electromagnetic fields can increase DNA synthesis,[43] GAG content,[44-46] and protein synthesis[47] by isolated chondrocytes[43] or chondrocytes in explant organ culture.[44,47] A recent study[48] also showed that an electric field can induce migration of isolated chondrocytes, which may have implications regarding cartilage remodeling and regeneration. Electric streaming currents are known to be coupled to mechanical deformation and fluid transport within cartilage due to electrokinetic interactions associated with the highly charged proteoglycan constituents of the ECM.[3] These findings can have implications for cartilage remodeling and regeneration.

We recently studied the effects of applied sinusoidal electric current densities in the 10 Hz to 10 kHz range, 25 mA/cm$^2$ amplitude on ECM and DNA synthesis in a chondrocyte-seeded agarose gel culture.[49] Bovine calf chondrocytes isolated from femoral condyle cartilage were cultured in 2% agarose gel samples that had been cast in Teflon holders (Fig. 3) at $1.5 \times 10^7$ cells/mL in 10% FBS up to 25 days prior to stimulation. Samples were stimulated in special chambers (Fig. 3) that were separated from platinum electrodes by 1-inch-long agarose salt-bridges. Electric current densities of 25 mA/cm$^2$, 0.01 kHz to 10 kHz, were applied across test specimens for up to 20 hours at 37°C using a feedback-controlled constant current source. Selected samples were flash frozen immediately poststimulation for real-time PCR. Chambers were controlled for pH, electrode byproducts, and temperature. Control and test chambers were compared using null fields in the latter. Western analysis showed additionally that there was no elevation in heat shock protein 70 caused by the applied electric field over the range of amplitudes and frequencies tested.

The applied electric currents caused a statistically significant increase in protein synthesis as assessed by $^3$H-proline incorporation at all frequencies tested.[49] Chromatography confirmed that ~84% of this $^3$H-proline was incorporated into newly synthesized collagen macromolecules, and essentially all the $^{35}$S-sulfate was incorporated into macromolecular GAG. GAG synthesis and proliferation, as measured by $^{35}$S-sulfate and $^3$H-thymidine incorporation respectively, was also significantly increased by an electric current den-

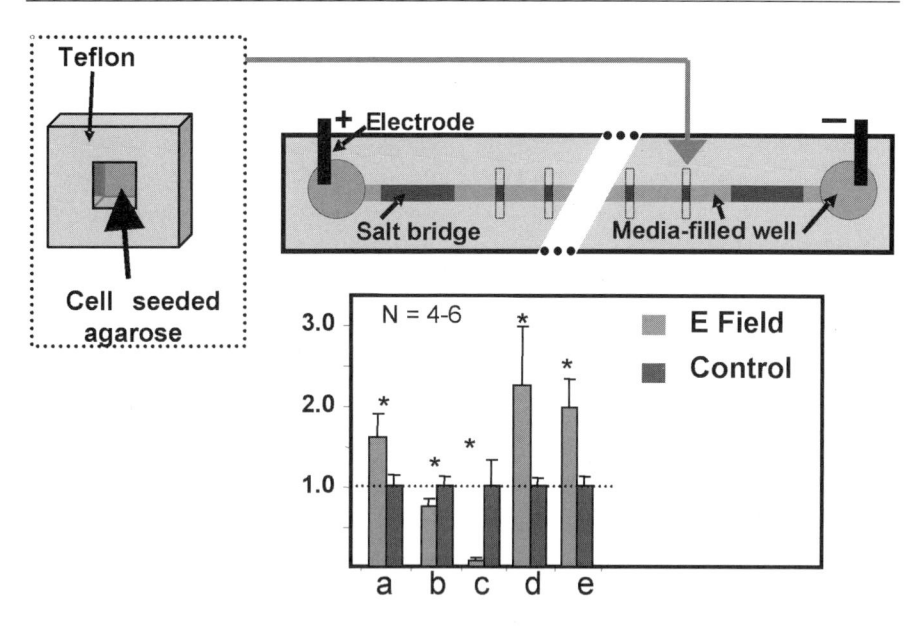

Figure 3 Schematic of Teflon specimen holder containing chondrocyte-seeded agarose specimen, which is inserted into the specialized chamber for electrical stimulation. Data are changes in mRNA levels measured by real-time PCR normalized to nonstimulated controls for **(a)** collagen 2a1; **(b)** link protein; **(c)** IGF-1; **(d)** fibromodulin; **(e)** MMP-3. *(Data adapted with permission from Szasz N, Hung H, Sen S, Grodzinsky AJ: Electric field regulation of chondrocyte biosynthesis in agarose gel constructs.* Trans Orthop Res Soc *2003;28:672.)*

sity of 25 mA/cm$^2$ at 1 kHz. Real-time PCR showed an increase in type 2 collagen, fibromodulin, and aggrecan transcription (Fig. 3), consistent here with the increased biosynthesis.[49] There was also an upregulation of catabolic agents (MMP-3, MMP-13, ADAMTS-4, TIMP-1, data not shown), which indicates the possibility of active matrix remodeling. It remains to be seen whether endogenous streaming currents (ie, local electric fields induced, for example, by mechanical compression of cartilage) may play an important role in regulation of chondrocyte metabolism. The possibility that endogenous electric fields can upregulate cell division while simultaneously upregulating ECM biosynthesis suggests a potential role for electrokinetic interactions as part of a coordinated cell signaling process within the tissue.

## Acknowledgment
Research funded by NIH grant AR33236.

## References
1. Guilak F, Mow VC: The mechanical environment of the chondrocyte: A biphasic finite element model of cell-matrix interactions in articular cartilage. *J Biomech* 2000;33:1663-1673.

2. Buschmann MD, Hunziker EB, Kim YJ, Grodzinsky AJ: Altered aggrecan synthesis correlates with cell and nucleus structure in statically compressed cartilage. *J Cell Sci* 1996;109:499-508.

3. Frank EH, Grodzinsky AJ: Cartilage electromechanics II: A continuum model of cartilage electrokinetics and correlation with experiments. *J Biomech* 1987;20:629-639.

4. Grodzinsky AJ, Lipshitz H, Glimcher MJ: Electromechanical properties of articular cartilage during compression and stress relaxation. *Nature* 1978;175:448-450.

5. Maroudas A: Physicochemical properties of articular cartilage, in Freeman MAR (ed): *Physicochemical Properties of Articular Cartilage*. Tunbridge Wells, England, Pitman Medical, 1979, pp 215-290.

6. Gray ML, Pizzanelli AM, Grodzinsky AJ, Lee RC: Mechanical and physiochemical determinants of the chondrocyte biosynthetic response. *J Orthop Res* 1988;6:777-792.

7. Urban JP, Hall AC, Gehl KA: Regulation of matrix synthesis rates by the ionic and osmotic environment of articular chondrocytes. *J Cell Physiol* 1993;154:262-270.

8. Eisenberg SR, Grodzinsky AJ: The kinetics of chemically induced nonequilibrium swelling of articular cartilage and corneal stroma. *J Biomech Eng* 1987;109:79-89.

9. Lai WM, Hou JS, Mow VC: A triphasic theory for the swelling and deformation behaviors of articular cartilage. *J Biomech Eng* 1991;113:245-258.

10. Sah RL, Kim YJ, Doong JY, et al: Biosynthetic response of cartilage explants to dynamic compression. *J Orthop Res* 1989;7:619-636.

11. Quinn TM, Grodzinsky AJ, Buschmann MD, Kim YJ, Hunziker EB: Mechanical compression alters proteoglycan deposition and matrix deformation around individual cells in cartilage explants. *J Cell Sci* 1998;111:573-583.

12. Torzilli PA, Grigiene R, Huang C, et al: Characterization of cartilage metabolic response to static and dynamic stress using a mechanical explant test system. *J Biomech* 1997;30:1-9.

13. Wong M, Siegrist M, Cao X: Cyclic compression of articular cartilage explants is associated with progressive consolidation and altered expression pattern of extracellular matrix proteins. *Matrix Biol* 1999;18:391-399.

14. Li KW, Williamson AK, Wang AS, Sah RL: Growth responses of cartilage to static and dynamic compression. *Clin Orthop* 2001;391:S34-S48.

15. Buschmann MD, Kim YJ, Wong M, et al: Stimulation of aggrecan synthesis in cartilage explants by cyclic loading is localized to regions of high interstitial fluid flow. *Arch Biochem Biophys* 1999;366:1-7.

16. Bonassar LJ, Grodzinsky AJ, Frank EH, et al: The effect of dynamic compression on the response of articular cartilage to insulin-like growth factor-I. *J Orthop Res* 2001;19:11-17.

17. Jin M, Frank EH, Quinn TM, Hunziker EB, Grodzinsky AJ: Tissue shear deformation stimulates proteoglycan and protein biosynthesis in bovine cartilage explants. *Arch Biochem Biophys* 2001;395:41-48.

18. Fitzgerald JB, Jin M, Dean D, Wood DJ, Zheng MH, Grodzinsky AJ: Mechanical compression of cartilage explants induces multiple time-dependent gene expression patterns and involves intracellular calcium and cyclic AMP. *J Biol Chem* 2004;279: 19502-19511.

19. Hodge WA, Fijan RS, Carlson KL, et al: Contact pressures in the human hip joint measured in vivo. *Proc Natl Acad Sci USA* 1986;83:2879-2883.

20. Herberhold C, Faber S, Stammberger T, et al: In situ measurement of articular cartilage deformation in intact femoropatellar joints under static loading. *J Biomech* 1999; 32:1287-1295.

21. Ragan P, Badger A, Cook M, et al: Down-regulation of chondrocyte aggrecan and type-II collagen gene expression correlates with increases in static compression magnitude and duration. *J Orthop Res* 1999;17:836-842.

22. Fanning P, Emkey G, Grodzinsky AJ, Trippel SD: Mechanical regulation of mitogen-activated protein kinase signaling in articular cartilage. *J Biol Chem* 2003;278: 50940-50948.

23. Parkkinen JJ, Lammi MJ, Pelttari A, et al: Altered Golgi apparatus in hydrostatically loaded articular cartilage chondrocytes. *Ann Rheum Dis* 1993;52:192-198.

24. Grodzinsky AJ, Levenston ME, Jin M, Frank EH: Cartilage tissue remodeling in response to mechanical forces. *Ann Rev Biomed Eng* 2000;2:691-714.

25. Dougherty ER, Barrera J, Brun M, et al: Inference from clustering with application to gene-expression microarrays. *J Comput Biol* 2002;9:105-126.

26. Eisen MB, Spellman PT, Brown PO, Botstein D: Cluster analysis and display of genome-wide expression patterns. *Proc Natl Acad Sci USA* 1998;95:14863-14868.

27. Alter O, Brown PO, Botstein D: Singular value decomposition for genome-wide expression data processing and modeling. *Proc Natl Acad Sci USA* 2000;97: 10101-10106.

28. Holter NS, Mitra M, Maritan A, Cieplak M, Banavar JR, Fedoroff NV: Fundamental patterns underlying gene expression profiles: Simplicity from complexity. *Proc Natl Acad Sci USA* 2000;97:8409-8414.

29. Kaarniranta K, Holmberg CI, Lammi MJ, Eriksson JE, Sistonen L, Helminen HJ: Primary chondrocytes resist hydrostatic pressure-induced stress while synovial cells and fibroblasts show modified Hsp70 response. *Osteoarthritis Cartilage* 2001;9:7-13.

30. Takahashi K, Kubo T, Kobayashi K, et al: Hydrostatic pressure influences mRNA expression of transforming growth factor-1 and heat shock protein 70 in chondrocyte-like cell line. *J Orthop Res* 1997;15:150-158.

31. Wilkins RJ, Browning JA, Ellory JC: Surviving in a matrix: Membrane transport in articular chondrocytes. *J Membr Biol* 2000;177:95-108.

32. Guilak F: Compression-induced changes in the shape and volume of the chondrocyte nucleus. *J Biomech* 1995;28:1529-1541.

33. Jortikka MO, Parkkinen JJ, Inkinen RI, et al: The role of microtubules in the regulation of proteoglycan synthesis in chondrocytes under hydrostatic pressure. *Arch Biochem Biophys* 2000;374:172-180.

34. Lee DA, Knight MM, Bolton JF, et al: Chondrocyte deformation within compressed agarose constructs at the cellular and sub-cellular levels. *J Biomech* 2000;33:81-95.

35. Lohmander LS, Hascall VC, Yanagishita M, Kuettner KE, Kimura JH: Post-translational events in proteoglycan synthesis: Kinetics of synthesis of chondroitin sulfate and oligosaccharides on the core protein. *Arch Biochem Biophys* 1986;250:211-227.

36. Kim YJ, Grodzinsky AJ, Plaas AH: Compression of cartilage results in differential effects on biosynthetic pathways for aggrecan, link protein, and hyaluronan. *Arch Biochem Biophys* 1996;328:331-340.

37. Wang N, Butler JP, Ingber DE: Mechanotransduction across the cell surface and through the cytoskeleton. *Science* 1993;260:1124-1127.

38. Hung CT, Henshaw DR, Wang CC, et al: Mitogen-activated protein kinase signaling in bovine articular chondrocytes in response to fluid flow does not require calcium mobilization. *J Biomech* 2000;33:73-80.

39. Robinson KR: The responses of cells to electrical fields: A review. *J Cell Biol* 1985;101:2023-2027.

40. Soong HK, Parkinson WC, Bafna S, Sulik GL, Huang SC: Movements of cultured corneal epithelial cells and stromal fibroblasts in electric fields. *Invest Ophthalmol Vis Sci* 1990;31:2278-2282.

41. Barker AT, Jaffe LF, Vanable JW Jr: The glabrous epidermis of cavies contains a powerful battery. *Am J Physiol Regul Integr Comp Physiol* 1982;242:R358-R366.

42. Weiss TF: *Cellular Biophysics: Electrical Properties.* Cambridge, MA, MIT Press, 1996.

43. Rodan GA, Bourret LA, Norton LA: DNA synthesis in cartilage cells is stimulated by oscillating electric fields. *Science* 1978;199:690-692.

44. Liu H, Abbott J, Bee JA: Pulsed electromagnetic fields influence hyaline cartilage extracellular matrix composition without affecting molecular structure. *Osteoarthritis Cartilage* 1996;4:63-76.

45. Ciombor DM, Lester G, Aaron RK, Neame P, Caterson B: Low frequency EMF regulates chondrocyte differentiation and expression of matrix proteins. *J Orthop Res* 2002;20:40-49.

46. Aaron RK, Wang S, Ciombor DM: Upregulation of basal TGF-b1 levels by EMF coincident with chondrogenesis: Implications for skeletal repair and tissue engineering. *J Orthop Res* 2002;20:233-240.

47. MacGinitie LA, Gluzband YA, Grodzinsky AJ: Electric field stimulation can increase protein synthesis in articular cartilage explants. *J Orthop Res* 1994;12:151-160.

48. Chao PHG, Roy R, Mauck RL, Liu W, Valhmu WB, Hung CT: Chondrocyte translocation response to direct current electric fields. *J Biomech Eng* 2002;122:261-267.

49. Szasz N, Hung H, Sen S, Grodzinsky AJ: Electric field regulation of chondrocyte biosynthesis in agarose gel constructs. *Trans Orthop Res Soc* 2003;28:672.

Chapter 10
# Mechanical Regulation of Osteocyte Function

*Jenneke Klein-Nulend, PhD*
*Peter J. Nijweide, PhD*
*Elisabeth H. Burger, PhD*

## The Osteocyte Syncytium

Mature osteocytes are stellate cells enclosed within the lacunocanalicular network of bone. The lacunae contain the cell bodies. Long slender cytoplasmic processes ("fingers") radiate from the cell bodies in all directions (Fig. 1), with the highest density perpendicular to the bone surface. These processes run through the bone matrix via small canals, the canaliculi. The more mature osteocytes are connected by these cell processes to neighboring osteocytes. The most recently incorporated osteocytes are connected to neighboring osteocytes as well as to the cells lining the bone surface. However, some of the processes oriented to the bone surface appear not to connect with the lining cells but pass through this cell layer, establishing contact between the osteocyte syncytium and the extraosseous space.[1] This finding suggests the existence of a signaling system between the osteocyte and the bone marrow compartments (osteoblast stem cells) without intervention of the osteoblasts/lining cells.

The typical morphology of the osteocyte was originally thought to be enforced on differentiating osteoblasts during their incorporation in the bone matrix. Osteocytes remain in contact with neighboring osteocytes and with bone surface cells to ensure the access of oxygen and nutrients. In vitro experiments with isolated osteocytes have shown, however, that although the cells lose their stellate shape in suspension, they express this typical morphology again as soon as they settle on a support[2] (Fig. 1). In bone, gap junctions are present between the tips of the cell processes of connecting osteocytes.[3] Within each osteon, therefore, osteocytes form a syncytium of gap junction-coupled cells. The lacunae within each osteon are also connected with each other via the canaliculi; therefore, the osteocyte syncytium represents both an intracellular and an extracellular network system.

Because of the osteocyte's location within the bone and its morphology, the question arises as to which stimuli are capable of "exciting" the osteocytes. The answer to this question will come from studies in which biomechanical concepts and techniques are applied to bone cell biology. Over the last decade, both theoretical and experimental data have led to the general notion that osteocytes are the pivotal cells in the biomechanical regulation of bone mass and structure.[4-11] The development of osteocyte isolation techniques, the use of highly sensitive immunocytochemical and in situ hybridiza-

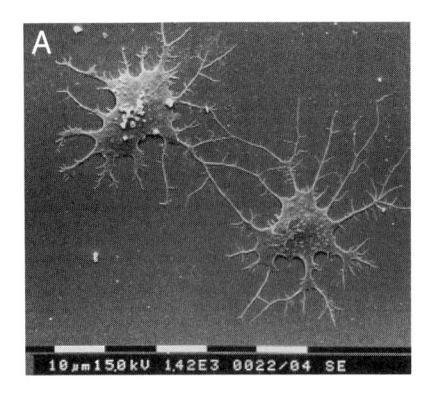

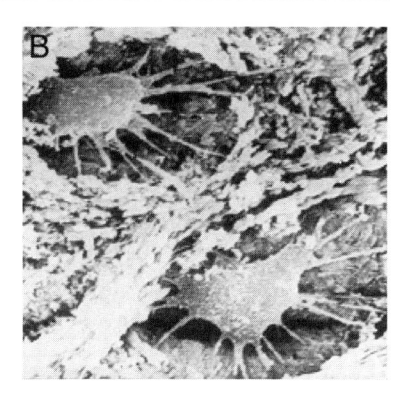

**Figure 1** Osteocyte morphology. **A,** isolated osteocytes in culture. Osteocytes were isolated by an immunodissection method using mAb OB7.3-coated magnetic beads. After isolation, the cells were seeded on a glass support, cultured for 24 hours, and studied with a scanning electron microscope. After attachment, osteocytes form cytoplasmic extrusions in all directions. **B,** Osteocytes embedded in calcified bone matrix. Note the many cell processes radiating from the osteocyte cell bodies as visualized using scanning electron microscopy (magnification, ×1000).

tion procedures, and molecular biologic methods applicable even when only small numbers of cells are available will most likely result in increased knowledge about the osteocyte, the least understood bone cell type. This chapter focuses on the role of osteocytes in the physiology of bone, with an emphasis on its role in determining the bone's structure.

## Osteocyte Isolation

Because osteocytes are postmitotic and embedded in hard matrix, they are difficult to study. The technique of osteocyte isolation and culture offered a major step forward. This technique became possible by the development of osteocyte-specific antibodies directed to antigens on the cytoplasmic membrane.[12] Using an immunodissection method, Van der Plas and Nijweide[2] succeeded in the isolation and purification of chicken osteocytes from mixed bone cell populations isolated from fetal bones by enzymatic digestion. Isolated osteocytes appeared to behave in vitro as they do in vivo, ie, in vitro osteocytes reacquired a stellate morphology and formed a network of cells coupled to each other by long, slender cell processes. As is the case in vivo, isolated osteocytes were postmitotic.[13]

## Osteocyte Markers

Osteocytes are fully defined by their location within the bone matrix and their typical stellate morphology. Related to this morphology is the cytoskeletal organization of the osteocytes. The prominent actin bundles in the osteocytic processes in combination with the abundance of the actin-bundling protein fimbrin are typical for osteocytes.[14] Furthermore, osteocytes express osteocalcin, osteonectin, and osteopontin but show little alkaline phosphatase activity.[15]

At present, the best markers for isolated osteocytes are their typical morphology, which they reacquire in culture[2] in combination with their reaction with monoclonal antibodies, which have been proved to be osteocyte-specific in tissue sections.[12] The identities of antigens involved in mAb OB7.3 were recently elucidated.[16]

# The Function of Osteocytes

## Osteocytes as Mechanosensor Cells

Several arguments can be raised in favor of osteocytes as the mechanosensory cells par excellence of bone.[4] First, consider their anatomic characteristics. In all types of bone, the osteocytes are dispersed throughout the mineralized matrix and are connected with their neighbor osteocytes via long slender cell processes running in slightly wider canaliculi of unmineralized matrix. The cell processes contact each other via gap junctions,[3] thereby allowing direct cell-to-cell coupling. The superficial osteocytes are connected with the lining cells covering most of the bone surface, as well as with the osteoblasts that cover the bone surface where new bone is deposited. Bone tissue is thus a three-dimensional network of cells, most of which are surrounded by a very narrow sheath of unmineralized matrix, followed by a much wider layer of mineralized matrix. There is an intracellular as well as an extracellular route for the rapid passage of ions and signal molecules, allowing cellular signaling from osteocytes lying deep within the bone tissue to surface lining cells and vice versa.

Several studies indicate that osteocytes are indeed sensitive to stress applied.[17-22] These studies show that intermittent loading at physiologic strain magnitude produces rapid changes of metabolic activity in osteocytes and suggest that osteocytes function as mechanosensors in bone. Finite element simulation of bone remodeling, assuming this to be a self-organizational control process, also predicted a role for osteocytes as stress sensors of bone.[5]

If osteocytes are mechanosensor cells, how do they sense mechanical loading? Over the last few years, a number of theoretical and experimental studies have appeared that agree that flow of interstitial fluid is probably the stress-derived factor that informs the bone cells about mechanical loading. In this view, the canaliculi form the necessary porous network, and the osteocytes act as the mechanosensor cells.

## Interstitial Fluid Flow in Bone

Early evidence of stress-induced fluid flow in bone was produced by Piekarski and Munro.[23] Subsequently, Dillaman[24] found experimental evidence for a substantial flow of fluid through the mineralized portion of bone. Using a mathematical model, Kufahl and Saha[25] found that the diameter of the canaliculi precisely allows the stress-derived fluid flow to reach even the outermost osteocytes of an osteon. These studies emphasized the importance of mechanically induced flow for the transport of metabolites to and from osteocytes in an osteon to ensure osteocyte viability.

## Effects of Fluid Flow on Osteocytes

Separation among osteocytes, osteoblasts, and fibroblasts became feasible when an osteocyte-specific antibody was produced by Nijweide and Mulder.[12] Using this antibody, an immunoseparation method was developed that allowed investigators to obtain populations of chicken calvarial bone cells enriched (90% to 95% pure) in osteocytes, osteoblasts, or periosteal fibroblasts.[2]

Klein-Nulend and associates[7] subjected these different cell populations to two stress regimes, intermittent hydrostatic compression and pulsatile fluid flow. Under both stress regimes, osteocytes appeared more sensitive than osteoblasts, and osteoblasts more sensitive than periosteal fibroblasts. In addition, osteocytes were particularly sensitive to fluid shear stress, more so than to hydrostatic stress. These conclusions are remarkably in agreement with the theory developed by Cowin and associates[4,6,26] that osteocytes are the professional mechanosensory cells of bone and that they detect mechanical loading events by the canalicular flow of interstitial fluid that results from that loading event.

How the mechanical signal is detected and converted in a chemical, intracellular response has yet to be established. The composition and structure of the matrix in the periosteocytic sheath and the adherence of osteocytes to their surrounding matrix are very important. The matrix composition and structure determines the bone's porosity for fluid flow and therefore the magnitude of the fluid shear stress.[6] Osteocytes are still capable of producing matrix proteins and proteoglycans; therefore, they might even modify their responsiveness to mechanical loading by adapting the matrix around them and thereby the porosity of the lacunocanalicular system.

Osteocytes adhere to their surrounding matrix by specific receptors on the cytoplasmic membrane, such as integrins and CD44 receptors. Both are coupled to the cytoskeleton. Therefore, it is likely that these receptors are the first step of intracellular signal transduction after mechanical stimulation. Regulation of the number of adhesion sites and/or their coupling to intracellular signal transduction pathways might provide a mechanism by which endocrine modulation of the mechanoregulation of bone occurs.

## Signal Transduction in Mechanosensing

To respond to mechanical stimuli with the production of signal molecules that modulate the activities of osteoblasts and osteoclasts, the mechanosensor cells, ie, the osteocytes, have to convert the mechanical stimuli into intracellular signals (mechanotransduction). Extracellular matrix receptors, such as integrins and CD44 receptors located in the osteocyte membrane, are attached to the extracellular matrix as well as to the cytoskeleton. They are prime candidates as mechanotransducers.[27] It is likely that the known intracellular signal transduction pathways, such as the intracellular $Ca^{2+}$-, IP-3-, or cAMP-dependent pathways known to play a role in other mechanosensitive cells, are involved.[28] Through these pathways, signal molecules such as prostaglandins and nitric oxide (NO) are produced and secreted.

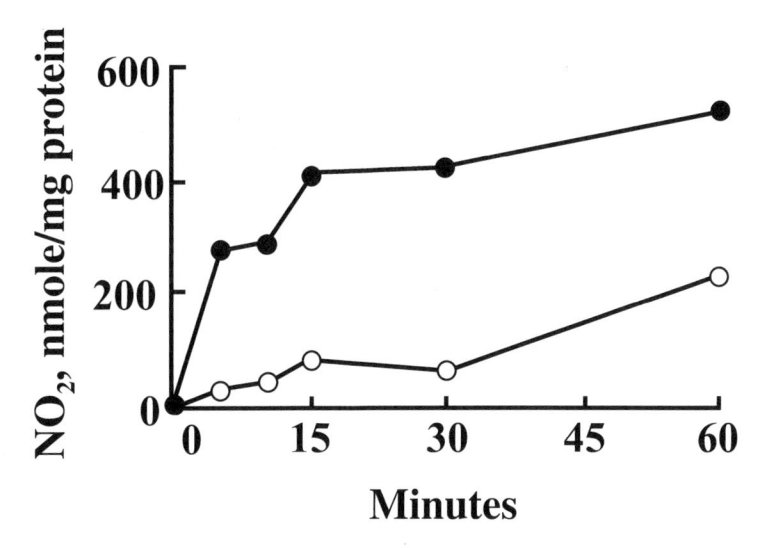

**Figure 2** Effect of pulsating fluid flow (5 Hz sigmoidal pulses, 0.6 +/- 0.03 Pa shear stress) on NO production by cultured human bone cells obtained from a transiliac bone biopsy. Cells were treated for 1 hour with or without flow, and the cell culture medium was assayed for NO, measured as $NO_2$. Black dots represent the stressed cells and white dots represent the nonstressed controls. Note that after 15 minutes, the initial rapid stimulation stops.

Prostaglandins play a predominant role in the response of bone tissue and cells to stress.[29-33] Animal studies have shown that both bone resorption caused by immobilization and bone formation caused by mechanical loading are inhibited by treating the animals with indomethacin.[34]

The early upregulation of prostaglandin release in response to mechanical stress is associated with a subsequent induction of cyclooxygenase-2 (COX-2).[35] Induction of COX-2 by stress may explain why prostaglandin production continues for several hours after stress is stopped,[7,36] and could be related to the memory phenomenon described in vivo. In animal studies, a limited number of stress cycles per day is sufficient to induce an adaptive response, suggesting that bone is able to memorize stress events over a period of several hours.[37]

NO produced by NO synthase is an important mediator of the response of bone to stress. Several studies[22,35,36,38,39] have shown that NO production is rapidly increased in response to mechanical stress in bone cells, including isolated osteocytes (Fig. 2). This rapid release by mechanically stressed bone cells makes NO an extremely interesting candidate for intercellular communication within the three-dimensional network of bone cells.

## Strain-dependent Regulation of Osteoclast Activity During Bone Remodeling

Bone tissue renews itself throughout life by means of basic multicellular units (BMUs). These groups of osteoclasts and osteoblasts act in a coordi-

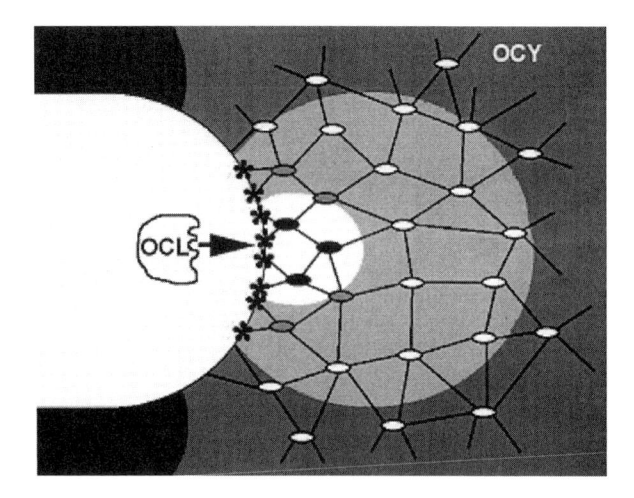

Section Three   Biophysical Regulation of Skeletal Cells and Tissues

**Figure 3** Illustration of the cutting cone tip of a bone multicellular unit showing the relation between apoptotic osteocytes and a progressing osteoclast. Osteocyte apoptosis (indicated as black lacunae) is caused by canalicular stasis, which directly results from the volumetric strain pattern caused by cyclic loading in the normal direction. As osteoclasts are attracted towards apoptotic osteocytes because of changes on the apopoptic cell surface (indicated by asterisks), the direction of the osteoclastic attack follows the direction of loading. OCY, osteocyte network; OCL, osteoclast.

nated fashion to first resorb existing bone tissue and subsequently refill the gap with new bone tissue.

BMUs literally move through existing bone tissue during the process of bone renewal. Osteoclasts appear first and dig a tunnel through compact bone or a trench along the surface of trabecular bone. The tunnel or trench is subsequently refilled with bone tissue by osteoblasts that appear to follow the osteoclasts. In the case of osteons, a central canal of connective tissue with blood vessels and neurons is always kept open: the Haversian channel. In the case of trabecular bone, the bone marrow sinusoids fulfill the function of the Haversian channel by providing a supply of blood vessels and neurons. The question of how osteoclasts and osteoblasts, which are cells of completely different origin and function, are able to collaborate to produce hemiosteons that run along the direction of dominant strain of the particular piece of bone remains a mystery.

How the resorbing osteoclasts find their way through the preexisting bone matrix during remodeling remains unexplained. The alignment of secondary osteons and trabecular hemiosteons along the dominant loading direction suggests that remodeling is guided by mechanical strain. This means that mechanical adaptation occurs throughout life at each remodeling cycle. It has been proposed that alignment during remodeling occurs as a result of different canalicular flow patterns around the cutting cone and reversal zone during loading.[9] Low canalicular flow around the tip of the cutting cone

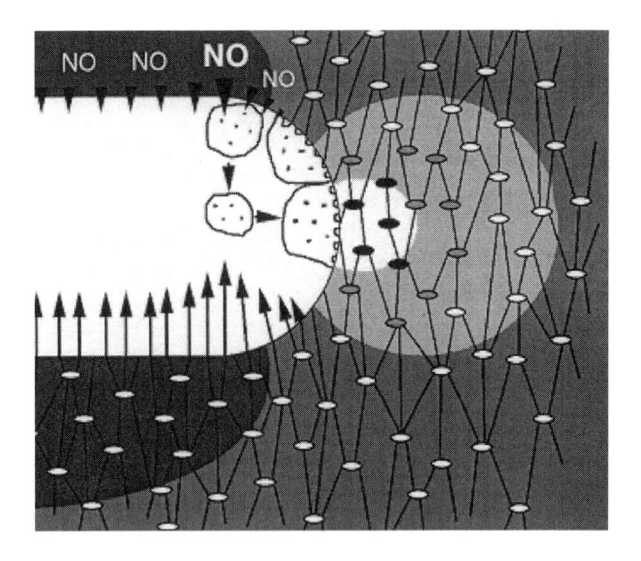

**Figure 4** Illustration of postulated events in the cutting cone of a progressing bone multicellular unit. Osteoclasts are attracted by apoptotic osteocytes in the cutting cone tip but are forced to withdraw again from the bone surface at the cutting cone base as a result of high amounts of NO produced by well-stressed osteocytes. Because NO production remains high further down the reversal zone, osteoclasts remain within the cutting cone and may even reenter the resorption cycle, leading to a treadmill of active and inactive osteoclasts that together dig the resorption tunnel or trench. Vertical arrows indicate direction and magnitude of canalicular fluid flow; vertical arrowheads indicate release of NO by well-stressed osteocytes.

reduces NO production by local osteocytes, thereby causing their apoptosis (Fig. 3). Osteocyte apoptosis attracts osteoclasts, leading to further excavation of bone in the direction of loading. At the transition between the cutting cone and reversal zone, enhanced canalicular flow stimulates osteocytes to release NO, which induces osteoclast retraction and detachment from the bone surface. Together this leads to a treadmill of attaching and detaching osteoclasts in the tip and the periphery of the cutting cone respectively and the digging of a tunnel or trench in the direction of loading (Fig. 4).

The question remains how the different strains around the cutting and closing cone are sensed by osteoclasts and osteoblasts. We have described mechanosensing in bone as primarily a task for the osteocytes, the mature, long-lived, terminal differentiation stage of the osteoblasts that lie buried in the mineralized bone matrix.[8]

Mechanotransduction then includes the translation by osteocytes of canalicular flow into cell signals that recruit osteoclasts and osteoblasts. Therefore, if local strain differences around the cutting and closing cone of a BMU regulate the activity of osteoclasts and osteoblasts, then these strain gradients must produce local canalicular flow differences that are related to the recruitment of these two cell types. We have related volumetric strain in the bone around a BMU cutting cone to canalicular fluid flow.[10,11] Using this data, we have proposed a mechanism that explains the behavior of the team of osteoclasts in the cutting cone.[9] This mechanism is based on the effect of different flow patterns on the osteocytes. In cell culture experiments, it has been shown that osteocytes produce high levels of NO in response to fluid shear stress.[22,36,40] Interestingly, endothelial cell nitric oxide synthase (eNOS) is the NO-producing enzyme isoform specifically involved in the cellular response to fluid shear stress that occurs in the endothelium of blood vessels in response to blood flow.[41] The findings that osteocytes also express eNOS and that the bone cell enzyme is also activated by fluid shear stress suggest that there may be common functions for eNOS in the endothelium and osteocytes. NO production in response to adequate shear stress protects the endothelial cells against apoptosis.[42] We have proposed that such a mechanism also operates in bone and that osteocytes are also protected against apoptosis by a basal amount of NO production under normal canalicular shear stress. At the tip of the cutting cone of a BMU, therefore, osteocytes enter apoptosis as a result of insufficient NO production that is due to insufficient fluid flow in the canaliculi[9] (Fig. 4).

In the endothelium, apoptosis of endothelial cells attracts monocyte/macrophages that phagocytose the dying cells.[43] In bone, the apoptotic osteocytes at the tip of the cutting cone attract osteoclasts that resorb the bone matrix, as well as phagocytose the dying osteocyte. Evidence that osteoclastic attack is directed towards apoptotic osteocytes has been reported in the growing skeleton,[44] in relation to bone renewal,[45] and under pathologic conditions.[46] Similar to macrophages, osteoclasts are attracted to apoptotic cells that expose phosphatidylserine on their outer cell surface at an early stage of apoptosis.[47] In osteoclasts, the apoptotic cells that attract them are osteocytes and hypertrophic chondrocytes of the growth plate.[47] Exposure of phosphatidylserine on osteocytic cell "fingers" in canaliculi abutting the wall of the cutting cone therefore may be the signal that urges the osteoclasts to continue resorption in that direction.

The mechanism discussed above explains why osteoclasts move in the direction of loading, which is the first key issue that must be solved for a cellular explanation of Wolff's law. A second question is why osteoclasts stop resorbing at the base of the cutting cone. Here too, NO production in response to canalicular flow may play an important role. At the base of the cutting cone and further down the reversal zone, osteocytes receive enhanced fluid shear stress during loading. NO production therefore will be even higher than normal. In particular, the superficial osteocytes will produce much NO because shear stress is highest close to the surface. The high NO level prevents further osteocyte apoptosis but also may have another effect—that of promoting the retraction and detachment of osteoclasts from the bone surface. In cell culture experiments, NO rapidly reduced the osteoclast spread area, followed by retraction of the cells from the tissue culture support.[48] A similar response may be expected at the base of the cutting cone, where osteocytes produce high levels of NO. NO has a short half-life of only a few minutes and therefore must always act locally when functioning as a paracrine cell modulator. This characteristic perfectly suits a role as a very local inhibitor of further osteoclastic attack.

These two mechanisms—attraction of osteoclasts to the cutting cone tip and induction of osteoclast detachment from the cutting cone base—together explain the mechanically meaningful behavior of osteoclasts during remodeling.

## Summary

Adult human bone contains approximately 10 times as many osteocytes as osteoblasts, and the number of osteoclasts is only a fraction of the number of osteoblasts. Although the osteocyte is the most abundant bone cell type, our current knowledge of the role of osteocytes in bone metabolism is far behind our insight into the properties and functions of osteoblasts and osteoclasts. The striking structural design of bone, however, predicts an important role for osteocytes in the determination of bone structure. Over the last several years, the role of osteocytes as the professional mechanosensory cells of bone has become clear, as has the role of the lacunocanalicular porosity as the structure that mediates mechanosensing. Strain-derived flow of interstitial fluid through this porosity appears to mechanically activate the osteocytes as well as ensure transport of cell signaling molecules, nutrients, and waste products. This concept allows explanation of local bone gain and loss, as well as remodeling in response to fatigue damage, as processes supervised by mechanosensitive osteocytes. Alignment during remodeling appears to occur as a result of the osteocyte's sensing different canalicular flow patterns around the cutting cone and reversal zone during loading, thus determining the bone's structure.

## Conclusions

Important progress has been made over the last few years regarding the understanding of the role of osteocytes in bone metabolism and turn-over. Theoretical as well as experimental in vivo and in vitro studies[4-7,10,11,17,22,26,35,37,49,50] agree that the network of osteocytes, perhaps in conjunction with the bone lining cells, provides the cellular structure that allows bone organs to determine local needs for bone augmentation or reduction in response to mechanical demands.

## References

1. Kamioka H, Honjo T, Takano-Yamamoto T: A three-dimensional distribution of osteocyte processes revealed by the combination of confocal laser scanning microscopy and differential interference contrast microscopy. *Bone* 2001;28:145-149.

2. Van der Plas A, Nijweide PJ: Isolation and purification of osteocytes. *J Bone Miner Res* 1992;7:389-396.

3. Doty SB: Morphological evidence of gap junctions between bone cells. *Calcif Tissue Int* 1981;33:509-512.

4. Cowin SC, Moss-Salentijn L, Moss ML: Candidates for the mechanosensory system in bone. *J Biomed Eng* 1991;113:191-197.

5. Mullender MG, Huiskes R: Proposal for the regulatory mechanism of Wolff's law. *J Orthop Res* 1995;13:503-512.

6. Weinbaum S, Cowin SC, Zeng Y: A model for the excitation of osteocytes by mechanical loading-induced bone fluid shear stresses. *J Biomech* 1994;27:339-360.

7. Klein-Nulend J, Van der Plas A, Semeins CM, et al: Sensitivity of osteocytes to biomechanical stress in vitro. *FASEB J* 1995;9:441-445.

8. Burger EH, Klein-Nulend J: Mechanotransduction in bone: Role of the lacuno-canalicular network. *FASEB J* 1999;13:S101-S112.

9. Burger EH, Klein-Nulend J, Smit TH: Strain-derived canalicular fluid flow regulates osteoclast activity in a remodeling osteon: A proposal. *J Biomech* 2003;36:1453-1459.

10. Smit TH, Burger EH: Is BMU coupling a strain-regulated phenomenon? A finite element analysis. *J Bone Miner Res* 2000;15:301-307.

11. Smit TH, Burger EH, Huyghe JM: A case for strain-induced fluid flow as a regulator of BMU-coupling and osteonal alignment. *J Bone Miner Res* 2002;17:2021-2029.

12. Nijweide PJ, Mulder RJP: Identification of osteocytes in osteoblast-like cultures using a monoclonal antibody specifically directed against osteocytes. *Histochemistry* 1986; 84:343-350.

13. Van der Plas A, Aarden EM, Feyen JHM, et al: Characteristics and properties of osteocytes in culture. *J Bone Miner Res* 1994;9:1697-1704.

14. Tanaka-Kamioka K, Kamioka H, Ris H, Lim SS: Osteocyte shape is dependent on actin filaments and osteocyte processes are unique actin-rich projections. *J Bone Miner Res* 1998;13:1555-1568.

15. Aarden EM, Wassenaar AM, Alblas MJ, Nijweide PJ: Immunocytochemical demonstration of extracellular matrix proteins in isolated osteocytes. *Histochem Cell Biol* 1996;106:495-501.

16. Westbroek I, De Rooij KE, Nijweide PJ: Osteocyte-specific monoclonal antibody MAb OB7.3 is directed against Phex protein. *J Bone Miner Res* 2002;17:845-853.

17. Skerry TM, Bitensky L, Chayen J, Lanyon LE: Early strain-related changes in enzyme activity in osteocytes following bone loading in vivo. *J Bone Miner Res* 1989;4:783-788.

18. El-Haj AJ, Minter SL, Rawlinson SCF, Suswillo R, Lanyon LE: Cellular responses to mechanical loading in vitro. *J Bone Miner Res* 1990;5:923-932.

19. Lean JM, Jagger CJ, Chambers TJ, Chow JW: Increased insulin-like growth factor I mRNA expression in rat osteocytes in response to mechanical stimulation. *Am J Physiol* 1995;268:E318-E327.

20. Westbroek I, Ajubi NE, Alblas MJ, et al: Differential stimulation of Prostaglandin G/H Synthase-2 in osteocytes and other osteogenic cells by pulsating fluid flow. *Biochem Biophys Res Commun* 2000;268:414-419.

21. Westbroek I, Van der Plas A, de Rooij K, Klein-Nulend J, Nijweide PJ: Expression of serotonin receptors in bone. *J Biol Chem* 2001;276:28961-28968.

22. Klein-Nulend J, Semeins CM, Ajubi NE, Nijweide PJ, Burger EH: Pulsating fluid flow increases nitric oxide (NO) synthesis by osteocytes but not periosteal fibroblasts-correlation with prostaglandin upregulation. *Biochem Biophys Res Commun* 1995;217: 640-648.

23. Piekarski K, Munro M: Transport mechanism operating between blood supply and osteocytes in long bones. *Nature* 1977;269:80-82.

24. Dillaman RM: Movement of ferritin in the 2-day-old chick femur. *Anat Rec* 1984; 209:445-453.
25. Kufahl RH, Saha S: A theoretical model for stress-generated flow in the canaliculi-lacunae network in bone tissue. *J Biomech* 1990;23:171-180.
26. Cowin SC, Weinbaum S, Zeng Y: A case for bone canaliculi as the anatomical site of strain generated potentials. *J Biomech* 1995;28:1281-1296.
27. Wang N, Butler JP, Ingber DE: Mechanotransduction across the cell surface and through the cytoskeleton. *Science* 1993;260:1124-1127.
28. Watson PA: Function follows form: Generation of intracellular signals by cell deformation. *FASEB J* 1991;5:2013-2019.
29. Binderman I, Shimshoni Z, Somjen D: Biochemical pathways involved in the translation of physical stimulus into biological message. *Calcif Tissue Int* 1984;36:S82-S85.
30. Ajubi NE, Klein-Nulend J, Nijweide PJ, et al: Pulsating fluid flow increases prostaglandin production by cultured chicken osteocytes: A cytoskeleton-dependent process. *Biochem Biophys Res Commun* 1996;225:62-68.
31. Klein-Nulend J, Burger EH, Semeins CM, Raisz LG, Pilbeam CC: Pulsating fluid flow stimulates prostaglandin release and prostaglandin G/H synthase mRNA expression in primary mouse bone cells. *J Bone Miner Res* 1997;12:45-51.
32. Klein-Nulend J, Sterck JGH, Semeins CM, et al: Donor age and mechanosensitivity of human bone cells. *Osteoporosis Int* 2002;13:137-146.
33. Rawlinson SC, El-Haj AJ, Minter SL, et al: Loading-related increases in prostaglandin production in cores of adult canine cancellous bone in vitro: A role for prostacyclin in adaptive bone remodeling? *J Bone Miner Res* 1991;6:1345-1351.
34. Thompson DD, Rodan GA: Indomethacin inhibition of tenotomy-induced bone resorption. *J Bone Miner Res* 1988;3:409-414.
35. Klein-Nulend J, Helfrich MH, Sterck JGH, et al: Nitric oxide response to shear stress by human bone cell cultures is endothelial nitric oxide synthase dependent. *Biochem Biophys Res Commun* 1998;250:108-114.
36. Pitsillides AA, Rawlinson SCF, Suswillo RFL, et al: Mechanical strain-induced NO production by bone cells: A possible role in adaptive bone (re)modeling. *FASEB J* 1995;9:1614-1622.
37. Sterck JGH, Klein-Nulend J, Lips P, Burger EH: Response of normal and osteoporotic human bone cells to mechanical stress in vitro. *Am J Physiol* 1998;274:E1113-E1120.
38. Rubin CT, Lanyon LE: Regulation of bone formation by applied dynamic loads. *J Bone Joint Surg Am* 1984;66:397-410.
39. Turner CH, Owan I, Takano Y, Madalli S, Murrell GAC: Nitric oxide plays a role in bone mechanotransduction. *J Bone Miner Res* 1995;10:S235.
40. Zaman G, Pitsillides AA, Rawlinson SC, et al: Mechanical strain stimulates Nitric oxide production by rapid activation of endothelial nitric oxide synthase in osteocytes. *J Bone Miner Res* 1999;14:1123-1131.
41. Busse R, Fleming I: Pulsatile stretch and shear stress: Physical stimuli determining the production of endothelium derived relaxing factors. *J Vasc Res* 1998;35:73-84.
42. Rossig L, Haendeler J, Hermann C, et al: Nitric oxide down-regulates MKP-3 mRNA levels: Involvement in endothelial cell protection from apoptosis. *J Biol Chem* 2000;275:2552-2557.

43. Dimmeler S, Zeiher AM: Nitric oxide and apoptosis: Another paradigm for the double-edged role of nitric oxide. *Nitric Oxide* 1997;1:275-281.

44. Bronckers AL, Goei SW, Luo G, et al.: DNA fragmentation during bone formation in neonatal rodents assessed by transferase-mediated end labeling. *J Bone Miner Res* 1996;11:1281-1291.

45. Verborgt O, Gibson GJ, Schaffler MB: Loss of osteocyte integrity in association with microdamage and bone remodeling after fatigue in vivo. *J Bone Miner Res* 2000; 15:60-67.

46. Noble BS, Stevens H, Loveridge N, Reeve J: Identification of apoptotic changes in osteocytes in normal and pathological human bone. *Bone* 1997;20:273-282.

47. Bronckers AL, Goei W, Van Heerde WL, et al: Phagocytosis of dying chondrocytes by osteoclasts in the mouse growth plate as demonstrated by annexin-V labeling. *Cell Tissue Res* 2000;301:267-272.

48. MacIntyre I, Zaidi M, Alam ASMT, et al: Osteoclast inhibition: An action of nitric oxide not mediated by cyclic GMP. *Proc Natl Acad Sci USA* 1991;88:2936-2940.

49. Huiskes R, Ruimerman R, van Lenthe GH, Janssen JD: Effects of mechanical forces on maintenance and adaptation from in trabecular bone. *Nature* 2000;405:704-706.

50. Bakker AD, Soejima K, Klein-Nulend J, Burger EH: The production of nitric oxide and prostaglandin E2 by primary mouse bone cells is shear stress dependent. *J Biomech* 2001;34:671-677.

# Chapter 11
# Mechanical Signals Repress Osteoclast Formation In Vitro

*Janet Rubin, MD*
*Xian Fan, MD*

## Introduction

Biophysical input generated during normal physiologic loading is a major determinant of bone mass and morphology. Imposing load increases bone strength and size, as in the dominant radius of tennis players.[1] In states in which skeletal loading is decreased, such as prolonged bed rest or in paraplegics, bone resorption is initiated. During microgravity, astronauts lose bone mineral in the lower skeleton at a rate more than tenfold what a postmenopausal woman experiences. These examples show that the skeleton reads its mechanical environment, interpreting the decreased loading as a need for less structure and concluding with an integrated decision to decrease bone mass. Unloading has been studied in the more controlled environment of the laboratory. In perhaps the best-studied model, the mechanically isolated turkey ulnae (whose cortical morphology is similar to that of human cortical bone) retains neurologic and muscle attachments but is isolated from mechanical loads. Significant endosteal and intracortical resorption can be visualized and measured in the unloaded ulnar bones within weeks.[2] Also, raising the hind limbs of rodents so that the animal bears weight only on the front limbs results in bone loss in the unweighted hind limbs. In all these cases, the bone resorption that results from the unloading condition requires the local recruitment and activity of bone osteoclasts. Thus, it is clear that physiologic loading represses either the recruitment of osteoclasts from the hematopoietic precursor pool or represses the activity of osteoclasts that are already present.

Substantial literature exists regarding the mechanical factors that are stimulated by loading the skeleton. External mechanical loading leads to a multiplicity of events at the level of the cell, including strain as the cell adjusts itself to the substrate surface, surface shear as interstitial fluid passes through canaliculae, transient pressure waves, and dynamic electric fields.[3] It is not possible to separate one of these factors from another in vivo; for instance, loading a long bone causes bending and thus strain of the hard tissue, the cells fixed to the tissue, and their extended processes throughout the canalicular network. The bending leads to increased pressure within the intramedullary space, with fluid flow in advance of the pressure wave and continuing throughout the bone. Fluid flow is associated with shear as well as the generation of streaming potentials as the interstitial fluid moves past charged bone crystals. Fluid flow also causes cell deformation, or strain, at cell surfaces. Scientists have tried to separate these multiple mechanical factors to identify whether one or another has specific effects on bone cells. Bone cells have been shown to respond to strain,[4] electric fields,[5] shear stress,[6] and intramedullary pressure waves,[7] to cite only a few of the many publications dealing with bone cell responses to mechanical factors.

The goal of our laboratory has been to identify mechanical factors that repress osteoclast formation or activity and to understand the mechanisms whereby physical factors are transformed into chemical signals that regulate cell function. Our approach is to recreate aspects of the mechanical environment, applying them to osteoclast-generating systems in vitro.

## Osteoclast Formation

We began our studies with the gold standard for generating osteoclasts in the laboratory, the murine bone marrow culture system, which has led to much insight into osteoclast differentiation. Murine marrow contains two of the necessary elements for osteoclast formation: the osteoclast progenitor cell and the bone stromal progenitor cell. The osteoclast derives from the hematopoietic stem cell, which progresses into the myeloid lineage and then into the macrophage lineage. The colony-forming unit for macrophages (CFU-M) has the capability to become an osteoclast if exposed to bone elements. The bone stromal cell supplies the bone element but must first be stimulated to produce a pro-osteoclastic, or resorptive, environment—thus a third element is required in osteoclast-generating systems, which is a stimulatory factor that makes the interaction between the stromal and stem cells one that is pro-osteoclastic. The pro-osteoclastic environment can be induced by many osteoactive factors, including the active metabolite of vitamin D (1,25 dihydroxyvitamin D3), parathyroid hormone, or certain interleukins.

Our initial experiments investigated the effect of dynamic electric fields on the regulation of osteoclast formation. Both pulsed electromagnetic fields and more defined low-frequency, low-intensity electric fields have been shown to inhibit bone resorption in the isolated turkey ulna model.[8] A coil system was designed to induce a uniform electric field of 60 Hz, and 10 µV could be applied to murine marrow culture. A sham coil, which delivered the same heating and environmental effects, was used to create the control condition. Osteoclast formation was stimulated in marrow cultures by adding 1,25 dihydroxyvitamin D3, and after 7 days, osteoclast numbers were assayed by counting osteoclast-like cells (multinuclear tartrate-resistant acid phosphatase-positive cells). We found a statistically significant effect of the applied electric field to reduce osteoclast numbers at culture end by nearly 25%.[9] The difficulties of applying uniform electric fields to these cultures, as well as the complicating effects of heating in the culture media, however, suggested that we needed to develop a new method of applying mechanical factors in vitro.

The next iteration of our work involved applying constant hydrostatic pressure at levels up to two atmospheres to osteoclast-generating cultures. In this work we found a greater and reliable effect: hydrostatic pressure decreased osteoclast formation by 30%.[10] The consistency of the hydrostatic effect allowed us to begin to pinpoint mechanisms. An important finding in this series of experiments was that the mechanical factor needed to be applied during the early part of culture and was ineffective if applied only during late culture. This confirmed that the mechanical factor affected events involved in early entry of CFU-M into the osteoclast pathway. In contrast, later differentiation events, such as fusion of mononuclear osteoclasts into the mature osteoclast polykaryons, did not appear to be targeted by either electric fields or hydrostatic pressure.

The availability of reliable instrumentation to deliver deformation, or strain, to monolayer cells by stretching the substrate to which cells attached at integrin fixation points was an important step for our laboratory. Straining cells maximally 1.8% (or 18,000 µε) at 10 cycles per minute robustly inhibited osteoclastogenesis by 40% when applied during early culture.[4] In this first generation Flexcell device, the marrow cells adhered to a collagen-coated thick elastic platen and a vacuum applied to the bottom of the dish stretched the elastic membrane above it. To complicate matters, deformation of the platen membrane was nonuniform, with highest strains achieved in the circumference of the plate, decreasing towards the central bullseye where the mechanical effect was to compress this area.[11] We used the nonuniformity of the applied deformation to some advantage by dividing the well into three parts as we counted osteoclasts—the outer ring with highest strain magnitude, the middle ring with lower strain, and the central bull's-eye with compression equivalent to the outer ring. In this way we showed that osteoclast formation was sensitive to the local strain, ie, the higher the strain, the higher the inhibitory effect.[4] Also, conditioned media from the strained plate transferred to unstrained plates was unable to reproduce the inhibitory effect of strains. Taken together with the "localized" strain magnitude effect, it became increasingly clear that mechanical inhibition of osteoclastogenesis involved a target that was fixed in location on the plate and transmitted the inhibitory signal to adjacent cells. In the late 1990s, RANKL (receptor activator of NFκB ligand) was identified as the critical element that caused CFU-M to differentiate along the osteoclast pathway. RANKL is a transmembrane molecule expressed by bone stromal cells, and resorptive hormones/cytokines such as vitamin D increase RANKL expression. The initial descriptions of RANKL showed that adding a soluble form of RANKL to cultures of hematopoetic osteoclast precursors could obviate the requirement for bone stromal cells and resorptive factors.[12] As we shall see, RANKL expression is a primary means whereby mechanical input can modulate the numbers of progenitors entering the osteoclast differentiation pathway.

Using a new instrument that allowed application of uniform equibiaxial strain across a thinner silastic membrane, we showed that strains under 2% magnitude decreased the expression of RANKL in mixed marrow culture.[13] Replacing soluble RANKL in cultures where strain was applied returned osteoclast numbers to levels equivalent with unstrained controls. Although osteoclast precursors respond to RANKL activation of their RANK receptors (which induces entry into osteoclast lineage), the precursors themselves do not express RANKL. Hence, as expected, when osteoclast precursors and other nonadherent cells retaining only the stromal elements of marrow were excluded from culture, application of the resorptive 1,25 dihydroxyvitamin D was able to increase RANKL expression in the culture equivalent to those cultures where osteoclast progenitors were present. Mechanically straining cultures of purified stromal cells caused an inhibition of RANKL by at least 40% as assessed by both Northern analysis and real-time PCR. This inhibition occurred rapidly within the first 24 hours after initiation of the strain. Concurrently, we measured the expression of another factor essential for osteoclast formation, macrophage colony stimulating factor (MCSF), which is both secreted and displayed on bone stromal cell membranes. Strain application caused no change in the expression of MCSF mRNA. Thus, at this point we had identified the following targets for the inhibitory effect of strain on osteoclast formation: the target cell was the RANKL-expressing bone stromal cell, and the target molecule was RANKL.

## Mechanotransduction

We then wanted to understand what intracellular pathways were stimulated by mechanical strain in the bone stromal cell, in particular those that specifically affected the ability of that cell to express RANKL. Cells involved in the vascular endothelium—both endothelial cells and smooth muscle cells—exist in a highly mechanically active environment. This environment includes shear, deformation, and pressure changes at magnitudes considerably higher than those thought to be present in bone, and it is perhaps this magnitude that allowed vascular scientists to explore mechanical signal transduction in the 1990s. Fluid shear of endothelial cells causes activation of three members of the MAP kinase family: N-terminal c-jun kinase (JNK),[14] extracellular signal-regulated kinases 1 and 2 (ERK 1/2), and Big MAP kinase.[15] Applying substrate strain to attached cells also activates members of the MAPK superfamily. In vascular smooth muscle cells, strain rapidly activates both ERK 1/2 and JNK.[16] These studies and many others on vascular cells have suggested that similar signals might be activated by shear, deformation, and pressure in bone cells. Because the cellular components in bone respond to shear and strain,[13,17] we considered that MAPK activation might be involved in transducing mechanical force in the skeleton.

We wanted to assess a possible causal relationship between MAPK activation and downregulation of RANKL expression. First, substrate strain (0.25% to 2%) indeed induced ERK 1/2 activation in adherent bone stromal cells.[18] Straining stromal cells also stimulated the activation of JNK and probably many other signals that we did not measure. However, a connection between strain-induced activation of ERK 1/2 and strain inhibition of RANKL expression was uncovered with the use of the ERK 1/2 inhibitor PD98059. Treatment of cells with ERK 1/2 inhibitor during the strain period abrogated the reduction in RANKL mRNA. Use of a JNK inhibitor, on the other hand, did not prevent RANKL downregulation during strain.[19] To further confirm the relationship of ERK 1/2 to mechanical strain inhibition of RANKL, we prepared an adenovirus encoding a constitutively activated MEK that specifically activates ERK 1/2. Infection of stromal cell cultures with this virus not only activated ERK 1/2 but also caused a significant decrease in RANKL expression.

Application of both shear and deformation (strain) had been shown to increase nitric oxide (NO) production by osteoblasts and osteocytes.[17,20] NO's effects on bone are complex, but many studies show that it decreases bone loss in animals. Loading rat vertebrae and ulnae caused immediate increases in NO release.[21] Collin-Osdoby and associates[22] have shown that reducing NO levels increases osteoclast recruitment and bone resorption. We have confirmed this work and have further shown that NO reduces RANKL expression by bone stromal cells, which suggests an alternate pathway (to ERK 1/2) by which RANKL can be regulated. Because of this finding, we were interested in the effects of strain on NO production in bone stromal cells.

We found that straining primary bone stromal cells causes a late increase in nitric oxide production associated with an increase in expression of endothelial nitric oxide synthase (eNOS).[19] This response also requires the activation of ERK 1/2, as pharmacologic inhibition of this kinase during substrate strain will prevent strain-induced increases in eNOS expression. Importantly, nitric oxide generation is not necessary either for the strain activation of ERK 1/2 or for ERK 1/2's inhibitory effect on RANKL expression. Thus, the effect of increasing eNOS expression and NO generating capacity is a secondary effect of strain activation of the ERK 1/2 kinase, interestingly in an entirely divergent direction from the ERK 1/2 effect on RANKL. The effects of strain-induced ERK 1/2 on RANKL and eNOS are strain-magnitude dependent, diverging from each other in a reciprocal manner. The anti-osteoclastogenic effect of increased NO through strain-induced eNOS should then be additive to the direct inhibitory effect of strain on RANKL expression.

## Discussion

Scientists working in vitro must always take into consideration what might be physiologic levels of the factors they sprinkle into their culture dishes. In the case of mechanical factors, achieving physiologic environments is almost impossible. Culture plates lack many of the dimensions that are present in bone as well as the architectural and physiochemical aspects of marrow, trabecular, or cortical environments. Thus one can only hope to model the strain environment. What kinds of strain does a bone cell experience? The hard tissue of long bones is within the range of a fracture threshold at 4,000 με and certainly can respond to lower levels of strain with restraint of resorption (see Chapter 5). The strain, or deformation, across any portion of a cell attached to the hard surface of bone is harder to judge. Theoreticians have judged bone cells to be exposed to strains between 100 and 50,000 με (eg, the long processes of osteocytes). By contrast, we have strained murine stromal cells at low-magnitude level, at least compared to the types of strain applied in vivo to vascular tissues. Indeed, while 0.25% strain activates ERK 1/2 kinase maximally in bone stromal cells, endothelial cells do not even start to respond until nearly 5% strain and continue to increase activation to

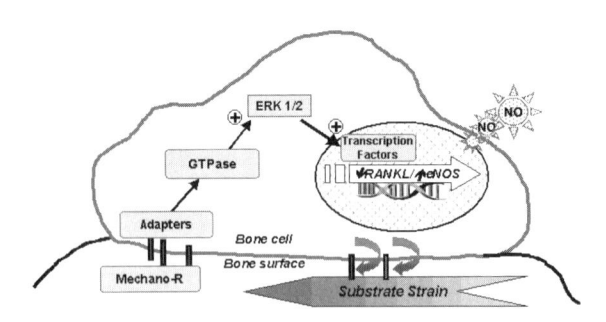

**Figure 1** Substrate strain controls the expression of at least two osteoactive genes through the activation of MAPK signaling.

levels of 20% strain. Both RANKL and eNOS are sensitive to very low levels of strain and respond in a strain magnitude dose-dependent fashion.[19]

What have we learned regarding physical loading and control of the bone remodeling cycle? By using in vitro models we have shown that at least three types of physically generated factors—electric fields, pressure, and strain—decrease osteoclast formation when applied at levels achievable in the skeleton. Because osteoclasts are the cell responsible for starting the activation cycle, this finding suggests that loading the skeleton can prevent bone turnover. Furthermore, strain limits osteoclast formation by decreasing the local expression of RANKL. Finally, strain inhibition of RANKL requires activation of a specific MAPK, ERK 1/2. Interestingly, strain activation of ERK 1/2 also induces the expression of endothelial nitric oxide synthase, suggesting many pathways by which strain might have an anabolic effect on bone cells through NO generation.

In summary, in vitro studies attempting to reproduce and understand the mechanical environment that is necessary for the healthy, well-adapted skeleton can inform us about target cells, molecules, and signal transduction pathways. Our work has shown that mechanical input can tightly regulate two molecules, RANKL and eNOS, in entirely divergent fashions through the same signal transduction pathway with critical effects on bone remodeling (Fig. 1). The promise of this research is that it may one day allow understanding of the as-yet-undiscovered mechanotransducer(s) turning mechanical into chemical signals as well as enable regulation of the genes that are associated with the complex response of the skeleton to its loading environment.

## Acknowledgments
Both the NIH and the VA supported this work.

# References

1. Haapasalo H, Kontulainen S, Sievanen H, Kannus P, Jarvinen M, Vuori I: Exercise-induced bone gain is due to enlargement in bone size without a change in volumetric bone density: A peripheral quantitative computed tomography study of the upper arms of male tennis players. *Bone* 2000;27:351-357.

2. Rubin C, Lanyon L: Regulation of bone formation by applied dynamic loads. *J Bone Joint Surg Am* 1984;66:397-402.

3. Rubin J, Rubin CT, McLeod KJ: Biophysical modulation of cell and tissue structure and function. *Crit Rev Eukaryot Gene Expr* 1995;5:177-191.

4. Rubin J, Fan X, Biskobing D, Taylor W, Rubin C: Osteoclastogenesis is repressed by mechanical strain in an *in vitro* model. *J Orthop Res* 1999;17:639-645.

5. Spadaro JA: Mechanical and electrical interactions in bone remodeling. *Bioelectromagnetics* 1997;18:193-202.

6. Smalt R, Mitchell FT, Howard RL, Chambers TJ: Mechanotransduction in bone cells: Induction of nitric oxide and prostaglandin synthesis by fluid shear stress, but not by mechanical strain. *Adv Exp Med Biol* 1997;433:311-314.

7. Qin YX, Lin W, Rubin C: The pathway of bone fluid flow as defined by in vivo intramedullary pressure and streaming potential measurements. *Ann Biomed Eng* 2002;30:693-702.

8. Rubin CT, Donahue HJ, Rubin JE, McLeod KJ: Optimization of electric field parameters for the control of bone remodeling: Exploitation of an indigenous mechanism for the prevention of osteopenia. *J Bone Miner Res* 1993;8:S573-S581.

9. Rubin J, McLeod KJ, Titus L, Nanes MS, Catherwood BD, Rubin CT: Formation of osteoclast-like cells is suppressed by low frequency, low intensity electric fields. *J Orthop Res* 1996;14:7-15.

10. Rubin J, Biskobing D, Fan X, Rubin C, McLeod K, Taylor WR: Pressure regulates osteoclast formation and MCSF expression in marrow culture. *J Cell Physiol* 1997; 170:81-87.

11. Gilbert JA, Weinhold PS, Banes AJ, Link GW, Jones GL: Strain profiles for circular cell culture plates containing flexible surfaces employed to mechanically deform cells in vitro. *J Biomech* 1994;27:1169-1177.

12. Yasuda H, Shima N, Nakagawa N, et al: Osteoclast differentiation factor is a ligand for osteoprotegerin/osteoclastogenesis-inhibitory factor and is identical to TRANCE/RANKL. *Proc Natl Acad Sci USA* 1998;95:3597-3602.

13. Rubin J, Murphy T, Nanes MS, Fan X: Mechanical strain inhibits expression of osteoclast differentiation factor by murine stromal cells. *Am J Physiol Cell Physiol* 2000; 278:C1126-C1132.

14. Chen KD, Li YS, Kim M, et al: Mechanotransduction in response to shear stress: Roles of receptor tyrosine kinases, integrins, and Shc. *J Biol Chem* 1999;274: 18393-18400.

15. Yan C, Takahashi M, Okuda M, Lee JD, Berk BC: Fluid shear stress stimulates big mitogen-activated protein kinase 1 (BMK1) activity in endothelial cells: Dependence on tyrosine kinases and intracellular calcium. *J Biol Chem* 1999;274:143-150.

16. Li C, Hu Y, Mayr M, Xy Q: Cyclic strain stress-induced MAP kinase phosphatase 1 expression in vascular smooth muscle cells is regulated by Ras/Rac-MAPK pathways. *J Biol Chem* 1999;274:25273-25380.

17. Smalt R, Mitchell F, Howard R, Chambers T: Induction of NO and prostaglandin E2 in osteoblasts by wall-shear stress but not mechanical strain. *Am J Phys* 1997;273: E751-E758.
18. Rubin J, Murphy T, Fan X, Goldschmidt M, Taylor W: Mechanical strain inhibits RANKL expression through activation of ERK1/2 in bone marrow stromal cells. *J Bone Miner Res* 2002;17:1452-1460.
19. Rubin J, Murphy TC, Zhu L, Roy E, Nanes MS, Fan X: Mechanical strain differentially regulates endothelial nitric-oxide synthase and receptor activator of nuclear kappa B ligand expression via ERK1/2 MAPK. *J Biol Chem* 2003;278:34018-34025.
20. Klein-Nulend J, Helfrich MH, Sterck JG, et al: Nitric oxide response to shear stress by human bone cell cultures is endothelial nitric oxide synthase dependent. *Biochem Biophys Res Commun* 1998;250:108-114.
21. Pitsillides AA, Rawlinson SC, Suswillo RF, Bourrin S, Zaman G, Lanyon LE: Mechanical strain-induced NO production by bone cells: A possible role in adaptive bone (re)modeling? *FASEB J* 1995;9:1614-1622.
22. Collin-Osdoby P, Rothe L, Bekker S, Anderson F, Osdoby P: Decreased nitric oxide levels stimulate osteoclastogenesis and bone resorption both in vitro and in vivo on the chick chorioallantoic membrane in association with neoangiogenesis. *J Bone Miner Res* 2000;15:474-488.

Chapter 12

# Chemomechanical Coupling in Articular Cartilage: IL-1α and TGF-β$_1$ Regulate Chondrocyte Synthesis and Secretion of Proteoglycan 4

*Tannin A. Schmidt, MS*
*Barbara L. Schumacher, BS*
*Eun Hee Han, BS*
*Travis J. Klein, PhD*
*Michael S. Voegtline, PhD*
*Robert L. Sah, MD, ScD*

## Introduction

Articular cartilage is the low-friction, wear-resistant, load-bearing tissue at the ends of long bones in skeletal joints.[1] This tissue is composed of three zones: superficial, middle, and deep. Each zone has distinct properties, with a matrix composition and macromolecular organization that vary gradually with depth from the articular surface and confer specialized mechanical properties to these tissue regions.[2] In the superficial zone, the collagen network is arranged in a tangential orientation relative to the articular surface, imparting a relatively high tangential tensile stiffness and strength to this zone. Proteoglycan content is relatively low, conferring a relatively low compressive stiffness and allowing the opposing surfaces to distribute forces over a broad area and thereby reduce contact stress. In contrast, the collagen network in the middle and deep zones is predominantly arranged in oblique and radial orientations respectively, imparting a relatively low tangential tensile stiffness and strength. Proteoglycan content in the middle and deep zones is relatively high, conferring a relatively high compressive stiffness. Finally, attached to the articular surface of the superficial zone are molecules, including superficial zone protein (SZP),[3] that appear to provide cartilage with its exquisite low-friction properties.[4]

The depth-varying metabolic activity of chondrocytes in cartilage appears to a large extent to govern the depth-varying composition, structure, and function of cartilage, and these metabolic properties, along with chondrocyte shape, size, and organization, further define the zones of articular cartilage.[5] In the superficial zone, chondrocytes synthesize and secrete SZP, with this specialized metabolic function distinguishing these cells from chondrocytes of the middle and deep zones.[3] Chondrocytes in the superficial zone are discoid, relatively small, and arranged in horizontal clusters.[6] In the middle and deep zones, chondrocytes synthesize proteoglycan at relatively high rates. In the middle zone, the cells are spherical, somewhat larger, and arranged in obliquely oriented clusters. In the deep zone, chondrocytes are oblong, even larger, and arranged in vertical columns. Adult articular cartilage is relatively acellular[5] and transport of macromolecules within cartilage is relatively slow;[7] therefore, chondrocyte metabolism has a large influence over the pericellular and intraterritorial tissue regions near individual cells.

The proteoglycan 4 (PRG4) gene encodes for proteins that have been termed megakaryocyte-stimulating factor, SZP, lubricin, and PRG4.[8] Lubricin, a metabolic product of synovial fibroblasts, is abundant in synovial fluid and highly homologous to SZP.[9] PRG4 molecules appear to play a critical role in facilitating low-friction properties of a variety of tissue surfaces. In this chapter, we refer to these molecules with a common immunoreactivity as PRG4. A thin layer of PRG4 is present at the articular surface in normal healthy joints as a discrete covering over the articular surface, colocalizing with the lamina splendens.[3] The presence of PRG4 at the articular surface, the abundance of PRG4 in synovial fluid, and the mechanical motion of the joint and joint loading provide an efficient system for boundary lubrication and low-friction articulation. In addition, mutations of the PRG4 gene cause dysfunction of tissues in which it is normally expressed, including the pericardium and pleura as well as cartilage.[10] In the camptodactyly-arthropathy-coxa vara-pericarditis syndrome in humans, joints exhibit camptodactyly, noninflamatory arthropathy, and hypertrophic synovitis with coxa vara deformity; the heart is afflicted with pericarditis; and the lung demonstrates a pleural effusion. Thus, the lubrication system involving PRG4 present in synovial joints appears to be operative and functionally important in other regions that require the relative sliding of opposing tissue surfaces.

Chemical and mechanical factors are coupled in articular cartilage in a number of ways[11] (Fig. 1). Chondrocyte functions and cartilage matrix metabolism are regulated by imposed mechanical[12] and chemical stimuli, with the latter including growth factors and cytokines.[13] The mechanical and transport properties of cartilage determine how such mechanical and chemical stimuli present at the surfaces or boundaries of cartilage tissue are transduced into signals at the microenvironmental level. The cellular microenvironment regulates cell synthesis of various molecules—including matrix components and matrix-modifying enzymes—as well as cell fate, which may be to proliferate, apoptose, necrose, or differentiate. The extracellular microenvironment may directly affect the assembly and loss of extracellular matrix components. The resultant balance between synthesis, assembly, and loss of matrix components determines the tissue content of specific molecules. Accordingly, the accretion of the bulk of the tissue—including proteoglycan, collagen, and other matrix molecules—as well as of the surface of the tissue—including lubricating molecules—is regulated through a number of metabolic mechanisms. In turn, the quantity and structure of specific matrix molecules determine the mechanical and transport properties of cartilage. Thus, a key to understanding dynamic processes of cartilage, such

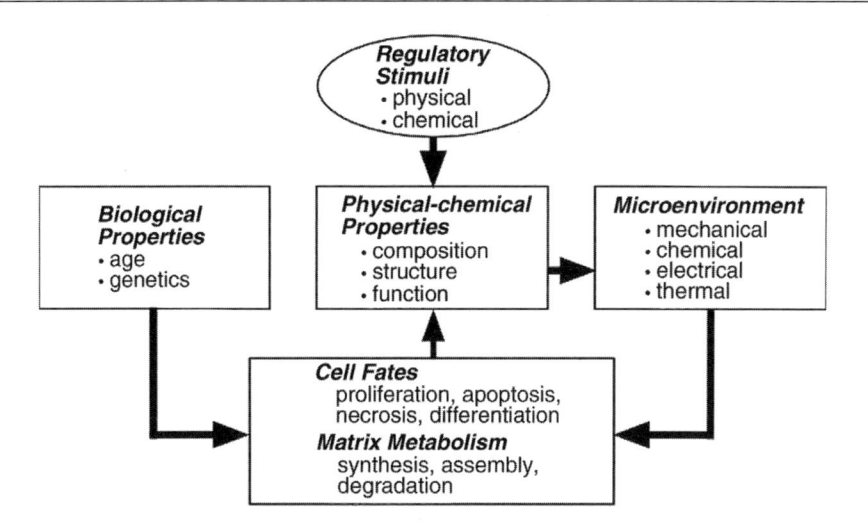

**Figure 1** Model of cartilage dynamics. Block diagram shows the influence of environmental regulatory stimuli and biologic properties on cartilage remodeling, which may lead to cartilage growth, degeneration, or repair.

as growth, maturation, homeostasis, and degeneration, is elucidating at various levels of detail the chemomechanical coupling processes that exist in and govern articular cartilage.

In joint injury and arthritis, transforming growth factor-beta 1 (TGF-$\beta_1$) and interleukin-1 alpha (IL-1$\alpha$) are present at relatively high levels[14] and may regulate chondrocyte synthesis of PRG4 as well as turnover of PRG4 adhered to the articular surface. Cytokines in general appear to play a major role in disease states of cartilage, where an imbalance of synthesis and degradation exists. Certain cytokines, such as IL-1, exhibit net catabolic effects on chondrocytes and cartilage by both inhibiting synthesis of extracellular matrix and stimulating degradation.[15] Certain growth factors, including TGF-$\beta$,[16] exhibit net anabolic effects on cartilage, stimulating synthesis of matrix and inhibiting degradation. Simulating pathologic conditions can be helpful in understanding the effects on specific functional molecules. Previous qualitative studies of PRG4 regulation by TGF-$\beta_1$[17,18] and IL-1$\alpha$[18] have examined chondrocytes from full-thickness cartilage in terms of mRNA expression in monolayer culture[17] and protein secretion in agarose culture from chondrocyte subpopulations.[18] These studies suggest that PRG4 expression in chondrocyte cultures is inhibited by IL-1$\alpha$ and stimulated by TGF-$\beta_1$. However, it is unclear if these factors also regulate PRG4 in the native cartilage environment. Explant cultures maintain a number of characteristic features of cartilage, including cell-matrix interactions and biosynthetic phenotype.[19]

The objective of the present study was to determine if TGF-$\beta_1$ and IL-1$\alpha$ regulate PRG4 metabolism in explant cultures of cartilage in terms of (1) synthesis and secretion by chondrocytes in their native superficial (S) and middle (M) zones, and (2) localization at the articular cartilage surface.

# Methods

## Cartilage Explant Harvest and Culture

Cartilage explants were isolated from regions of cartilage that either included or were devoid of the superficial zone, essentially as described previously.[20] Osteochondral cores were harvested from the patellofemoral groove of immature (1 to 3 weeks old) bovine knees. These cores were cut in a sledge microtome to obtain slices (0.3 mm thick) from the superficial (S, 0 to 0.3 mm) and middle (M, 0.6 to 0.9 mm) layers. These layers of cartilage were then punched into smaller 3-mm diameter disks. During harvest, cartilage was maintained hydrated by irrigation with phosphate-buffered saline supplemented with antibiotics and antimycotic (100 units/mL penicillin, 100 µg/mL streptomycin, and 0.25 µg/mL amphotericin B).

Cartilage disks were then incubated with or without serum, and with various levels of IL-1α or TGF-$β_1$ alone or in sequence. Disks were incubated in a basal medium (Dulbecco's modified Eagle's medium [DMEM], 10 mM HEPES buffer, 0.1 mM nonessential amino acids, 0.4 mM L-proline, 2 mM L-glutamine, 100 units/mL penicillin, 100 µg/mL streptomycin, and 0.25 µg/mL amphotericin B) at 37°C in an atmosphere of 5% $CO_2$, supplemented with 25 µg/mL ascorbic acid, 0.01% BSA (0% FBS), or 10% FBS, as well as graded levels (0, 0.1, 1, 10 ng/mL) of either recombinant human IL-1α or porcine TGF-$β_1$. Every 2 days, medium (0.360 mL per S disk and 0.175 mL per M disk) was replaced, and the spent medium collected for subsequent analysis. These amounts of medium were chosen to achieve a medium volume of 1 mL per million cells per day, with S disks given more medium due to their higher cell density.[20] Some disks were analyzed for the reversibility of effects of IL-1α by TGF-$β_1$ by first treating on days 0 to 6 with graded levels of IL-1a, rinsing on day 8 with basal medium over 48 hours, and then treating during days 8 to 12 with medium supplemented with 10 ng/mL of TGF-$β_1$.

## PRG4 Secretion

PRG4 expression from cartilage disks was quantified in spent medium by indirect ELISA as described previously,[21] using the monoclonal antibody (mAb) 3-A-4 (a gift from Bruce Caterson, PhD).[3] Briefly, medium samples were diluted serially, adsorbed, and then reacted with mAb 3-A-4, horseradish peroxidase-conjugated secondary antibody, and 2,2-azino-di(3-ethyl-benzthiozoline-sulfonate-[6]) substrate, with three washes with PBS + 0.1% between each step. PRG4 levels were calculated using purified bovine standards.[3]

## PRG4 Immunolocalization

The presence of PRG4 at the articular surface and within chondrocytes was determined qualitatively in freshly explanted disks and also in cultured disks that were terminated at day 6. To visualize PRG4 as a function of depth from the articular surface, samples were analyzed by immunohistochemistry using the monoclonal antibody (mAb) 3-A-4, essentially as described previously.[21] Here, samples were incubated overnight in medium supplemented

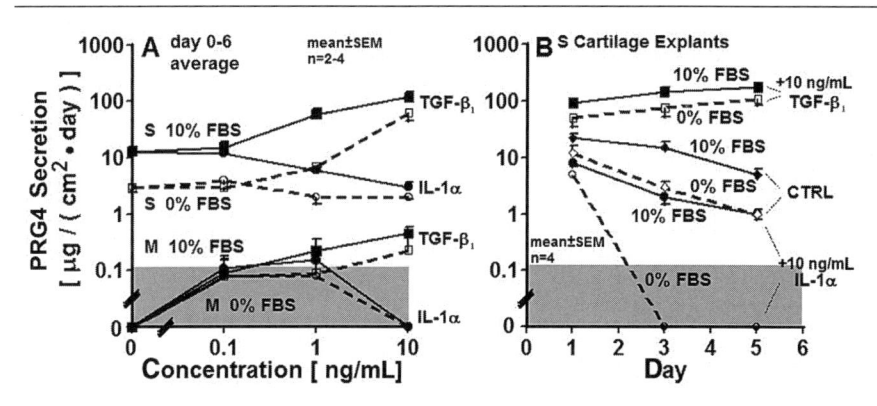

**Figure 2** PRG4 secretion by chondrocytes in cartilage explant cultures. Articular cartilage disks (0.3 mm thick, 3 mm diameter) from the superficial (S, 0 to 0.3 mm), and middle (M, 0.6 to 0.9 mm) zones of the patellofemoral groove of immature (1 to 3 weeks old) bovine knees were incubated as explants for 6 days at 37°C in an atmosphere of 5% $CO_2$ with medium (DMEM +25 µg/mL ascorbic acid) with 0.01% BSA (0% FBS) or 10% FBS as well as graded levels (0, 0.1, 1, 10 ng/mL) of either recombinant human IL-1α or porcine TGF-$β_1$. Culture medium was changed every 2 days and collected for PRG4 analysis by indirect ELISA using the monoclonal antibody 3-A-4. **A**, Effect of recombinant human IL-1α and porcine TGF-$β_1$ concentration on the average rate of PRG4 secretion by explants during the culture. **B**, Effect of days in culture on the PRG4 secretion rate by S explants with 10 ng/mL of recombinant human IL-1α or porcine TGF-$β_1$. Shaded regions indicate levels at or below assay sensitivity.

with 0.1 µM monensin and then rinsed with PBS. Cryosections of a thickness of 5 µm were prepared, reacted with mAb 3-A-4, and detected with a peroxidase-based system. The stained samples were viewed to identify immunoreactive cells, indicating synthesis of PRG4, as well as to assess the presence of adherent PRG4 at the articular surface. Results were documented by photomicroscopy. To visualize PRG4 macroscopically at the sample surfaces, disks were rinsed in PBS, fixed with 4% paraformaldehyde, reacted with mAb 3-A-4, and detected with a peroxidase-based system essentially as described above. Results were documented by digital photography. As negative controls, some samples were probed with a nonspecific isotype-matched antibody.

## Statistical Analysis

Quantitative data are expressed as the mean ± SEM. Effects of cartilage layer, medium components, and culture duration on PRG4 secretion were assessed by repeated-measures ANOVA of the data after log transformation (to improve the uniformity of variance among the experimental groups).

## Results

### PRG4 Secretion

The average rate of secretion of PRG4 over the first 6 days of culture (Fig. 2, *A*) was much higher for S disks than M disks ($P < 0.01$), much higher in the presence of FBS ($P < 0.05$), and markedly affected by the presence of TGF-$\beta_1$ or IL-1$\alpha$ ($P < 0.05$) at different doses ($P < 0.001$). Several interaction effects were also apparent. The dose-dependent effect depended on the tissue layer, being marked for S disks but not M disks ($P < 0.01$). In addition, the dose-dependent effects were distinct for TGF-$\beta_1$ and IL-1$\alpha$, with the former causing a stimulation and the latter causing an inhibition ($P < 0.001$). Also, the effect of serum depended on the tissue layer, being marked for S disks but not M disks ($P < 0.05$). The PRG4 secretion rate by S disks cultured in medium with 10% FBS was $13 \pm 3$ µg/(cm$^2$/day) and was upregulated by TGF-$\beta_1$ and downregulated by IL-1$\alpha$ in a dose-dependent manner, reaching a high of $118 \pm 26$ µg/(cm$^2$/day) with 10 ng/mL TGF-$\beta_1$ and a low of $3 \pm 1$ µg/(cm$^2$/day) with 10 ng/mL IL-1$\alpha$. For S disks cultured in medium without FBS, the trends in regulation of PRG4 secretion were similar, although the rates were lower, being $3 \pm 1$ µg/(cm$^2$/day) in basal medium and $62 \pm 18$ and $2 \pm 1$ µg/(cm$^2$/day) with 10 ng/mL of TGF-$\beta_1$ and 10 ng/mL IL-1$\alpha$ respectively.

The time course of alteration of PRG4 secretion in S disks was fairly rapid (Fig. 2, B). The secretion rate varied with days in culture ($P < 0.01$) as well as the presence of serum ($P < 0.05$) and cytokine ($P < 0.001$) as noted overall for the 6-day period. PRG4 secretion rates were already clearly different within the first 2 days of treatment with TGF-$\beta_1$ or IL-1$\alpha$ and changed gradually in the subsequent days (2 to 4 and 4 to 6). There was a significant interaction between the effect of cytokine and days in culture ($P < 0.01$), as indicated by the secretion rates of cultures treated with the maximum dose of TGF-$\beta_1$ increasing with culture duration while decreasing in cultures treated with IL-1$\alpha$, and also decreasing (to a lesser extent) without any IL-1$\alpha$. For S disks cultured in medium without FBS, the trends in regulation of PRG4 secretion were similar, although the rates of secretion were lower. Secretion rates from M disks (Fig. 2, A) were only slightly above the threshold of detectability, 0.1 µg/(cm$^2$/day), even when cultured with 10 ng/mL TGF-$\beta_1$.

The inhibitory effect of IL-1$\alpha$ on S disks was partially reversible. After IL-1$\alpha$ treatment for the first 6 days of culture, the secretion rate from S disks during days 8 to 12 was $2.4 \pm 1.4$ µg/(cm$^2$/day) in basal medium with or without 10% FBS, $0.2 \pm 0.2$ µg/(cm$^2$/day) with 10 ng/mL IL-1$\alpha$, and back up to $12.9 \pm 4.4$ µg/(cm$^2$/day) with 10 ng/mL TGF-$\beta_1$.

## PRG4 Immunolocalization

PRG4 was localized differentially in cartilage samples depending on the culture conditions. In all samples, PRG4 staining was only evident for S disks in regions at or near the articular surface, and was absent from the deeper regions of S disks and also absent from M disks. The number of chondrocytes staining positive for PRG4 generally was consistent with the observed levels of PRG4 appearing in the medium (Fig. 2). Vertical sections of freshly isolated (Fig. 3, A) and cultured control samples (0 or 10% FBS, Fig. 3, Ciii, Civ) showed many PRG4 positive chondrocytes, as did samples treated with TGF-$\beta_1$ (Fig. 3, Cvii, Cviii). In contrast, samples treated with IL-1$\alpha$ showed relatively few PRG4 positive chondrocytes (Fig. 3, Cv, Cvi). PRG4

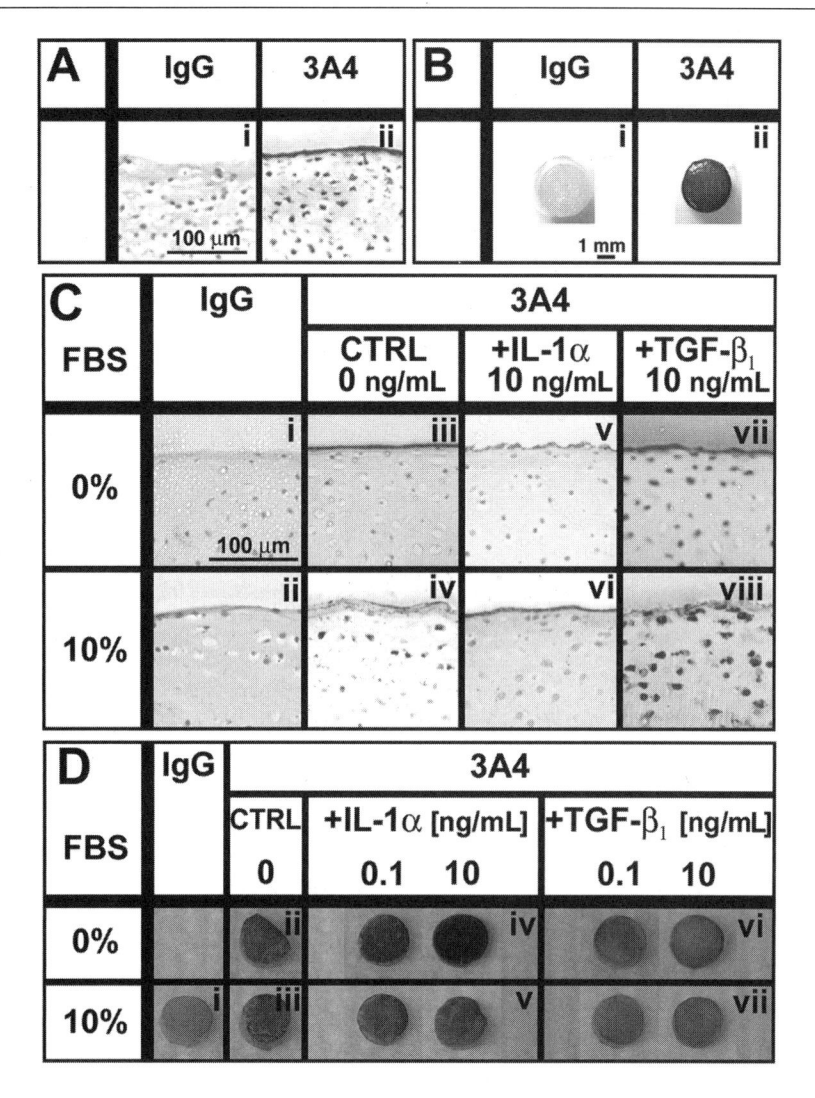

**Figure 3** PRG4 immunolocalization in fresh and cultured superficial (S, 0 to 0.3 mm) 3-mm cartilage explants with the monoclonal antibody 3-A-4 (a nonspecific IgG antibody was used as a negative control). **A,** Vertical cryosections of fresh S disks after overnight incubation in medium with 0.1 µM monensin to identify cells synthesizing PRG4. **B,** Macroscopic en face views of the articular surface of fresh S cartilage disks. **C,** Vertical cryosections of S disks cultured as explants for 6 days at 37°C in an atmosphere of 5% $CO_2$ with medium (DMEM +25 µg/mL ascorbic acid) with 0.01% BSA (0% FBS) or 10% FBS as well as 0 (iii, iv) or 10 ng/mL of either recombinant human IL-1α (v, vi) or porcine TGF-$β_1$ (vii, viii) after overnight incubation in medium with 0.1 µM monensin, to identify cells synthesizing PRG4. **D,** Macroscopic en face views of the articular surface of S disks cultured as explants for 6 days at 37°C in an atmosphere of 5% $CO_2$ with medium (DMEM +25 µg/mL ascorbic acid) with 0.01% BSA (0% FBS) or 10% FBS as well as graded levels (0 (ii, iii), 0.1, 10 ng/mL) of either recombinant human IL-1α (iv, v) or porcine TGF-$β_1$ (vi, vii).

was immunolocalized macroscopically at the articular surface of all the intact disks, both freshly isolated (Fig. 3, *B*) and cultured (Fig. 3, *D*). Vertical sections of freshly isolated (Fig. 3, *A*) and cultured control samples (0 or 10% FBS, Fig. 3, *Ciii, Civ*) showed a fairly regular staining for PRG4 at the articular surface, as did samples treated with IL-1α (Fig. 3, *Cv, Cvi*). Samples treated with TGF-β$_1$ showed a variable staining for PRG4 at the articular surface (Fig. 3, *Cvii, Cviii*). Control samples using nonspecific primary antibody were appropriately PRG4 negative.

## Discussion

These findings demonstrate that PRG4 secretion by chondrocytes near the articular surface is highly regulated by IL-1α and TGF-β$_1$ in explant cultures of cartilage. IL-1α had an inhibitory effect that was partially reversible, whereas TGF-β$_1$ was stimulatory, both in a dose-dependent manner (Fig. 2, *A*). The pattern of secretion in different culture conditions also varied, decreasing with time in cultures supplemented with IL-1α and increasing with time in those supplemented with TGF-β$_1$ (Fig. 2, *B*). The secretion rate also decreased in control cultures as previously described,[22] although not nearly as much as in cultures treated with IL-1α (Fig. 2, *B*). The trends in regulation of secretion were similar for S disks cultured in medium without FBS, although the rates were lower. PRG4 was immunolocalized to the articular surface and/or in S cells in all culture conditions, both histologically (Fig. 3, *C*) and macroscopically (Fig. 3, *D*). The finding that PRG4 expression is so modulated in explant cultures of cartilage represents a step toward understanding the regulated role of PRG4 in cartilage during normal growth, homeostasis, and pathology.

The interpretation of the results of the present study is affected by a number of factors. The amount of PRG4 secreted by the explants during the first two days of culture (Fig. 2, *B*) was much more than that adherent initially at the surface.[22] This indicates that the PRG4 accumulation in the medium represents molecules that predominantly were synthesized during culture. The pattern of PRG4 staining (Fig. 3) provides additional information about the source and location of PRG4 in cartilage explants. After treatment overnight with monensin to inhibit secretion, it is readily possible to identify cells synthesizing PRG4 at relatively high amounts in vertical immunohistochemical preparations because such cells are stained intensely. In contrast, the staining for PRG4 at the articular surface in macroscopic preparations and also in vertical sections showed graded levels of staining, which may not be directly representative of the amounts of PRG4 that are present in this location. Thus, the current studies provide information primarily about chondrocyte synthesis and secretion of PRG4.

These results agree with and extend previous qualitative studies of PRG4 regulation in chondrocytes by TGF-β$_1$[17,18] and IL-1α.[18] In those studies, full-thickness populations and subpopulations of chondrocytes were used in various culture systems, and qualitative analyses indicated that PRG4 expression was inhibited by IL-1α and upregulated by TGF-β$_1$. The current study quantifies the extent of regulation on chondrocytes in their native S and M zones within cartilage explants by measuring the secretion rate into culture medium. The localization of PRG4 in chondrocytes in the superficial region suggests that regulation is primarily of cells residing in this region of cartilage. The reversibility of the inhibitory effect of IL-1α after a relatively short-term treatment suggests that the effects on individual cells are not permanent.

The marked regulation in PRG4 expression may alter the homeostatic balance of PRG4 at the surface of articular cartilage and in joints. The amount of PRG4 present at articulating surfaces is most likely dependent on a balanced system of synthesis, deposition, and removal. Sources of PRG4 include synovial fibroblasts[9] and S chondrocytes,[3] and PRG4 has been localized to the surfaces of cartilage,[3] meniscus,[23] and tendon.[24] The synthesis and retention of PRG4 may be inhibited or altered under pathologic conditions. Variant forms of the molecule may also be present, possibly due to splice variants or proteolysis,[10,24] and mechanical stimuli may remove PRG4 from the articulating surfaces as well. It is likely that turnover of PRG4 at the surface of articular cartilage is affected by not only the synthesis rate of S chondrocytes but also the presence of PRG4 in the synovial fluid from the various other sources, all of which may be subject to regulation under pathologic conditions.

Because PRG4 normally functions as a boundary lubricant,[4,9,25] the inhibition of PRG4 secretion by IL-1α may contribute to the pathogenesis of arthritis. The apparent presence of PRG4 at the surface, even after 6 days of IL-1α treatment, may reflect the inability of induced proteases[26] to cleave this molecule from the surface. In osteoarthritis, it is possible that the extent of mechanical removal of the surface layer is in excess of the synthesis and deposition of PRG4 at the articular surface, with the net result that the normal low-friction wear-resistant function of cartilage is diminished. Conversely, the stimulation of PRG4 secretion by TGF-$\beta_1$ may be beneficial for normal cartilage function.

Identifying and quantifying the various chemomechanical coupling processes is critical for understanding the dynamic processes of articular cartilage growth, maturation, homeostasis, and degeneration. As with the dynamic regulation of extracellular matrix components in general, the synthesis and presence of PRG4 at the articular surface are likely to be important determinants of the low-friction and wear-resistant properties of articular cartilage. In turn, these mechanical properties may affect the way in which external stimuli, especially mechanical stimuli, affect the cellular microenvironment and ultimately cell functions, including the synthesis and presence of PRG4. Therefore, the ability to modulate the dynamic regulation of the putative lubricant PRG4, whether in homeostasis or degeneration, may ultimately be useful in prolonging the maintenance or slowing the deterioration of articular cartilage's critical mechanical functions at the end of long bones.

## Acknowledgments

This work was supported by the Arthritis Foundation, NASA, NIH, and NSF.

# References

1. Stockwell RA: *Biology of Cartilage Cells.* New York, NY, Cambridge University Press, 1979.

2. Schinagl RM, Gurskis D, Chen AC, Sah RL: Depth-dependent confined compression modulus of full-thickness bovine articular cartilage. *J Orthop Res* 1997;15:499-506.

3. Schumacher BL, Hughes CE, Kuettner KE, Caterson B, Aydelotte MB: Immunodetection and partial cDNA sequence of the proteoglycan, superficial zone protein, synthesized by cells lining synovial joints. *J Orthop Res* 1999;17:110-120.

4. Schmid T, Soloveychik V, Kuettner K, Schumacher B: Superficial zone protein (SZP) from human cartilage has lubrication activity. *Trans Orthop Res Soc* 2001;26:178.

5. Hunziker EB, Quinn TM, Hauselmann H: Quantitative structural organization of normal adult human articular cartilage. *Osteoarthritis Cartilage* 2002;10:564-572.

6. Schumacher BL, Su J-L, Lindley KM, Kuettner KE, Cole AA: Horizontally oriented clusters of multiple chondrons in the superficial zone of ankle, but not knee articular cartilage. *Anat Rec* 2001;266:241-248.

7. Quinn TM, Grodzinsky AJ, Buschmann MD, Kim YJ, Hunziker EB: Mechanical compression alters proteoglycan deposition and matrix deformation around individual cells in cartilage explants. *J Cell Sci* 1998;111:573-583.

8. Ikegawa S, Sano M, Koshizuka Y, Nakamura Y: Isolation, characterization and mapping of the mouse and human PRG4 (proteoglycan 4) genes. *Cytogenet Cell Genet* 2000;90:291-297.

9. Jay GD, Tantravahi U, Britt DE, Barrach HJ, Cha CJ: Homology of lubricin and superficial zone protein (SZP): Products of megakaryocyte stimulating factor (MSF) gene expression by human synovial fibroblasts and articular chondrocytes localized to chromosome 1q25. *J Orthop Res* 2001;19:677-687.

10. Marcelino J, Carpten JD, Suwairi WM, et al: CACP, encoding a secreted proteoglycan, is mutated in camptodactyly-arthropathy-coxa vara-pericarditis syndrome. *Nat Genet* 1999;23:319-322.

11. Sah RL: The biomechanical faces of articular cartilage, in Kuettner KE, Hascall VC (eds): *The Many Faces of Osteoarthritis.* New York, NY, Raven Press, 2002, pp 409-422.

12. Guilak F, Sah RL, Setton LA: Physical regulation of cartilage metabolism, in Mow VC, Hayes WC (eds): *Basic Orthopaedic Biomechanics,* ed 2. New York, NY, Raven Press, 1997, pp 179-207.

13. Lotz M, Blanco FJ, von Kempis J, et al: Cytokine regulation of chondrocyte functions. *J Rheumatol* 1995;22:104-108.

14. Moos V, Fickert S, Muller B, Weber U, Sieper J: Immunohistological analysis of cytokine expression in human osteoarthritic and healthy cartilage. *J Rheumatol* 1999;26:870-879.

15. Malfait AM, Verbruggen G, Veys EM, Lambert J, De Ridder L, Cornelissen M: Comparative and combined effects of interleukin 6, interleukin 1 beta, and tumor necrosis factor alpha on proteoglycan metabolism of human articular chondrocytes cultured in agarose. *J Rheumatol* 1994;21:314-320.

16. Lafeber FP, Vander Kraan PM, Huber-Bruning O, Vanden Berg WB, Bijlsma JW: Osteoarthritic human cartilage is more sensitive to transforming growth factor beta than is normal cartilage. *Br J Rheum* 1993;32:281-286.

17. Benya PD, Qiao B, Padilla SR: Synthesis of superficial zone protein/lubricin is synergistically stimulated by TGF-beta and adenoviral expression of TAK1a in rabbit articular chondrocytes. *Trans Orthop Res Soc* 2003;28:135.

18. Flannery CR, Hughes CE, Schumacher BL, et al: Articular cartilage superficial zone protein (SZP) is homologous to megakaryocyte stimulating factor precursor and is a multifunctional proteoglycan with potential growth-promoting, cytoprotective, and lubricating properties in cartilage metabolism. *Biochem Biophys Res Commun* 1999;254: 535-541.

19. Sokoloff L: In vitro culture of joints and articular tissues, in Sokoloff L (ed): *The Joints and Synovial Fluid*. New York, NY, Academic Press, 1980, pp 1-27.

20. Li KW, Williamson AK, Wang AS, Sah RL: Growth responses of cartilage to static and dynamic compression. *Clin Orthop* 2001;391:S34-S48.

21. Klein TJ, Schumacher BL, Schmidt TA, et al: Tissue engineering of articular cartilage with stratification using chondrocyte subpopulations. *Osteoarthritis Cartilage* 2003;11: 595-602.

22. Schmidt TA, Schumacher BL, Klein TJ, Voegtline MS, Sah RL: Synthesis of proteoglycan 4 by chondrocyte subpopulations in cartilage explants, monolayer cultures, and resurfaced cartilage cultures. *Arthritis Rheum* 2004;50:2849-2857.

23. Schumacher BL, Schmidt TA, Voegtline MS, Chen AC, Sah RL: Proteoglycan 4 (PRG4) synthesis and immunolocalization in bovine meniscus. *J Orthop Res* 2005;In Press.

24. Rees SG, Davies JR, Tudor D, et al: Immunolocalisation and expression of proteoglycan 4 (cartilage superficial zone proteoglycan) in tendon. *Matrix Biology* 2002;21: 593-602.

25. Jay GD, Haberstroh K, Cha C-J: Comparison of the boundary-lubricating ability of bovine synovial fluid, lubricin, and Healon. *J Biomed Mater Res* 1998;40:414-418.

26. Billinghurst RC, Wu W, Ionescu M, et al: Comparison of the degradation of type II collagen and proteoglycan in nasal and articular cartilages induced by interleukin-1 and the selective inhibition of type II collagen cleavage by collagenase. *Arthritis Rheum* 2000;43:664-672.

# Consensus Panel 3
# Evaluation of Biophysical Regulation of Skeletal Cells and Tissues

**Dr. Mark Bolander:** All the presentations at this meeting have been superb, and I think that's certainly true of the presentations this morning. I think Alan Grodzinsky's talk gave a wonderful overview. There's obviously a lot of clarity of thought. He showed how the models can be very cleverly used to elucidate different aspects and methods. Bob Sah went on and added the concept of the coordination between chemical and mechanical signaling. Jenneke Klein-Nulend added the concept that in the musculoskeletal system there are unique anatomic features, such as the canalicular system. We need to make sure that we incorporate those concepts in our understanding of how the signaling processes take place. And then Janet Rubin concluded with something that shed light on cellular mechanisms when she showed how we can take information from another system, the endothelial cell system. We can incorporate these ideas into our thinking; we can build paradigms of action and include other systems that are indeed relevant to the musculoskeletal system as well as unique musculoskeletal signal molecules, such as the RANKL (receptor activator of NFκB ligand) system. So in that brief summary, I think you can see the tremendous amount of information that was presented and the real value of that. Now, my concern is frankly that there's so much information and there's so many important things to talk about that the conversation will be all over the map. And when it's done, we really may not have a sense of having had a meaty discussion about central issues. And so I'm going to do something that I hadn't planned on until I started listening to talks this morning. I'm going to try to focus the discussion on what I think is perhaps of greatest value in in vivo studies, and that's our ability to develop models. I'd like to focus on a specific aspect of the models, and that is how they help us organize our thinking about the signal transduction mechanisms. And I'm going to use that focus to develop a number of questions. For example, I'm going to pose to the panel four specific questions: (1) Are the signaling mechanisms the same in different musculoskeletal tissues? (2) Are the responses to mechanical signaling unique, or would we expect them to be unique? (3) Do we have reason to think that there is cross-talk among different systems? (4) Can we always expect that the paradigms that we develop from other tissues are indeed relevant to the musculoskeletal system; and perhaps most important, to what extent can we use models that have been developed in one tissue to inform our thinking about signal transduction models in another tissue? To kick this off, I've asked the speakers to draw a depiction of the mechanistic model that they propose. I've asked them to try to capture the salient features of their thinking, and I'm hoping that this will form the starting point for discussion. In Alan Grodzinsky's model, he has emphasized the importance of the intracellular processes, the signal going into the nucleus, the posttranscriptional translational processes that are involved, and the concept that there are signals that can be damaging to the cell.

**Dr. Alan Grodzinsky:** Signaling isn't just an initiating of events at the membrane. There may be, in the case of cartilage and chondrocytes, important responses to mechanical forces at the intracellular level where perturbations may occur in the intracellular organelles.

**Dr. Mark Bolander:** Bob Sah's model shows that mechanical and chemical signaling is very complex at the membrane level, so we need to organize our thinking in a way that focuses on this very exquisite anatomic structure. Jenneke Klein-Nulend's model incorporates a lot of the anatomic features of bone and points out the roles of nitric oxide and prostaglandin $E_2$. The osteocyte canalicular structure responds to fluid flow. And then Janet Rubin's model is one that focuses very much on the roles of integrin regulation of intracellular signaling. Extracellular signal-regulated kinase is the central component in this and regulates RANKL and osteoprotegerin. Now I'm going to ask the consensus panel members to comment on how we can use these models of cartilage and of bone to improve our understanding of mechanisms, and perhaps to focus on two specific questions: first, where are there opportunities to take information from one model and understand something about the other models? And second, are these models robust enough to answer the questions that we have?

**Dr. Hari Reddi:** I'm going to be somewhat reductionist. So as far as the cartilage is concerned, one of the key issues is, what are the endogenous physical signals? According to Alan Grodzinsky, there is electromechanical coupling, and he made the point that some of the electric signals will cause physical deformation of cells and perhaps matrix. But I have a problem as a simple biologist: you talk about physical signals, and then we have at least electric, mechanical, and ultrasound. What do they have in common? Do they all go to one final pathway? I would like to have comments from all the speakers because I'm not enlightened. In fact I'd like to ask, perhaps, with your permission, Sol Pollack to chime in. These are three different signals; do they work through distinct or common receptors?

**Dr. Mark Bolander:** I think, Mone, you had a question and I'm hoping it's going to be about the cross-talk.

**Dr. Mone Zaidi:** There is a well-defined preclinical paradigm now that is emerging in the literature, and many of you may not be privy to that information, but I certainly am. And the information is that if in an osteoarthritis model you give a bisphosphonate—the function of which is to cure osteoporosis by acting on the osteoblast—you can actually prevent the progression of osteoarthritis. Now the question is, is the bisphosphonate actually acting directly on the cartilage, or is the bisphosphonate acting to stabilize the subchondral bone, which then speaks for the cartilage in some way or other? I think what needs to be clarified is whether there is a chemical signal that could be transmitted from the bone to the cartilage—for example, a bone morphogenetic protein (BMP) or a transforming growth factor-beta (TGF-$\beta$) that would then stabilize the cartilage. Or is this simply a mechanical effect to stabilize the subchondral bone and hence prevent degenerative joint disease? So one question is, are there also soluble signals?

**Dr. Mark Bolander:** Considering Janet Rubin's point that there is an attachment here to the matrix, can we assume that there might be some type of attachment between the cartilage and the bone that would also regulate that?

**Dr. Mone Zaidi:** There are a lot of integrins on bone cells that could do that. Somebody needs to define what is going on in the interaction between bone and cartilage.

**Dr. Mark Bolander:** So perhaps the way that these models can be used to answer mechanistic questions is to focus on the soluble factors and consider the attachment to extracellular matrix molecules. Janet, when you look at information about the effect in cartilage, do you think there are reasons to believe that the mechanisms that are central to mechanical signaling in osteoclasts would also be central to the signaling in these other types of physical stimuli?

**Dr. Janet Rubin:** I think there are so many signal transduction pathways and redundancies that it surprises me that if you knock out one, any signal will be interrupted. I do want to disagree with Dr. Reddi if I could about hormones and their specific actions. The signaling world is now finally attacking the fact that signal transduction mechanisms, whether it be a BMP receptor, TGF-$\beta$ receptor, or others, are linked to their signaling benefits through scaffolds, and we know that if you change the scaffold that a signaling molecule sits on, it will then activate a different distal cellular mechanism. Mechanical strain can do the same thing.

**Dr. Hari Reddi:** Unfortunately, what you said is absolutely wrong. TGF-$\beta$ has its own receptors, as you know. Inside the cell it phosphorylates SMAD-2 and -3. And its common partner is SMAD-4. You don't need scaffolds inside the cytoplasm. I'm sorry to disagree with you because I generally don't like to disagree with ladies.

**Dr. Mark Bolander:** Here's your chance to disagree with another lady.

**Dr. Barbara Boyan:** I'm going with Janet Rubin on this. Not against you but with Janet. The point here is that signaling pathways really are complicated. And they all do turn out the same master molecules. In fact, TGF-$\beta$ activates protein kinase C. It's much more complicated and there are lots of synergistic effects.

**Dr. Stephen Trippel:** Everyone who has made comments on this area is correct and I agree with everybody. The issue that everybody is addressing here, which we're not going to solve today, is that specificity in signal transduction mechanisms is very complicated. It's multifactorial and it involves all of the things that we've been hearing about. It may be a little bit of an overstatement to say that it's the Holy Grail for a lot of work that is going on in endocrinology and cell biology, but if it is an overstatement, it's probably not too much of one. The data just aren't there to solve that problem now, and we shouldn't try to solve a problem without that kind of data.

**Speaker:** I'd like to extend what Steve Trippel said. We've seen evidence from the talks today that there are maturation effects with respect to the cell and its specialized extracellular matrix. We still don't know enough about what the pericellular environment is. There are heparan sulphate proteoglycans that are co-receptors. Janet Rubin alluded to the fact that there is specific scaffolding, and that specific scaffolding is just now being unraveled. If you think Ras is complicated, there are domains on the different Ras with respect to SHS-3 and -2 that actually dictate what phosphorylation kinetics will occur on the target molecule, and these we haven't even touched on. So I believe from the point of view of mechanical reception that that's probably going to be more hardwired than we're actually prepared to talk about now. And it may very well be tied back to specific integrins working in concert with growth factor receptors. I think Bob Sah's data make it clear that soluble ligands binding receptors can have huge effects on the cells, as we know is the case with interleukin-1 (IL-1). One molecule of IL-1 sitting on one receptor is about all you would need. I would also like to say that, at the level of the pericellular matrix in the case of the osteocyte where there seem to be the canaliculi, people are actually looking at the level of nanoprotein organization, which may be as important as protein conformation and fluid flow. This could be an issue in other cells as well, particularly chondrocytes. Certainly in human osteoarthritic sites, when we culture chondrocytes, they send out processes that we don't see in normal cells. So there may be morphologic changes over time that impact upon the mechano- or extracellular reception mechanism.

**Dr. Mark Bolander:** Bob, a question for you if I may. Jenneke Klein-Nulend has elegantly combined the microarchitecture of the osteocyte and histologic architecture. And you've done some of the same thing in dividing your cartilage into three different regions. Are there opportunities to expand this organization? And if there are, how would you do it?

**Dr. Robert Sah:** I think one issue that that model and depiction really brought out very nicely is the dynamic nature of models and how we can look at them over different time and length scales. So the model that I sketched up there is one that I think is useful for looking at cartilage in a certain state, but if you look at growth, then the cells get farther apart as we age and tissue undergoes changes in geometry, which Marjolein van der Meulen made reference to in her talk. Then, in disease, the structure changes and the signals coming in may also change. So I think there are opportunities to look at whatever phenomenon we are looking at in different length scales—for example, the very detailed model that Alan Grodzinsky has of a cell responding to physical forces. On the other hand, in the area of growth or arthritis, maybe that level of the model isn't needed in so much detail.

**Dr. Charles Turner:** Actually, Sol Pollack would probably be able to answer the first part of Dr. Reddi's question. He asked for commonalities and differences in the various physical stimulation technologies. Two years ago, Dr. Brighton and Sol published a paper in which they looked at mechanical stimulation, capacitive coupling, biomagnetic fields, and pulsed electromagnetic fields (PEMF) on osteoblast proliferation. They also looked at specific blockers of various pathways, including release of calcium from intracellular stores and certain calcium channels. The common modality that came out of it was that, if you block calmodulin, the effects of all the signals go away. So there is a common upregulation in intracellular calcium through the calcium calmodulin pathway that is necessary for an effect, but an increase in intracellular calcium is different for the different physical signals. Certainly in capacitive coupling, you could block the intracellular calcium by blocking voltage-gated calcium channels with verapamil, so the calcium is coming in from the outside. With PEMF and combined magnetic fields, there was no effect of verapamil, but if you block calcium released from intracellular stores, you blocked the effect. Mechanical stimulation was blocked by blocking inositol phosphate-3.

**Dr. Solomon Pollack:** The point of that paper was that just because it's biophysical doesn't mean there's going to be a single transduction site. All the things we talked about so far this week demonstrate that there are so many ways for a cell to recognize the presence of a biophysical signal. It then has all of these different cascading pathways available to it in order to respond. There are the integrated pathways, as Janet Rubin was describing. I think we're not looking just for a single site. I think we're looking for the way biophysical stimuli interact, perhaps with a family of receptors. Any one of these physical stimuli could just slightly alter the conformation of one of the receptors and change its binding kinetics.

**Speaker:** I don't see at the membrane level anything that is unifying. There may be some unifying ways in which the cascading events occur and there may not be, just as there may not be with all the different drugs that you get. But it's an important thing to look for, and from a basic science point of view, it's very exciting. It ought to be something that encourages far more research than actually takes place, because that's where the first step in the basic science of transduction is going to take place.

**Dr. Randall Duncan:** There are a lot of different responses to calcium. There are subcellular domains within the cell that will achieve different responses, and we hope to show that tomorrow. I think that buffering and providing a barrier between these different sections would produce different types of signals. And I think there are two different responses to mechanical stimulation. One is a signal amplification response, in which you have things like nitric oxide and prostaglandins that release to stimulate other surrounding cells and present an amplified signal to the lining cells of the osteoblast.

**Dr. Mark Bolander:** So there are two signal transduction concepts. One is that the calcium signal can also be specific in terms of its location. And the other concept is that amplification of a signal actually has several components to it. One is amplification of the signal inside the cell. And the other is the application by activities that recruit other cells.

**Dr. Mone Zaidi:** I had a comment enlarging that concept. When you deform the cell, you also deform the intranuclear compartment, and you also deform the other organelles. And one of the interesting fields that is emerging is how nuclear transport is regulated. The nucleus has the capacity to generate its own calcium signals. So if you deform the nucleus, you could get a completely different profile of calcium signaling within the nucleus as opposed to what gets transmitted from the exterior. So I think we've got to also focus on the intracellular messengers for the membrane system.

**Dr. Mark Bolander:** These ideas seem to be suggesting that a signal that is a general signal can acquire some type of specificity, although we don't know how specificity occurs.

**Dr. Farshid Guilak:** I think Randy Duncan and Mone Zaidi brought up some of the points that I was going to mention, and that's kind of polarized the room. How can you have the same signaling molecule that has varied end results? For calcium, at least, it's pretty well understood, and it's sort of the same way that we can all pick up a cell phone and talk on a different channel even if we're talking on the same frequency, because the signal is encoded. For calcium, it can be encoded by frequency, magnitude, and space. So a short calcium burst is different than a long calcium burst, and it's different than an oscillating calcium. And in the same manner, some of these signaling molecules can be included within the cell so that even though you're running on the same pathway, you can have very different end results and signals.

## Future Directions

- We need to define whether there is cross-talk among various tissues exposed to biophysical signals.

- There may be secondary signaling among cells or tissues in response to biophysical perturbations, and this signaling may take the form of soluble mediators, extracellular matrix, or integrins.

- Cellular transduction mechanisms of biophysical signals are extremely complicated, and commonalities and differences among transduction of different biophysical signals need to be explored.

- The specificity and amplification of signal transduction mechanisms remain important areas to investigate.

# Section Four
## Biophysical Regulation of Growth Factor Synthesis

# Chapter 13
# Stimulation of Growth Factors by Physical Agents: An Intermediary Mechanism of Action

*Deborah McK. Ciombor, PhD*

Genetic factors both permit and constrain the range of expression of skeletal features; however, these features are also influenced by environmental factors. In the 19th century, Wilhelm Roux[1] proposed that mechanical factors played a central role in the morphogenesis of musculoskeletal tissues. He referred to the collective physiochemical processes influencing developmental morphogenesis as "developmental mechanics" or *entwicklungsmechanik*. In modern biochemical and molecular terms, this concept can be expressed as genetic potential modified by epigenetic factors. Considerable evidence exists that intermittent physical forces affect cell differentiation, particularly the formation of cartilage and bone. More to the point, it is well accepted that the physical environment exerts regulatory influences on gene expression for and synthesis of structural (extracellular matrix, or ECM) and signaling proteins.

In developing endochondral tissues, the differentiation of chondroprogenitor cells and subsequent bone formation are most likely regulated by local growth factors expressed in spatial and temporal gradients. The therapeutic intervention for the repair and cartilage of bone requires an understanding of the regulatory effects of these gradients on bone and cartilage cells. However, the therapeutic efficacy of growth factors in bone and cartilage repair is limited by diffusion of material away from the desired site. Several solutions to this problem have been proposed, including the use of (1) carriers (either a biologic matrix or a constructed polymer), (2) engineered three-dimensional scaffolds, or (3) gene therapy. Another possibility is the upregulation of growth factor gene expression and protein synthesis by biophysical mechanisms.

## Biomechanical Forces

Mechanical strain—the most obvious of physical forces—affects the overall physical environment of tissues, including pH, $pO_2$, hydrostatic pressure fluid flow, osmotic pressure, and electrokinetic phenomena. The physical environment, in turn, exerts regulatory influences on gene expression and synthesis of a variety of proteins, including those constituting extracellular matrix and regulatory proteins, and therefore has an overall influence on morphogenesis.

Rubin and associates[2-6] published data indicating that osteoclast differentiation was suppressed by physical forces associated with skeletal loading,

**Table 1 Mechanical Strain Upregulates TGF-β/BMP**

| Study | Model | Observations |
|---|---|---|
| Claes et al[13] 1998 | Osteoblasts | TGF-β |
| Neidlinger-Wilke et al[14] 1995 | Osteoblasts | TGF-β |
| Helms et al[12] 1998 | Fracture | BMP/IHH |
| Bostrom and Asnis[11] 1998 | Fracture | TGF-β |
| Wu et al[15,16] 2001 | Chondrocytes | IHH/BMP |
| Yamashiro et al[17] 2001 | Osteocytes | CTGF |

Furthermore, they showed that hydrostatic pressure also suppresses osteoclastogenesis, and that dynamic mechanical strain suppresses osteoclast differentiation from marrow stromal cells through a regulation of RANKL following activation of ERK 1/2 MAP kinase and nitric oxide (NO). Other groups have published data confirming these findings. Ogata[7] showed that osteoblast-like cells in culture responded to mechanical stimuli by increasing the phosphorylation of ERK 1/2 as well as enhancing the expression of early response genes for c-fos or egr-1, which results in the increase of epidermal growth factor concentration. Jin and associates[8] and Tzima and associates[9] showed that biomechanical stimulation may have different effects on cell function but use similar signaling pathways. Those pathways include the integrins interacting with the extracellular matrix and receptor tyrosine kinase phosphorylation. Weiss and associates[10] subsequently demonstrated that allowing mechanical stimulation during distraction osteogenesis produced a cascade of biochemical factors compared with a rigid osteotomy. A systemic regulation of increases in bFGF, TGF-β, IGF-1, and IGFBP-3 was seen. Further, a correlation was found between osteoblastic markers and increases in TGF-β and bFGF. The authors suggest that strain-activated osteoblasts were the major source of the systemically elevated growth factors.

Several groups have shown an upregulation of the TGF-β/BMP pathway by mechanical strain.[11-17] Claes and associates[13] demonstrated that in vitro osteoblasts grown under the effects of mechanical strain upregulated TGF-β$_1$. In a fracture model, Carter and associates[12] showed an upregulation of BMP-2 and -4 and Indian Hedgehog (IHH); Bostrom and Asnis,[11] in another fracture model, demonstrated an upregulation of TGF-β$_1$ produced by mechanical strain. The findings of these groups are summarized in Table 1.

Zhen and associates[15] and Wu and associates[16] showed that conditioned medium from mechanically stretched chondrocytes had a stimulatory effect on resting chondrocytes, resulting in increased proliferation. When exposed to conditioned medium from stretched chondrocytes, resting chondrocytes had an increase in cell number of nearly 40% by day 2. This work led to the identification of a stress-activated proliferation factor (SAPF), which is released by mechanically stretched chondrocytes, and confirmed that SAPF stimulates chondrocyte proliferation. Mechanical stimulation of the collagen type X promoter was shown to occur through a BMP-responsive element, and mechanical stimulation of collagen type X transcription has been confirmed to be mediated through an IHH/BMP-dependent pathway. The mechanical signal transduction pathway following stretch-induced matrix deformation appears to have a direct stimulation on the chemical mediator IHH, which in turn regulates BMP-2 and -4 to sustain and amplify proliferation, a final biologic response for many systems.

Goldspink and Yang[18,19] discovered a second isoform of IGF-1, mechano-growth factor (MGF), that only occurs in muscle following mechanical stimulation. Further experiments showed that stretch and stretch combined with electrical stimulation, rather than electrical stimulation alone, are important in inducing MGF expression.

The effect of exercise on the concentration of both systemic and bone growth factors was studied in the rat.[20] The effect of additional weight bearing during exercise was tested in relation to the systemic response of IGF-1 and local bone concentrations of IGF-1 and TGF-$\beta$. Serum growth hormone concentration was modulated by running and exercise. Hering and associates[21] also showed that circulating TGF-$\beta_1$ is elevated in humans following extensive exercise. The baseline level of TGF-$\beta_1$ in the plasma of resting individuals was 525 pg/mL; however, TGF-$\beta_1$ concentrations rose to 710 pg/mL after 2 weeks of training. Levels slowly declined to 650 pg/mL after 2 weeks and 440 pg/mL after 4 weeks with no exercise.

Finally, the dramatic effect of a loss of mechanical information to a biologic system was shown by Ontiveros and McCabe[22] using MC3T3 osteoblasts grown on microcarrier beads for 14 days and then placed in rotating wall vessels to simulate microgravity for 24 hours. In addition to Runx2 and activator protein-1 (AP-1) transactivation, key regulators of osteoblast differentiation and bone formation were reduced by more than 60%.

It is clear that biomechanical forces affect a range of connective tissue responses. Although the underlying mechanisms are still not fully understood, it is clear from the studies presented above as well as many others that the activation of gene expression and upregulation of protein synthesis of growth factors are of central importance.

## Ultrasound

Ultrasound is transmitted through biologic tissues as acoustic pressure. The application of ultrasound may induce conformational changes in the cell membrane and therefore alter ionic permeability. Additionally, activation of second messengers has been observed that could lead to downstream changes in gene expression. Two placebo-controlled, randomized, double-blind clinical studies regarding fracture healing with ultrasound have been published,[23,24] and other clinical studies with ultrasound have been summarized. In a meta-analysis of 138 potential studies, only six met inclusion criteria, and the information of three trials was pooled in the final data.[25,26]

Ryaby and associates[27] have indicated that the MC3T3/TE 85 osteoblastic cell line increased adenylate cyclase activity when exposed to ultrasound. Additionally, the cells increased their expression of TGF-$\beta_1$ following exposure. Ito and associates[28] showed that both the SaOS-2 osteoblastic cell line and HUVEC endothelial cells increase PDGF-$\alpha$/$\beta$ secretion following exposure to ultrasound.

Mechanical perturbation of osteoblastic cells in culture by ultrasound has been studied in several laboratories. Naruse and associates[29] showed a distinct anabolic response in osteoblasts exposed to low-intensity pulsed ultrasound. Young primary osteoblasts reacted by transiently increasing the message levels of immediate early genes as well as those of osteocalcin and IGF-1. Conversely, mature osteocytes responded to a lesser extent. Sun and associates[30] showed in rat alveolar mononuclear cell-calvaria osteoblasts that osteoblast cell number was increased while that of osteoclasts was decreased. The total alkaline phosphatase amount in the culture medium was increased, as was tumor necrosis factor-$\alpha$. The authors suggest that this may be the biologic mechanism by which ultrasound positively effects fracture repair. The data of Kokubu and associates[31] indicate that the expression of cyclooxygenase-2 (COX-2) mRNA was rapidly upregulated in a time-dependent manner following the exposure of a mouse osteoblast cell line to ultrasound. The result was a threefold increase in $PGE_2$ at 60 minutes in comparison to unexposed control cells.

Warden and associates[32,33] demonstrated that low-intensity ultrasound induces an osteogenic mechanical stimuli in both isolated bone cells and fractured bone. The results of this study indicate that ultrasound may not be a beneficial treatment for osteoporosis and that intact bone may be less sensitive to ultrasound than fractured bone or in vitro bone cell systems. These studies may point to a biophysical mechanism of ultrasound involving ultrasound-responsive growth factors. Mechanistic considerations are complicated by potential thermal effects, unresolved questions of piezoelectric effects, and conflicting $Ca^{+2}$ data. Reviews by Warden and associates[32] and Nelson and associates[34] provide a comprehensive presentation.

## Electromagnetic Fields

Because other biophysical events occur coincidentally with mechanical strain, it is difficult if not impossible to isolate the effects of the mechanical environment from those caused by accompanying fluid flow such as ion movement and electrokinetic events, and it is difficult to implicate any individual force as having a regulatory function in connective tissues. The exogenous application of pulsed electromagnetic fields (PEMF) induces an electric field in the tissue and permits the isolation of this physical force as a regulator of connective tissue function. It is of interest in clinical medicine as a technique to regulate repair and in more basic terms as a probe with which to perturb and examine cell behavior.

Several groups have shown that electromagnetic and pulsed magnetic fields have an impact on growth factor regulation.[35-42] Pulsed electric and magnetic fields (inductive coupling) and capacitive coupling induce fields through soft tissue and bone, resulting in low voltage and currents in the exposed tissues. Increases in proliferation; increases in TGF-$\beta$, mRNA, and mRNA for BMP-2, -4, and -7; and an increase in differentiation of progenitor cells to chondrocytes have been shown (Table 2).

In some of the earliest studies implicating growth factors, Fitzsimmons and associates[43] and Ryaby and associates[44] showed an increase in IGF-2

**Table 2 Growth Factor Regulation by Electromagnetic and Pulsed Magnetic Fields**

| Study | Technique | Model | Result |
|---|---|---|---|
| Zhuang et al[35] | CC | MC3T3 | Proliferation, TGF-$\beta_1$ mRNA |
| Bodamyali et al[36] | IC | Osteoblasts | Proliferation, BMP-2, -4 mRNA |
| Nagai and Ota[37] | IC | Osteoblasts | BMP-2, -4 mRNA |
| Yajima et al[38] | IC | Osteoblasts | BMP-2, -4, -7 mRNA |
| Aaron et al[39] | IC | EO in vivo | Differentiation, TGF-$\beta$ mRNA + Protein |
| Lohmann et al[40] | IC | MG 63 | Differentiation, TGF-$\beta$ |
| Guerkov et al[41] | IC | Nonunions | TGF-$\beta$ |
| Aaron et al[42] | IC | EO in vivo | Differentiation, TGF-$\beta$ |

mRNA and protein and suggested that IGF-2 may in part mediate proliferation of osteoblast-like cells. Combined magnetic field exposure of both human osteoblast-like and rat fracture callus cells demonstrated increases in IGF-2 levels after 30 minutes of exposure.[44]

In studies examining isolated mesenchymal stem cells exposed to a clinically relevant PEMF, Guerkov and associates[41] showed that 8 hours of exposure affects the levels of both TGF-$\beta_1$ and PGE$_2$. The magnitude and time course of this effect is dependent on the maturational state of the cell at the time of exposure. This laboratory also examined the MG63 human osteoblast-like cell line. Under PEMF exposure, there was decreased proliferation; increased alkaline phosphate activity and collagen synthesis; and increased osteocalcin, TGF-$\beta_1$, and PGE$_2$ at early time points. However, with the osteocyte-like cell line MLO-Y4, there was no change in cell number and in osteocalcin, despite an increase in TGF-$\beta_1$ and PGE$_2$. NO concentration in the cells was altered. In vitro cultures of human nonunion cells exposed to PEMF resulted in a time-dependent increase in TGF-$\beta_1$ levels on day 2 in hypertrophic nonunion cells but required exposure to day 4 in atrophic nonunion cells. Confluent cultures at various stages of maturation were exposed to a PEMF consisting of a burst of 20 pulses repeating at 15 Hz for 8 hours per day for 1, 2, or 4 days. Controls were cultured under identical conditions without exposure to PEMF. Because the mechanisms by which PEMF mediates its effects on the cells are not known, physiologic responses of the cells were measured rather than mRNA levels alone. These included cell proliferation determined by cell number and [$^3$H]-thymidine incorporation; differentiation determined as a function of alkaline phosphatase-specific activity of isolated cells as well as of the cell layer; extracellular matrix production based on collagen synthesis and [$^{35}$S]-sulfate incorporation; and local factor production using levels of total TGF-$\beta_1$, PGE$_2$, and NO$^{2-}$ in the conditioned media as indicators. This method provides a general quantitative assessment of cell response. The examination of terminally differentiated MLO-Y4 osteocyte-like cells did not show an effect of PEMF. Neither cell number nor osteocalcin levels were changed; however, TGF-$\beta_1$ and PGE$_2$ levels were increased and NO$^{2-}$ concentration was altered. These studies suggest that the effect of PEMF on TGF-$\beta_1$ levels in this system was mediated through a prostaglandin-dependent mechanism involving COX-1 but not the COX-2 pathway. The PEMF-dependent increase in TGF-$\beta_1$ could be blocked by inhibition of prostaglandin production by indomethacin, which blocks both forms of cyclooxygenase.

Implantable direct current (DC) electrical stimulation has been shown to increase mRNA levels of BMP-2, -6, and -7, as well as BMP receptor ALK-2 compared with controls. By comparison, capacitively coupled electric fields (CCEF) increased mRNA levels of BMP-2, TGF-$\beta_1$, FGF-2, and vascular endothelial growth factor compared with controls. The time course of message expression was not disrupted in the exposed groups compared with controls. This study shows that both DC and CCEF induce a biologic response by upregulating a cascade of growth factors throughout the exposure, and that they do so by enhancing the normal expression of these factors.

Other laboratories have shown increases in growth factors of the TGF-$\beta_1$/ BMP and IGF-2 families by PEMF. Because PEMF can be applied over relatively long periods of time, a sustained increase in growth factor synthesis could be anticipated. If so, this would have significant advantages over single factor injection. Studies in our laboratory describe upregulation of TGF-$\beta_1$ in vivo, temporally coincident with chondrogenic differentiation in endochondral ossification. Following exposure to PEMF of an in vivo model of decalcified bone matrix-induced endochondral ossification, mRNA expression for and protein synthesis of TGF-$\beta_1$ were upregulated coincident with increases in extracellular matrix protein and gene expression. In response to a power frequency field, TGF-$\beta_1$ mRNA levels increased 68%, the active protein 25%, and number of immunopositive cells 119% in the actively stimulated group compared to controls in the same experimental model.[39] Further studies of endochondral bone formation demonstrated that PEMF used therapeutically for bone healing upregulated cell differentiation, extracellular matrix synthesis, and TGF-$\beta_1$ expression in chondroprogenitor and osteoprogenitor cells. The pattern of TGF-$\beta_1$ expression was preserved throughout the developmental sequence, suggesting that PEMF exposure enhances but does not disorganize the normal physiologic expression pattern of TGF-$\beta_1$.[42] These studies demonstrated no difference in DNA content between control and PEMF-exposed endochondral bone formation, indicating an absence of a proliferative response to field exposure. Chondrogenesis, however, was markedly stimulated, exhibiting a twofold increase in sulfate incorporation and a 64% increase in glycosaminoglycan content compared to controls. The glycosaminoglycan content expressed per unit of tissue, or per chondrocyte, and the chodrocyte:matrix ratios were not different between the groups, indicating that differentiation of chondrocytes in PEMF-exposed tissue was responsible for the observed increases. The total cell number was unchanged by PEMF exposure. This finding suggests that the increased number of chondrocytes comprised a greater fraction of the total cell content in PEMF-exposed compared to unexposed tissue. PEMF exposure both augmented and accelerated the levels of aggrecan and type II collagen mRNA and initiated the earlier appearance and deposition of cartilage-specific proteoglycans. Sustained increases in TGF-$\beta_1$ protein were observed in PEMF-stimulated tissues compared to control tissues throughout the developmental sequence. During early chondrogenesis, the normal

**Table 3 Quantitated Levels of mRNA and Protein Expression**

|  | Control | PEMF Exposed | *P* Value |
|---|---|---|---|
| Proteoglycan mRNA | 95.9 ± 10.8 | 150.2 ± 17.9 | 0.03 |
| Type II collagen mRNA | 24.5 ± 2.2 | 38.2 ± 5.2 | 0.04 |
| TGF-β mRNA (OD) | 189.7 ± 36.6 | 318.4 ± 37.6 | 0.03 |
| TGF-β active protein (pg/mg) | 66.8 ± 2.8 | 83.3 ± 4.4 | 0.005 |
| TGF-β immunopositive cells (n) | 227.7 ± 55.8 | 499.0 ± 6.1 | 0.005 |

peak expression of TGF-$β_1$ was observed also in PEMF-stimulated tissue, although it was quantitatively increased. Increases in TGF-$β_1$ protein ranged from 16.2 pg/mg on day 2 to an average of 9.8 pg/mg on days 4 to 10 of development. On day 6, the increase produced by PEMF was 0.08 pg/μg DNA. PEMF exposure resulted in an overall increase of 32% in TGF-$β_1$ protein compared with control. mRNA levels were increased 2.5-fold in PEMF-exposed tissues compared to unexposed tissues. Immunohistochemical studies demonstrated that TGF-$β_1$ was synthesized by chondrocytes. These data demonstrated that the transcription of TGF-$β_1$ mRNA and the accumulation of active TGF-$β_1$ protein are upregulated by PEMF coincident with accelerated chondrogenesis, suggesting that these PEMF effects may be mediated by TGF-$β_1$. Both mechanical forces and PEMF act early in the developmental cascade of endochondral ossification with the putative mechanism being an increase in growth factor gene expression and protein synthesis.[45]

The exposure of Hartley guinea pigs, which spontaneously develop osteoarthritis, to PEMF reduced the severity of osteoarthritis and preserved articular cartilage. A reduction in cartilage neoepitopes and suppression of the matrix metalloproteases (MMP-3 and collagenase) were observed in this study. Cells immunopositive to IL-1 were decreased in number, whereas the number of cells immunopositive to TGF-$β_1$ were increased. These studies in our laboratory suggested that exposure to PEMF not only alters gene expression for structural proteins of the extracellular matrix but also affects cytokine signaling[46] (Table 3).

A study of the effects of PEMF on angiogenesis, a process critical to the process of healing in connective tissues, showed a sevenfold increase in endothelial cell tubulization. In the same in vitro model, proliferation was enhanced threefold over control cultures. Angiogenic protein analysis showed that a fivefold increase in FGF-2 as well as a smaller but still significant increase in other angiogenic factors that were responsible for the observed biologic response.[47]

# A Unifying Signal Transduction Theme of Physical Forces: Activation of Stress-activated Protein Kinases

The physical environment exerts regulatory influences on gene expression for and synthesis of structural (ECM) and signaling proteins. The studies presented here all present similar responses to mechanical strain, ultrasound, and PEMF exposure, and the stimulation of growth factor gene expression

## EMF    US    Mechanical

↓

**MAPK**

↓

**Early Immediate Genes**

↓

**Growth Factors (Gene expression; Protein synthesis)**

↓

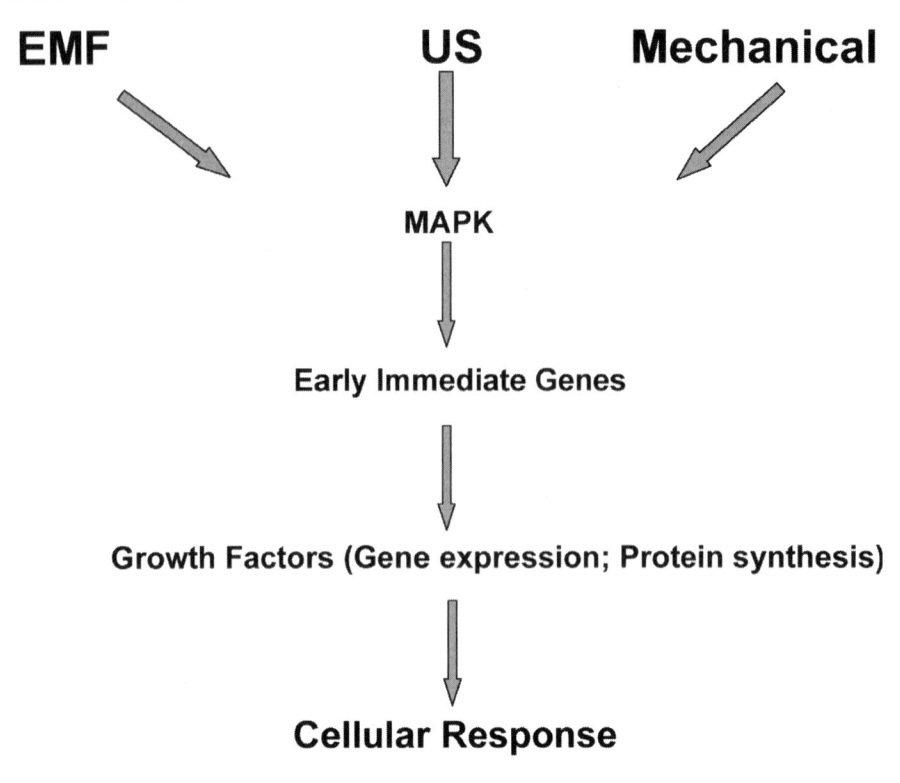

**Cellular Response**

**Figure 1** Proposed common mechanistic pathway as the unifying theme of tissue response to physical forces.

and protein synthesis may represent an intermediary signaling mechanism modulating the effect of biophysical input in general (Fig. 1).

Consideration of intracellular signaling suggests a testable hypothesis of cell responses to biophysical input. Our laboratory has shown that effects seen in endochondral ossification are due to changes in gene transcription and protein content for growth factors, particularly the multifunctional cytokine TGF-$\beta_1$, during the early stages of chondrogenesis. TGF-$\beta_1$ exerts its influence in repair through modulation of cell proliferation, differentiation, and the production of extracellular matrix components. The induction of TGF-$\beta_1$ gene transcription is mediated by binding of the AP-1 complex in the promoter. AP-1 is composed of DNA binding proteins belonging to the jun and fos families of early immediate response genes and plays a critical role in cell regulation, including cell proliferation and differentiation. AP-1 activity is required to initiate transcription of many genes that become activated during skeletal development and repair. Our data demonstrate that PEMF enhances binding to the AP-1 site in the TGF-$\beta_1$ promoter, increases c-Jun and c-Fos protein concentrations, and activates the MAP kinase signaling pathway JNK/SAPK. Western blot analysis showed no changes in the basal levels of JNK but rather that PEMF elevates phosphorylation events in a manner consistent with increases in c-Jun, leading to increased levels of AP-1 and binding to the high affinity AP-1 site of the TGF-$\beta_1$ promoter.

A phosphorylation event is responsible for the increases in c-Fos and c-Jun expression and protein concentration. Taken together, the data presented in this chapter support the hypothesis that the stimulation of gene expression for and the protein synthesis of growth factors is an underlying event that leads to the enhancement of bone and cartilage formation. The TGF-$\beta_1$ gene superfamily is the primary agent, although it is not unique. Furthermore, the regulation of the increase in synthesis is controlled by transcription factors in the MAP kinase pathways. These data extend mechanistic understanding of how physical forces change gene expression and will lead to an understanding of signal transduction mechanisms at the membrane level.

# References

1. Roux W: *Der Kampf der Teile im Organismus*. Leipzig, Germany, Engelmann, 1881.
2. Rubin J, Biskobing D, Fan X, et al: Pressure regulates osteoclast formation and MCSF expression in marrow culture. *J Cell Physiol* 1997;170:81-87.
3. Rubin J, Fan X, Biskobing D, Taylor W, Rubin C: Osteoclastogenesis is repressed by mechanical strain in an in vitro model. *J Orthop Res* 1999;17:639-645.
4. Rubin J, Murphy T, Fan X, Goldschmidt M, Taylor W: Activation of extracellular signal-regulated kinase is involved in mechanical strain inhibition of RANKL expression in bone stromal cells. *J Bone Miner Res* 2002;17:1452-1460.
5. Rubin J, Murphy T, Nanes M, Fan X: Mechanical strain inhibits expression of osteoclast differentiation factor by murine stromal cells. *Am J Physiol Cell Physiol* 2000;278:C1126-C1132.
6. Rubin J, Murphy T, Shu L, et al: Mechanical strain differentially regulates endothelial nitric-oxide synthase and receptor activator of nuclear kappa B ligand expression via ERK 1/2 MAPK. *J Biol Chem* 2003;278:34018-34025.
7. Ogata T: Increase in epidermal growth factor receptor protein induced in osteoblastic cells after exposure to flow of culture media. *Am J Physiol Cell Physiol* 2003; 285:C425-C432.
8. Jin G, Sah RL, Li YS, Lotz M, Shyy JY, Chien S: Biomechanical regulation of matrix metalloproteinase-9 in cultured chondrocytes. *J Orthop Res* 2000;18:899-908.
9. Tzima E, del Pozo M, Shattil S, Chien S, Schwartz M: Activation of integrins in endothelial cells by fluid shear stress mediates Rho-dependent cytoskeletal alignment. *EMBO J* 2001;20:4639-4647.
10. Weiss S, Baumgart R, Jochum M, Strasburger CJ, Bidlingmaier M: Systemic regulation of distraction osteogenesis: A cascade of biochemical factors. *J Bone Miner Res* 2001;17:1280-1289.
11. Bostrom MP, Asnis P: Transforming growth factor beta in fracture repair. *Clin Orthop* 1998;355:S124-S131.
12. Carter DR, Beaupre GS, Giori NJ, Helms JA: Mechanobiology of skeletal regeneration. *Clin Orthop* 1998;355:S41-S55.

13. Claes LE, Heigele CA, Neidlinger-Wilke C, et al: Effects of mechanical factors on the fracture healing process. *Clin Orthop* 1998;355:S132-S147.

14. Neidlinger-Wilke C, Stalla I, Claes L: Human osteoblasts from younger normal and osteoporotic donors shows different proliferation and TGF-beta release in response to cyclic strain. *J Biomechanics* 1995;28:1411-1418.

15. Zhen X, Wei L, Wu Q, Zhang Y, Chen Q: Mitogen-activated protein kinase p38 mediates regulation of chondrocyte differentiation by parathyroid hormone. *J Biol Chem* 2001;276:4879-4885.

16. Wu Q, Zhang Y, Chen Q: Indian hedgehog is an essential component of mechanotransduction complex to stimulate chondrocyte proliferation. *J Biol Chem* 2001;276:35290-35296.

17. Yamashiro T, Fukunaga T, Kobshi N, et al: Mechanical stimulation induces CTGF espression in rat osteocytes. *J Dent Res* 2001;80:461-465.

18. Goldspink G: Age-related muscle loss and progressive dysfunction in mechanosensitive growth factor signaling. *Ann NY Acad Sci* 2004;1019:294-298.

19. Yang S, Goldspink G: Different roles of the IGF-I Ec peptide (MGF) and mature IGF-I in myoblast proliferation and differentiation. *FEBS Lett* 2002;522:156-160.

20. Bravenboer N, Engelbergt MJ, Visser NS, Popp-Snijders C, Lips P: The effect of exercise on systemic and bone concentrations of growth factors in rats. *J Orthop Res* 2001;19:945-949.

21. Hering S, Jost C, Schulz H, et al: Circulating transforming growth factor beta1 (TGFbeta1) is elevated by extensive exercise. *Eur J Appl Physiol* 2002;86:406-410.

22. Ontiveros C, McCabe LR: Simulated microgravity suppresses osteoblast phenotype, Runx2 levels and AP-1 transactivation. *J Cell Biochem* 2003;88:427-437.

23. Heckman J, Ryaby J, McCabe J, Frey J, Kilcoyne R: Acceleration of tibial fracture-healing by non-invasive, low-intensity pulsed ultrasound. *J Bone Joint Surg Am* 1994;76:26-34.

24. Kristiansen T, Ryaby J, McCabe J, Frey J, Roe L: Accelerated healing of distal radial fractures with the use of specific low-intensity ultrasound: A multicenter, prospective, randomized, double-blind, placebo-controlled study. *J Bone Joint Surg Am* 1997;79:961-973.

25. Busse JW, Bhandari M, Kulkarni AV, Tunks E: The effect of low-intensity pulsed ultrasound therapy on time to fracture healing: A meta-analysis. *Can Med Assoc J* 2002;166:437-441.

26. Rubin C, Bolander M, Ryaby JP, Hadjiargyrou M: The use of low-intensity ultrasound to accelerate the healing of fractures. *J Bone Joint Surg Am* 2001;83:259-270.

27. Ryaby J, Matthew J, Duarte-Alves P: Low intensity pulsed ultrasound affects adenylate cyclase activity and transforming growth factor beta synthesis. *Trans Orthop Res Soc* 1992;7:590.

28. Ito M, Azuma Y, Ohta T, Komoriya K: Effects of ultrasound and 1,25 dihydroxyvitamin $D_3$ on growth factor secretion in co-culture of osteoblasts and endothelial cells. *Ultrasound Med Biol* 2000;26:161-166.

29. Naruse K, Miyauchi A, Itoman M, Mikuni-Takagaki Y: Distinct anabolic response of osteoblast to low-intensity pulsed ultrasound. *J Bone Miner Res* 2003;18:360-369.

30. Sun JS, Hong RC, Chang WH, et al: In vitro effects of low-intensity ultrasound stimulation on the bone cells. *J Biomed Mater Res* 2001;57:449-456.

31. Kokubu T, Matsui N, Fujioka H, Tsunoda M, Mizuno K: Low intensity pulsed ultrasound exposure increases prostaglandin $E_2$ production via the induction of cyclooxygenase-2 mRNA in mouse osteoblasts. *Biochem Biophys Res Comm* 1999;256: 284-287.

32. Warden SJ: A new direction in ultrasound therapy in sports medicine. *Sports Med* 2003;33:95-107.

33. Warden SJ, Bennell KL, Forwood MR, McKeeken JM, Wark JD: Skeletal effects of low-intensity pulsed ultrasound on the ovarectomized rodent. *Ultrasound Med Biol* 2001;27:989-998.

34. Nelson FR, Brighton CT, Ryaby J, et al: Use of physical forces in bone healing. *J Am Acad Orthop Surg* 2003;11:344-354.

35. Zhuang H, Wang W, Seldes R, Tahernia AD, Fan H, Brighton C: Electrical stimulation induces the level of TGF-b$_1$ mRNA in osteoblastic cells by a mechanism involving calcium/calmodulin pathway. *Biochem Biophys Res Comm* 1997;237:225-229.

36. Bodamyali T, Bhatt B, Hughes F, et al: Pulsed electromagnetic fields induce osteogenesis and upregulate transcription of bone morphogenetic proteins 2 and 4 in rat osteoblasts in vitro. *Biophys Biochem Res Comm* 1998; 250: 458-461.

37. Nagai M, Ota M: Pulsating electromagnetic field stimulates mRNA expression of bone morphogenetic proteins 2 and 4. *J Dent Res* 1994;73:1601-1605.

38. Yajima A, Ochi M, Hirose Y: Effects of pulsing electromagnetic fields on gene expression of bone morphogenetic proteins in human osteoblastic cell line in vitro. *J Bone Mineral Res* 1996;11(suppl):381.

39. Aaron RK, Ciombor DM, Keeping H, Wang S, Polk C: Power frequency fields promote cell differentiation coincident with an increase in transforming TGF-β$_1$ expression. *Bioelectromagnetics* 1999;10:453-458.

40. Lohmann C, Schwarz Z, Liu Y, et al: Pulsed electromagnetic field stimulation of MG63 osteoblast-like cells affects differentiation and local factor production. *J Orthop Res* 2000;18:637-646.

41. Guerkov H, Lohmann C, Liu Y, et al: Pulsed electromagnetic fields increase growth factor release by nonunion cells. *Clin Orthop* 2001;384:265-279.

42. Aaron RK, Wang S, Ciombor DM: Upregulation of basal TGF-b$_1$ levels by EMF coincident with chondrogenesis: Implications of skeletal repair and tissue engineering. *J Orthop Res* 2002;20:233-240.

43. Fitzsimmons RJ, Strong DD, Mohan S, Baylink DJ: Low-amplitude, low-frequency electric field-stimulated bone cell proliferation may in part be mediated by increased IGF-II release. *J Cell Physiol* 1992;150:84-89.

44. Ryaby J, Fitzsimmons RG, Khin NA, Baylink DJ: The role of insulin-like growth factor II in magnetic field regulation of bone formation. *Bioelectrochem Bioenerg* 1994; 35:87-91.

45. Aaron RK, Boyan B, Ciombor DM, Schwartz Z, Simon BJ: Stimulation of growth factor by electric and electromagnetic fields. *Clin Orthop* 2004;419:30-37.

46. Ciombor DM, Aaron RK, Wang S, Simon BJ: Modification of osteoarthritis by pulsed electromagnetic field: A morphological study. *Osteoarthritis Cartilage* 2003;11: 455-462.

47. Tepper OM, Callaghan MJ, Chang EI, et al: Electromagnetic fields increase in vitro and in vivo angiogenesis through endothelial release of FGF-2. *FASEB J* 2004;18: 1231-1233.

# Chapter 14

# Mechanical Loading and Growth Factor Effects on Connective Tissue Metabolism

*R. Lane Smith, PhD*

## Introduction

Connective tissues provide the support structures of the body and are continually subjected to mechanical loads that arise as the result of normal daily activities. Bone is the tissue responsible for the skeletal elements, whereas articular cartilage, tendons, and ligaments enable muscle-driven motion to occur between bony segments. Connective tissue metabolism relies on a dynamic interplay between primary and secondary stimulatory effects generated by mechanical loading and a diversity of physiologic mediators.

Connective tissues detect and process an "effector-stimulus" as a common requirement for mechanical loads and physiologic mediators to functionally alter cellular metabolism. Although the details remain unclear, mechanical loads act directly on connective tissue cells through a process of mechanotransduction with a resultant effect on tissue differentiation, function, and stability.[1,2] Physiologic mediators, such as hormones, growth factors and cytokines, act on connective tissue cells through relatively well-recognized membrane-receptors.[3,4] This chapter examines parameters by which mechanical stimulation and growth factors interact to modulate connective tissue gene expression and protein synthesis.

## Cellular Mechanotransduction

As is the case for all eukaryotic tissues, metabolic control of the cells within tendons, ligaments, bone, and cartilage is achieved through molecule-dependent, conformation-specific signaling pathways.[5,6] The signaling pathways serve to translate events occurring outside the cell into synthetic responses generated inside the cell. The signal recognition process relies on kinases, phosphatases, and nucleotide second messengers to chemically modify the cytoplasmic or nuclear proteins that regulate the genes determining tissue phenotype and metabolic activity. The details of the intracellular pathways vary with the cell type and represent unique aspects of tissue-specific differentiation.

Although the general organization and composition of the cellular membranes of eukaryotic cells are well characterized,[7,8] the precise mechanisms by which integral plasma membrane proteins transduce mechanical stimuli remain unclear. In connective tissues, membrane proteins must interconnect with macromolecules of the adjacent pericellular margin to macromolecules of the more distant extracellular matrix.[9,10] The distances are unlike those of the cardiovascular system, in which endothelial cells and smooth muscle cells react to shear stress or circumferential stress at the plasma membrane.[11] In most connective tissues, cells are isolated from the primary stimulus, being located within an abundant fibrillar collagen matrix in tendons and ligaments or within a mineralized organic matrix in bone. In connective tissues, interactions between plasma membrane receptors and extracellular matrix macromolecules act as conduits to transmit force to the cell and initiate mechanotransduction.

One important aspect of cellular reactivity to mechanical stimulation involves the activity of integrins, specialized integral membrane proteins that extend through the plasma membrane.[12,13] Integrin reactivity serves as a well-developed mechanosensory mechanism by virtue of the proteins having an extracellular domain and a cytoplasmic domain. Integrins consist of alpha and beta subunits assembled from a diverse family of subsets of alpha and beta subunits.[14] The individual integrin protein subunits may then interact selectively both with extracellular matrix molecules, such as fibronectin and laminin, and intracellular cytoskeletal components, such as actin.[15,16] The mixture of alpha and beta subunits may then convey a variety of cell-specific binding behaviors that support cross-talk between different signaling pathways.

One manifestation of integrin-mediated mechanosensory behavior occurs when cells establish focal adhesions.[17] The transmembrane integrin receptors link to the actin cytoskeleton at focal adhesion sites via cytoplasmic domains. Manipulation of the ability of the cells to establish focal adhesions through inhibitors, antibodies, or selective deposition of cell-adhesion binding proteins significantly alters cell viability and metabolism.[18]

## Connective Tissue Loading

Understanding how mechanical loads influence connective tissue metabolism requires categorization of the forces that generate the stress states that cells and tissues experience. Carter and Beaupre[19] described the origin of the forces as being due to intrinsic static forces arising from tissue growth, externally applied forces imposed on the organism, and forces generated by muscle contractions that act on tissues through specific attachments. At a tissue level, the mechanical loads may be characterized as either stress or strain. Stress represents the local intensity of load on a material and is typically expressed as a force per area, such as newtons per square millimeter. Strain represents the normalized measure of local deformation, which implies some change in shape or size.

When loads are applied to cells and tissues, the stress states can be resolved mathematically into two invariants, hydrostatic stress and shear stress.[20] Hydrostatic stress acts uniformly in either compression or tension. Shear stress acting on a tissue characteristically induces a deformation and change in shape. In finite element studies of tissues such as articular cartilage, hydrostatic pressure is distributed uniformly throughout the internal architecture of tissue, whereas shear stress occurs at the boundaries of the cartilage matrix, just adjacent to the underlying subchondral bone.[21] When used to predict and estimate the distribution of load at various anatomic regions, finite element studies show that the distribution of stress and strain correlates with specific tissue types.

The resulting mathematical solutions led Carter and associates[22] to generate a schematic representation in which hydrostatic stress and distortional strain are graphically related to patterns of differentiation of connective tissue. According to their analysis of load distributions, areas of high strain with accompanying compression coincide with the generation of fibrocartilage, whereas areas of only high tensile strain give rise to a purely fibrous tissue. In contrast, high compressive pressure in an environment of low distortional strain is associated with development of cartilage, and low distortional strain with some level of tension is associated with bone formation.

## Growth Factors and Cell Metabolism

Within a conceptual framework in which mechanical loading is recognized as a critical component for connective tissue differentiation, it is important to assess whether specific relationships also exist between the occurrence of different types of load and other physiologic mediators. An expanding array of growth factors and cytokines is currently associated with metabolic changes in bone, articular cartilage, and other connective tissues.[23] Although growth factors and cytokines are recognized as the primary mediators that determine and stabilize unique genetic states, the precise relationship between growth factor expression and the mechanical environment remains less well defined.[24]

Genetic studies confirm that a balance between active and inactive genes determines the cell-specific phenotypes distinguishing embryonic from differentiated tissues, developing from mature organ systems, and healthy from diseased organisms. The "effector-stimulus" for selective gene expression is achieved in part through the actions of tissue-specific growth factors. Growth factors are protein products of multiple gene families that are often relatively small peptides.[25] The active growth factor may or may not be a degradation product of larger precursor proteins. The low molecular weight of the growth factors contributes to their rapid synthesis, transport, and exchange by autocrine, paracrine, or endocrine processes.

Growth factors are now recognized to interact with specific integral membrane protein receptors.[26,27] Membrane receptor binding in turn triggers an intracellular signaling cascade that then alters the metabolic or differentiated state of the recipient cell. The bone-specific factors include the bone morphogenetic proteins (BMPs), insulin-like growth factor-1 (IGF-1), and fibroblast growth factors (FGFs), whereas articular cartilage has a more restricted profile with IGF-1 being most prominent.[28] In the early embryo, gradients of growth factors such as transforming growth factor-beta (TGF-$\beta$) are recognized as the active components setting regional variation, such as the animal and vegetal pole.[29] In the more mature embryo, growth factors are recognized as primary determinants of specialized tissues.

Multiple families of proteins influence connective tissue differentiation, including FGFs, IGFs, TGFs, platelet-derived growth factors, and connective tissue growth factors.[30] Within the transforming growth factor family, subsets of growth factors such as BMPs, TGFs, and growth and differentiation factors act on connective tissues.[31] How these multiple families of proteins shape and maintain connective tissue within different mechanical loading environments is an area of ongoing study.

## Mechanical Stimulation and Connective Tissue Metabolism

A fundamental characteristic of interactions between mechanical stimulation and growth factors on connective tissues is that force alone is sufficient to modify cellular metabolism. The presence of exogenously added growth factors is not absolutely necessary to influence connective tissue differentiation or metabolism. In experiments with bone marrow-derived cells, mechanical stimulation induced collagen type I fiber bundles characteristic of ligament morphology in the absence of exogenously added growth factors.[32] In this model, mRNA expression of collagen type I and III was accompanied by an increase in tenascin-C mRNA as a marker of ligament cells. However, it remains to be determined whether the extent to which loading exerts effects on cell metabolism may involve intracellular autocrine-like effects through endogenous growth factor expression. Within the context of applying homogeneous types of load, shear stress and hydrostatic pressure functionally alter the metabolism of articular chondrocytes. In vivo, altering the balance between each of these types of load may be a critical component in the shift from a normal cartilage phenotype to one characteristic of tissue damage observed in osteoarthritis.[33]

Onset and progression of cartilage degeneration appear to be associated with increased levels of stress when diarthrodial joints are subjected to inappropriate loading.[34] The cause may be traumatic injury, damage to normal joint structures, or misalignment. Experiments with chondrocytes in culture show that shear stress induces the expression of the proinflammatory cytokine interleukin-6, prostaglandin $E_2$ ($PGE_2$), and tissue inhibitor of metalloproteinase-1.[35,36] Analysis of dose-dependent effects of shear stress on bovine and human osteoarthritic chondrocytes showed that increased levels of shear stress are accompanied by increased release of nitric oxide (NO).[37,38] Induction of NO release from normal bovine chondrocytes by shear stress is blocked by inhibitors of the inducible form of NO synthase and by inhibitors of G-protein signaling.[37] However, NO release could not be completely reduced, suggesting that multiple signaling pathways are involved in the chondrocyte response to shear stress.

With human osteoarthritic chondrocytes in culture, shear stress at a level of 1.64 Pa increases NO release by 1.8-, 2.4-, and 3.5-fold at 2, 6, and 24 hours respectively.[38] Shear stress also increases NO synthase gene expression. Exposure of chondrocytes to shear stress for 2, 6, and 24 hours inhibits type II collagen mRNA signal levels by 27%, 18%, and 20% respectively after a constant postshear incubation period of 24 hours. Aggrecan mRNA signal levels were inhibited by 30%, 32%, and 41% under identical conditions. Addition of a NO antagonist increased type II collagen mRNA signal levels by an average of 1.8-fold (137% of the unsheared control) and reestablished the aggrecan mRNA signal levels by an average of 1.4-fold after shear stress (92% of the unsheared control) (ANOVA $P < 0.05$).

The application of shear stress to osteoarthritic chondrocytes in culture is accompanied by an increase in apoptosis as evidenced by presentation of membrane phosphatidylserine and nucleosomal degradation.[39] Increases in apoptosis are accompanied by a decrease in the expression of the antiapoptotic factor Bcl-2. NO antagonists L-N(5)-(1-iminoethyl) ornithine and N-omega-nitro-L-arginine methyl ester (L-NAME) reduce shear stress-induced nucleosomal degradation by 62% and 74% respectively. Inhibition of shear stress-induced NO release by L-NAME coincided with a 2.7-fold increase of Bcl-2 when compared with chondrocytes exposed to shear stress in the absence of L-NAME.

Studies of chondrocytes in cartilage explants from 2- to 3-year-old pigs exposed to unconfined intermittent compression show that the proinflammatory mediators $PGE_2$ and NO are unregulated in response to loading.[40] The release of both proinflammatory molecules follows the magnitude of applied stress. Addition of a cyclooxygenase-2 (COX-2) inhibitor effectively decreased the release of both proinflammatory mediators. In this system, addition of an inhibitor of NO synthase increased the release of $PGE_2$ and expression of the COX-2 enzyme. These data show that modulation of loading environment and addition of pharmacologic agents that act on soluble mediators effectively alter chondrocyte metabolism.

## Mechanical Loading and Bone Metabolism

Some of the earliest experiments addressing the interactions between loading and tissue differentiation used fetal mouse calvarial culture systems that were exposed to intermittent compressive forces.[41] The experiments showed that applying a compressive load induced increased release of collagenase-digestible protein and decreased osteoclastic precursor cells in bone marrow cultures. Similarly, an experiment carried out with rat osteocytes showed that a single 10-minute episode of mechanical stimulation in the vertebrae of rats was sufficient to induce IGF-1 mRNA in all osteocytes localized within the diaphysis cortex and metaphyseal trabecular bone.[42] The increase in the IGF-1 signaling preceded mRNA expression for type I collagen.

In other studies with isolated bone cells, osteocytes maintained under static loading and in low serum were sixfold more likely to undergo apoptosis when compared with periosteal fibroblasts or threefold more likely when compared with osteoblasts cultured under similar conditions.[43] Exposure of the osteocytes with shear stress reduced the number of serum-starved osteocytes that exhibited phosphatidylserine on the cell surface as a marker for onset of apoptosis. Exposure to shear stress also increased mRNA for the cell survival protein Bcl-2 in a dose-dependent manner. These data show that mechanical stimulation promotes osteocyte survival and supports the hypothesis that bone organization may be altered by the onset of cell death in the absence of loading.

Of particular interest with respect to bone cell metabolism, recent studies have shown that signaling centers in epithelial tissues express factors that participate in cranial facial growth and patterning.[44,45] The interactions between signaling proteins such as Sonic Hedgehog (SHH) and a cell surface receptor, patched, are necessary for cell survival. The regulation of cellular viability dictates in large part the morphogenetic pattern for the developing tissues. There is evidence that some of the signaling processes for the SHH pathway are sensitive to application of mechanical loading.[46,47] These pathways may involve a family of extracellular proteins, the Wnt proteins, whose occupancy of cell-surface receptors modulates bone cell differentiation.[48,49]

The process of distraction osteogenesis represents one of the most dramatic examples of the interplay between mechanical stimulation and bone metabolism. In distraction osteogenesis, bone lengthening follows a gradual longitudinal expansion of a fracture callus that is created by a resection of the bone outer cortex to create a fracture-like bony separation.[50,51] Although the technique is recognized to be dependent on preservation of periosteal tissue and the blood supply to the bone, recent studies show that the role of growth factors in the outcome is becoming increasingly apparent.[52,53] The rate at which the bones are pulled apart is generally 1 mm per day. This mechanical stretching of the tissues is hypothesized to induce a fibroblastic response by undifferentiated mesenchymal cells and to create a hypoxic environment. The change in the local tissue environment is then followed by differentiation of the cells into a bone phenotype so that mineralization of the tissue occurs. The mineralization of the tissue is associated with an increase in vascularity and a return to an aerobic environment.

Distraction osteogenesis is accompanied by the selective expression of growth factors that coincides with the appearance of distinct zones of tissue differentiation and localized protein concentration. Expression of BMP-2 and -4 occurs at the onset of distraction and during early callus elongation in a rat model of femoral lengthening.[54] In the rabbit, increased expression of BMP-2 and -4 in the fracture callus is accompanied by expression of BMP-7 in regions associated with precursor cells.[55] In contrast to the BMPs, other growth factors—such as FGF-2 and TGF-β—were associated with the primary mineralization front, where the osteoblastic activity was high. Growth factor expression is upregulated by mechanical strain with the level of expression influenced by the distraction rate.[56] In some systems, patterns of growth factor expression are overlapping with angiogenic factors—such as vascular endothelial growth factor—that are present in association with osteoblastic factors such as BMP-2 and BMP-4.[57]

Analysis of bone formation in distraction osteogenesis demonstrates the importance of mechanical stress as stimulus to the tissues surrounding fracture sites. The strain imposed on the cells alters the release of growth factors and contributes to progenitor cell recruitment, vessel formation, and mineralization. The extent to which the growth factors may be applied exogenously to accelerate or improve structural strength of the developing bone remains an area of investigation. Delivery of bone-specific growth factors either within an implantable matrix or through gene therapy appears to be a useful adjunctive therapy.[58,59]

The goal of these approaches is to accelerate the rate at which the bone lengthening process is conducted or to improve outcomes with compromised tissues, such as postinfection or traumatic nonunions. Not all mechanical stimulation is advantageous to connective tissue metabolism. In fracture healing, larger interfragmentary movements resulted in more fibrocartilage formation and less bone formation.[60] This observation is consistent with results showing that shear movement at diaphyseal osteotomy sites reduced bridging of the osteotomy fragments by 40% and reduced peripheral callus formation by 36% compared with axial movement.[61] Allowing only axial motion with fracture fixation increased mechanical rigidity threefold compared with fixation in which shear movement occurred.

The bone response to mechanical loading has long been associated with changes in morphology and strength. Lack of skeletal loading is associated with decreased bone mineral density and increased resorption.[62,63] The mechanism by which this occurs involves suppression of the bone-forming osteoblastic activity,[64,65] and when there is a concomitant increase in inflammation, the numbers of bone-resorbing cells—the osteoclasts—are also increased.[66] The bone cell reaction to changes in the mechanical environment depends in part on fluctuations in fluid flow that result in changes in intracellular calcium concentrations.[67] A prominent working hypothesis is that the canaliculi extending from osteocytes within the mineralized matrix are the conduits for transmission of the localized stress states.[68]

Effects of calcium on bone cell metabolism result from release of intracellular calcium in contrast to uptake of calcium through membrane channels.[69] A study on the effects of fluid-induced shear induction of COX-2 showed that translocation of NFκB into the nucleus was necessary for protein expression.[70] Prevention of calcium entry into the cells did not alter NFκB translocation. However, addition of an intracellular calcium chelator or inhibition of phospholipase-C-dependent intracellular calcium release completely blocked the effect of shear stress on NFκB translocation. Other intracellular signaling pathways implicated in bone mechanotransduction include membrane ion channels, nicotinamide adenine dinucleotide levels, adenosine triphosphate, prostanoid receptors, and NO.[71] Bone signaling pathways are hypothesized to involve a desensitization of cell receptors that reduces anabolism so that rest periods may be necessary to maintain bone strength.[72]

## Mechanical Stimulation of Articular Cartilage Metabolism

A number of experimental approaches document that cartilage cells respond to mechanical loads under in vitro testing conditions. Efforts to test the effects of repetitive loads that vary with magnitude and frequency of loading have applied forces by compression, stretching, or gas pressurization.[73,74] In explant culture, chondrocytes remain localized within the native cartilage matrix and react to both the type and the level of applied load.[75-77] In culture, static compression inhibits glycosaminoglycan synthesis and decreases amino acid uptake according to the geometry of loading.[78] In closely controlled companion trials, where effects of strictly static compressive loads were compared with effects of repetitive loads, the cartilage response correlated best with definite maxima and minima for cyclic loading.[79]

Intermittent compressive forces alter histomorphometric parameters of the chondrocytes, including intracellular parameters such as nuclear size and extracellular formation of cellular aggregates.[80] Isolated chondrocytes also respond to compressive forces with alteration in the uptake of $^3$H-thymidine incorporation, an indicator of changes in proliferative capacity of the cells.[81] Favorable effects of joint motion and loading on cartilage were observed in vivo using free autogenous periosteal grafts to repair full-thickness cartilage defects where continuous passive motion increased neochondrogenesis.[82] A general conclusion arising from experimental loading of chondrogenic tissue is that the cellular response, whether inhibitory or synthetic, varies directly with the type and level of stress applied, the age of the cells, and the presence or absence of growth factors.[83,84]

## Hydrostatic Pressure and Articular Chondrocyte Metabolism

Hydrostatic pressure is the predominant type of load to which chondrocytes are exposed in a normally loaded diarthrodial joint. Direct measurement has documented levels of hydrostatic pressure in the range of 7 to 8 MPa but can reach as high as 12 MPa during the walking cycle.[85] Hall and associates[86] established that hydrostatic pressure at levels of 5 to 15 MPa alters radiolabeled sulfate and proline incorporation rates in adult bovine articular cartilage in vitro. Finite element studies by Wong and Carter[87] and in vitro organ culture experiments of Klein-Nulend and associates[88] demonstrate that sites of proteoglycan production coincide with regions of pure hydrostatic pressure.

Normal bovine articular chondrocytes respond to application of intermittent hydrostatic pressure through an increase in expression of aggrecan and type II collagen.[89,90] When bovine articular chondrocytes in high-density monolayers or as aggregated clusters were exposed to intermittent hydrostatic pressure at a level of 10 MPa and at a frequency of 1 Hz, the results showed that type II collagen mRNA signal levels exhibited a biphasic pattern in response to continuously applied pressure for periods of 2, 4, 8, 12, and 24 hours. Type II collagen mRNA signal initially increased approximately fivefold at 4 and 8 hours and subsequently decreased by 24 hours. In contrast, aggrecan mRNA signal increased progressively up to threefold throughout the loading period. Changing the loading profile to 4 hours per day for 4 days increased the mRNA signal levels for type II collagen ninefold and for aggrecan 20-fold when compared with unloaded cultures.

In a separate set of experiments,[91] normal human articular chondrocytes were isolated from knee cartilage and maintained as primary, high-density monolayer cultures. Intermittent hydrostatic pressure was applied at magnitudes of 1, 5, and 10 MPa at 1 Hz for a duration of either 4 hours per day for 1 day (4 × 1) or 4 hours per day for 4 days (4 × 4). Total cellular RNA was isolated and analyzed for aggrecan and type II collagen mRNA signal levels using specific primers and reverse transcription polymerase chain reaction nested with beta-actin primers as internal controls. With the 4 × 1 loading regimen, aggrecan mRNA signal levels increased 1.3- and 1.5-fold relative to beta-actin mRNA after exposure to 5 and 10 MPa respectively when compared with unloaded cultures. With the 4 × 4 loading regimen, aggrecan mRNA signal levels increased 1.4-, 1.8-, and 1.9-fold at loads of 1, 5, and 10 MPa respectively. In contrast to the effects of hydrostatic pressure on aggrecan, type II collagen mRNA signal levels were only increased after exposure to 5 and 10 MPa with the 4 × 4 loading regimen. Detection of cell-associated proteins by Western blotting confirmed that aggrecan and type II collagen were increased in the chondrocyte extracts. In these experiments, both duration and magnitude of applied hydrostatic pressure differentially altered cartilage matrix protein expression.

Intermittent hydrostatic pressure also counteracts effects of shear stress and the inflammatory mediator bacterial lipopolysaccharide (LPS) on chondrocyte metabolism.[92,93] Intermittent hydrostatic pressure was applied at 10 MPa for 4 hours to human chondrocytes pretreated with LPS (1 µg/mL for 18 hours). LPS exposure decreased mRNA signal levels for type II collagen by 67% and aggrecan by 56%, and increased NO 3.1-fold. In addition, LPS increased monocyte chemotactic protein-1 mRNA signal levels 6.5-fold and matrix metalloproteinase-2 mRNA signal levels 1.3-fold. Application of IHP to shear stress- or LPS-activated chondrocytes decreased NO synthase mRNA signal levels and NO levels in the culture medium. Exposure of LPS-treated chondrocytes to hydrostatic pressure partially restored the type II collagen and aggrecan mRNA signal levels approximately 1.7-fold relative to chondrocytes treated with LPS and maintained without loading. In addition, application of hydrostatic pressure decreased mRNA signal levels of monocyte chemotactic factor-1 and matrix metalloproteinase-2 after LPS treatment by 45% and 15% respectively.

## Mechanical Loading and Intracellular Signaling Pathways in Chondrocytes

Mechanical loads alter chondrocyte metabolism through activation of specific intracellular kinase pathways depending on the type of load applied.[94] Compressive loading induces a phased phosphorylation of the extracellular regulated kinases 1 and 2 (ERK 1/2) where ERK 2 exhibits a persistent phosphorylated state for up to 24 hours.[95] Other kinases—p38 mitogen-activated kinase (p38) and a member of c-Jun N-terminal kinase pathway (SEK-1)—exhibited more transient responses (10 minutes to 1 hour). A similar pattern of ERK 1/2 activation has been demonstrated in other studies of chondrocyte responses to shear stress; this pattern coincides with an increase in expression of cytokines and a decrease in matrix protein synthesis.[96]

Mechanical signaling events that activate or suppress gene expression involve regulatory transcription factors that bind to the promoter sequences as enhancers or suppressors of protein expression.[97,98] Expression of type II collagen in growing cartilage is associated with the presence of the transcription factor SOX-9, but in adult tissue there is a shift in the dependence of type II collagen expression on this protein.[99,100] With respect to the chondrocyte response to mechanical loading, a limited series of transcription factors have been studied. Hydrostatic pressure increases transcription factor activation,[101] and shear stress is implicated in the translocation of the signal transducer and activator of transcription (STAT) proteins.[102] However, the major transcription factors studied in chondrocytes are those closely associated with the onset of proinflammatory mediator and matrix metalloproteinase release.

## Summary

The results reviewed here demonstrate that connective tissues react to and are dependent on appropriate and specific regimens of mechanical loading for normal differentiation and homeostasis. Major questions remain regarding the precise basis by which mechanotransduction influences the steady-state control of extracellular matrix stability. Other important questions concern the processes by which interacting effects of mechanical loads and growth factors drive the recruitment and maturation of early progenitor cells in development and in tissue repair following injury and disease. The advent of new protein targets as a result of information gained from genomic studies of human and animal models is expected to further expand our understanding of how mechanical loads and growth factors maintain connective tissue structure and function.

## Acknowledgments

This work was supported in part by NIH grant AR45788, a VA Medical Merit grant, and a VA Research Career Award.

## References

1. Silver FH, Siperko LM: Mechanosensing and mechanochemical transduction: How is mechanical energy sensed and converted into chemical energy in an extracellular matrix? *Crit Rev Biomed Eng* 2003;31:255-331.

2. Bershadsky AD, Balaban NQ, Geiger B: Adhesion-dependent mechanosensitivity. *Annu Rev Cell Dev Biol* 2003;19:677-695.

3. Schlessinger J: Common and distinct elements in cellular signaling via EGF and FGF receptors. *Science* 2004;306:1506-1507.

4. Janmey PA: The cytoskeleton and cell signaling: Component localization and mechanical coupling. *Physiol Rev* 1998;78:763-781.

5. Shi Y, Massague J: Mechanisms of TGF-beta signaling from cell membrane to the nucleus. *Cell* 2003;113:685-700.

6. Chang W, Tu C, Chen TH, et al: Expression and signal transduction of calcium-sensing receptors in cartilage and bone. *Endocrinology* 1999;140:5883-5893.

7. Vereb G, Szollosi J, Matko J, et al: Dynamic, yet structured: The cell membrane three decades after the Singer-Nicolson model. *Proc Natl Acad Sci USA* 2003;100: 8053-8058.

8. Jacobson K, Sheets ED, Simon R: Revisiting the fluid mosaic model of membranes. *Science* 1995;268:1441-1442.

9. Chen CS, Tan J Tien J: Mechanotransduction at cell-matrix and cell-cell contacts. *Annu Rev Biomed Eng* 2004;6:275-302.

10. Alahari SK, Reddig PJ, Juliano RL: Biological aspects of signal transduction by cell adhesion receptors. *Int Rev Cytol* 2002;220:145-184.

11. Chen KD, Li YS, Kim M, et al: Mechanotransduction in response to shear stress: Roles of receptor tyrosine kinases, integrins, and Shc. *J Biol Chem* 1999;274: 18393-18400.

12. Millward-Sadler SJ, Salter DM: Integrin-dependent cascades in chondrocyte mechanotransduction. *Ann Biomed Eng* 2004;32:435-446.

13. Loeser RF: Integrins and cell signaling in chondrocytes. *Biorheology* 2002;39:119-124.

14. Springer TA, Wang JH: The three-dimensional structure of integrins and their ligands, and conformational regulation of cell adhesion. *Cell Mol Life Sci* 2000;57:1272-1286.

15. Weyts FA, Li YS, van Leeuwen J, Weinans H, Chien S: ERK activation and alpha v beta 3 integrin signaling through Shc recruitment in response to mechanical stimulation in human osteoblasts. *J Cell Biochem* 2002;87:85-92.

16. Coussen F, Choquet D, Sheetz MP, Erickson HP: Trimers of the fibronectin cell adhesion domain localize to actin filament bundles and undergo rearward translocation. *J Cell Sci* 2002;115:2581-2590.

17. Wozniak MA, Modzelewska K, Kwong L, Keely PJ: Focal adhesion regulation of cell behavior. *Biochim Biophys Acta* 2004;1692:103-119.

18. Wehrle-Haller B, Imhof B: The inner lives of focal adhesions. *Trends Cell Biol* 2002;12:382-389.

19. Carter DR, Beaupre GS: *Skeletal Function and Form: Mechanobiology of Skeletal Development, Aging and Regeneration.* Cambridge, England, Cambridge University Press, 2001, pp 40-47.

20. Carter DR, Orr TE, Fyhrie DP, Schurman DJ: Influence of mechanical stress on prenatal and postnatal skeletal development. *Clin Orthop* 1987;219:237-250.

21. Beaupre GS, Stevens SS, Carter DR: Mechanobiology in the development, maintenance, and degeneration of articular cartilage. *J Rehabil Res Dev* 2000;37:145-151.

22. Carter DR, Beaupre GS, Giori NJ, Helms JA: Mechanobiology of skeletal regeneration. *Clin Orthop* 1998;355:S41-S55.

23. Wozney JM, Rosen V: Bone morphogenetic protein and bone morphogenetic protein gene family in bone formation and repair. *Clin Orthop* 1998;346:26-37.

24. Chubinskaya S, Kuettner KE: Regulation of osteogenic proteins by chondrocytes. *Int J Biochem Cell Biol* 2003;35:1323-1340.

25. Reddi AH: Interplay between bone morphogenetic proteins and cognate binding proteins in bone and cartilage development: noggin, chordin and DAN. *Arthritis Res* 2001;3:1-5.

26. van den Berg WB, van der Kraan PM, Scharstuhl A, van Beuningen HM: Growth factors and cartilage repair. *Clin Orthop* 2001;391:S244-S250.

27. Hoffmann A, Gross G: BMP signaling pathways in cartilage and bone formation. *Crit Rev Eukaryot Gene Expr* 2001;11:23-45.

28. Dupont J, Holzenberger M: Biology of insulin-like growth factors in development. *Birth Defects Res C Embryo Today* 2003;69:257-271.

29. Chan AP, Etkin LD: Patterning and lineage specification in the amphibian embryo. *Curr Top Dev Biol* 2001;51:1-67.

30. O'Connor WJ, Botti T, Khan SN, Lane JM: The use of growth factors in cartilage repair. *Orthop Clin North Am* 2000;31:399-410.

31. Buxton P, Edwards C, Archer CW, Francis-West P: Growth/differentiation factor-5 (GDF-5) and skeletal development. *J Bone Joint Surg Am* 2001;83:S23-S30.

32. Altman GH, Horan RL, Martin I, et al: Cell differentiation by mechanical stress. *FASEB J* 2002;16:270-272.

33. Wilson W, van Rietbergen B, van Donkelaar CC, Huiskes R: Pathways of load-induced cartilage damage causing cartilage degeneration in the knee after meniscectomy. *J Biomech* 2003;36:845-851.

34. Andriacchi TP, Munderman A, Smith RL, Alexander EJ, Dyrby CO, Koo S: A framework for the in vivo pathomechanics of osteoarthritis at the knee. *Ann Biomed Eng* 2004;32:447-457.

35. Smith RL, Donlon BS, Gupta MK, et al: Effects of fluid-induced shear on articular chondrocyte morphology and metabolism in vitro. *J Orthop Res* 1995;13:824-831.

36. Mohtai M, Gupta MK, Donlon B, et al: Expression of interleukin-6 in osteoarthritic chondrocytes and effects of fluid-induced shear on this expression in normal human chondrocytes in vitro. *J Orthop Res* 1996;14:67-73.

37. Das P, Schurman DJ, Smith RL: Nitric oxide and G proteins mediate the response of bovine articular chondrocytes to fluid-induced shear. *J Orthop Res* 1997;15:87-93.

38. Lee MS, Trindade MC, Ikenoue T, Schurman DJ, Goodman SB, Smith RL: Effects of shear stress on nitric oxide and matrix protein gene expression in human osteoarthritic chondrocytes in vitro. *J Orthop Res* 2002;20:556-561.

39. Lee MS, Trindade MC, Ikenoue T, Goodman SB, Schurman DJ, Smith RL: Regulation of nitric oxide and bcl-2 expression by shear stress in human osteoarthritic chondrocytes in vitro. *J Cell Biochem* 2003;90:80-86.

40. Fermor B, Weinberg JB, Pisetsky DS, Misukonis MA, Fink C, Guilak F: Induction of cyclooxygenase-2 by mechanical stress through a nitric oxide-regulated pathway. *Osteoarthritis Cartilage* 2002;10:792-798.

41. Klein-Nulend J, Semeins CM, Veldhuijzen JP, Burger EH: Effect of mechanical stimulation on the production of soluble bone factors in cultured fetal mouse calvariae. *Cell Tissue Res* 1993;271:513-517.

42. Lean JM, Jagger CJ, Chambers TJ, Chow JW: Increased insulin-like growth factor I mRNA expression in rat osteocytes in response to mechanical stimulation. *Am J Physiol* 1995;268:E318-E327.

43. Bakker A, Klein-Nulend J, Burger E: Shear stress inhibits while disuse promotes osteocyte apoptosis. *Biochem Biophys Res Commun* 2004;320:1163-1168.

44. Helms JA, Schneider RA: Cranial skeletal biology. *Nature* 2003;423:326-331.

45. Hu D, Helms JA: The role of sonic hedgehog in normal and abnormal craniofacial morphogenesis. *Development* 1999;126:4873-4884.

46. Helms JA, Kim CH, Hu D, Minkoff R, Thaller C, Eichele G: Sonic hedgehog participates in craniofacial morphogenesis and is down-regulated by teratogenic doses of retinoic acid. *Dev Biol* 1997;187:25-35.

47. Wu Q, Zhang Y, Chen Q: Indian hedgehog is an essential component of mechanotransduction complex to stimulate chondrocyte proliferation. *J Biol Chem* 2001;276: 35290-35296.

48. de Boer J, Siddappa R, Gaspar C, van Apeldoorn A, Fodde R, van Blitterswijk C: Wnt signaling inhibits osteogenic differentiation of human mesenchymal stem cells. *Bone* 2004;34:818-826.

49. Derfoul A, Carlberg AL, Tuan RS, Hall DJ: Differential regulation of osteogenic marker gene expression by Wnt-3a in embryonic mesenchymal multipotential progenitor cells. *Differentiation* 2004;72:209-223.

50. Ilizarov GA: The tension-stress effect on the genesis and growth of tissues: Part I. The influence of stability of fixation and soft-tissue preservation. *Clin Orthop* 1989;238: 249-281.

51. Ilizarov GA: The tension-stress effect on the genesis and growth of tissues: Part II. The influence of rate and frequency of distraction. *Clin Orthop* 1989;238:263-285.

52. Aronson J: Temporal and spatial increases in blood flow during distraction osteogenesis. *Clin Orthop* 1994;301:124-131.

53. Sato M, Ochi T, Nakase T, et al: Mechanical tension-stress induces expression of bone morphogenetic protein (BMP)-2 and BMP-4, but not BMP-6, BMP-7, and GDF-5 mRNA, during distraction osteogenesis. *J Bone Miner Res* 2000;14:1084-1095.

54. Cho T-J, Choi IH, Chung CY, Park SS, Park YK: Temporal and spatial expression of bone morphogenetic protein-2 and -4 mRNA in distraction osteogenesis and fracture healing. *J Korean Orthop Assoc* 1998;33:595-605.

55. Rauch F, Lauzier D, Croteau S, Travers R, Glorieux FH, Handy R: Temporal and spatial expression of bone morphogenetic protein-2, -4, and -7 during distraction osteogenesis in rabbits. *Bone* 2000;27:453-459.

56. Weiss S, Baumgart R, Jochum M, Strasburger CJ, Bidlingmaier M: Systemic regulation of distraction osteogenesis: A cascade of biochemical factors. *J Bone Miner Res* 2002;17:1280-1289.

57. Yeung HY, Lee KM, Fung KP, Leung KS: Sustained expression of transforming growth factor-beta1 by distraction during distraction osteogenesis. *Life Sci* 2002;71: 67-79.

58. Yang X, Tare RS, Partridge KA, et al: Induction of human osteoprogenitor chemotaxis, proliferation, differentiation, and bone formation by osteoblast stimulating factor-1/pleiotrophin: Osteoconductive biomimetic scaffolds for tissue engineering. *J Bone Miner Res* 2003;18:47-57.

59. Luk KD, Chen Y, Cheung KM, Kung HF, Lu WW, Leong JC: Adeno-associated virus-mediated bone morphogenetic protein-4 gene therapy for in vivo bone formation. *Biochem Biophys Res Commun* 2003;308:636-645.

60. Claes L, Eckert-Hubner K, Augat P: The effect of mechanical stability on local vascularization and tissue differentiation in callus healing. *J Orthop Res* 2002;20:1099-1105.

61. Augat P, Burger J, Schorlemmer S, Henke T, Perous M, Claes L: Shear movement at the fracture site delays healing in a diaphyseal fracture model. *J Orthop Res* 2003;21: 1011-1017.

62. Bikle DD, Sakata T, Halloran BP: The impact of skeletal unloading on bone formation. *Gravit Space Biol Bull* 2003;16:45-54.

63. Bailon-Plaza A, van der Meulen MC: Beneficial effects of moderate, early loading and adverse effects of delayed or excessive loading on bone healing. *J Biomech* 2003;36:1069-1077.

64. Halloran BP, Bikle DD, Harris J, et al: Skeletal unloading induces selective resistance to the anabolic actions of growth hormone on bone. *J Bone Miner Res* 1995;10:1168-1176.

65. Ontiveros C, McCabe LR: Simulated microgravity suppresses osteoblast phenotype, Runx2 levels and AP-1 transactivation. *J Cell Biochem* 2003;88:427-437.

66. Goldring SR: Inflammatory mediators as essential elements in bone remodeling. *Calcif Tissue Int* 2003;73:97-100.

67. Mullender M, El Haj AJ, Yang Y, van Duin MA, Burger EH, Klein-Nulend J: Mechanotransduction of bone cells in vitro: Mechanobiology of bone tissue. *Med Biol Eng Comput* 2004;42:14-21.

68. Weinbaum S, Cowin SC, Zeng Y: A model for the excitation of osteocytes by mechanical loading-induced bone fluid shear stresses. *J Biomech* 1994;27:339-360.

69. Jacobs CR, Yellowley CE, Davis BR, Zhou Z, Cimbala JM, Donahue HJ: Differential effect of steady versus oscillating flow on bone cells. *J Biomech* 1998;31:969-976.

70. Chen NX, Geist DJ, Genetos DC, Pavalko FM, Duncan RL: Fluid shear-induced NFkappaB translocation in osteoblasts is mediated by intracellular calcium release. *Bone* 2003;33:399-410.

71. Romanello M, Bicego M, Pirulli D, Crovella S, Moro L, D'Andrea P: Extracellular NAD+: A novel autocrine/paracrine signal in osteoblast physiology. *Biochem Biophys Res Commun* 2002;299:424-431.

72. Turner CH, Robling AG: Exercise as an anabolic stimulus for bone. *Curr Pharm Des* 2004;10:2629-2641.

73. Suh JK, Li Z, Woo SL: Dynamic behavior of a biphasic cartilage model under cyclic compressive loading. *J Biomech* 1995;28:357-364.

74. Kim YJ, Bonassar LJ, Grodzinsky AJ: The role of cartilage streaming potential, fluid flow and pressure in the stimulation of chondrocyte biosynthesis during dynamic compression. *J Biomech* 1995;28:1055-1066.

75. Guilak F, Meyer BC, Ratcliffe A, Mow VC: The effects of matrix compression on proteoglycan metabolism in articular cartilage explants. *Osteoarthritis Cartilage* 1994;2:91-101.

76. Kurz B, Jin M, Patwari P, Cheng DM, Lark MW, Grodzinsky AJ: Biosynthetic response and mechanical properties of articular cartilage after injurious compression. *J Orthop Res* 2001;19:1140-1146.

77. Li KW, Williamson AK, Wang AS, Sah RL: Growth responses of cartilage to static and dynamic compression. *Clin Orthop* 2001;391:S34-S48.

78. Ragan PM, Badger AM, Cook M, et al: Down-regulation of chondrocyte aggrecan and type-II collagen gene expression correlates with increases in static compression magnitude and duration. *J Orthop Res* 1999;17:836-842.

79. Sah RL, Kim YJ, Doong JY, Grodzinsky AJ, Plaas AH, Sandy JD: Biosynthetic response of cartilage explants to dynamic compression. *J Orthop Res* 1989;7:619-636.

80. Guilak F, Ratcliffe A, Mow VC: Chondrocyte deformation and local tissue strain in articular cartilage: A confocal microscopy study. *J Orthop Res* 1995;13:410-421.

81. Li KW, Falcovitz YH, Nagrampa JP, et al: Mechanical compression modulates proliferation of transplanted chondrocytes. *J Orthop Res* 2000;18:374-382.

82. O'Driscoll SW, Keeley FW, Salter RB: The chondrogenic potential of free autogenous periosteal grafts for biological resurfacing of major full-thickness defects in joint surfaces under the influence of continuous passive motion: An experimental investigation in the rabbit. *J Bone Joint Surg Am* 1986;68:1017-1035.

83. Bonasser LJ, Grodzinsky AJ, Frank EH, Davila SG, Bhaktav NR: The effect of dynamic compression on the response of articular cartilage to insulin-like growth factor-I. *J Orthop Res* 2001;19:11-17.

84. Bonasser LJ, Grodzinsky AJ, Srinivasan A, Davila SG, Trippel SB: Mechanical and physicochemical regulation of the action of insulin-like growth factor-I on articular cartilage. *Arch Biochem Biophys* 2000;379:57-63.

85. Hodge WA, Fijan RS, Carlson KL, Burgess RG, Harris WH, Mann RW: Contact pressures in the human hip joint measured in vivo. *Proc Natl Acad Sci USA* 1986;83:2879-2883.

86. Hall AC, Urban JP, Gehl KA: The effects of hydrostatic pressure on matrix synthesis in articular cartilage. *J Orthop Res* 1991;9:1-10.

87. Wong M, Carter DR: Theoretical stress analysis of organ culture osteogenesis. Bone 1990;11:127-131.

88. Klein-Nulend J, Veldhuijzen JP, van de Stadt RJ, van Kampen GP, Kuijer R, Burger EH: Influence of intermittent compressive force on proteoglycan content in calcifying growth plate cartilage in vitro. *J Biol Chem* 1987;262:15490-15495.

89. Smith RL, Rusk SF, Ellison BE, et al: In vitro stimulation of articular chondrocyte mRNA and extracellular matrix synthesis by hydrostatic pressure. *J Orthop Res* 1996;14:53-60.

90. Smith RL, Lin J, Trindade MC, et al: Time-dependent effects of intermittent hydrostatic pressure on articular chondrocyte type II collagen and aggrecan mRNA expression. *J Rehabil Res Dev* 2000;37:153-161.

91. Ikenoue T, Trindade MC, Lee MS, et al: Mechanoregulation of human articular chondrocyte aggrecan and type II collagen expression by intermittent hydrostatic pressure in vitro. *J Orthop Res* 2003;21:110-116.

92. Lee MS, Trindade MC, Ikenoue T, Schurman DJ, Goodman SB, Smith RL: Intermittent hydrostatic pressure inhibits shear stress-induced nitric oxide release in human osteoarthritic chondrocytes in vitro. *J Rheumatol* 2003;30:326-328.

93. Lee MS, Ikenoue T, Trindade MC, et al: Protective effects of intermittent hydrostatic pressure on osteoarthritic chondrocytes activated by bacterial endotoxin in vitro. *J Orthop Res* 2003;21:117-122.

94. Hung CT, Henshaw DR, Wang CC, et al: Mitogen-activated protein kinase signaling in bovine articular chondrocytes in response to fluid flow does not require calcium mobilization. *J Biomech* 2000;33:73-80.

95. Fanning PJ, Emkey G, Smith RJ, Grodzinsky AJ, Szasz N, Trippel SB: Mechanical regulation of mitogen-activated protein kinase signaling in articular cartilage. *J Biol Chem* 2003;278:50940-50948

96. Li KW, Wang AS, Sah RL: Microenvironment regulation of extracellular signal-regulated kinase activity in chondrocytes: Effects of culture configuration, interleukin-1, and compressive stress. *Arthritis Rheum* 2003;48:689-699.

97. de Crombrugghe B, Lefebvre V, Nakashima K: Regulatory mechanisms in the pathways of cartilage and bone formation. *Curr Opin Cell Biol* 2001;13:721-727.

98. Akiyama H, Chaboissier MC, Martin JF, Schedl A, de Crombrugghe B: The transcription factor Sox9 has essential roles in successive steps of the chondrocyte differentiation pathway and is required for expression of Sox5 and Sox6. *Genes Dev* 2002;16:2813-2828.

99. Stokes DG, Liu G, Dharmavaram R, Hawkins D, Piera-Velazquez S, Jimenez SA: Regulation of type-II collagen gene expression during human chondrocyte de-differentiation and recovery of chondrocyte-specific phenotype in culture involves Sry-type high-mobility-group box (SOX) transcription factors. *Biochem J* 2001;360:461-470.

100. Aigner T, Gebhard PM, Schmid E, Bau B, Harley V, Poschl E: SOX9 expression does not correlate with type II collagen expression in adult articular chondrocytes. *Matrix Biol* 2003;22:363-372.

101. Kaarniranta K, Elo MA, Sironen RK, Karjalainen HM, Helminen HJ, Lammi MJ: Stress responses of mammalian cells to high hydrostatic pressure. *Biorheology* 2003;40:87-92.

102. Wong M, Siegrist M, Goodwin K: Cyclic tensile strain and cyclic hydrostatic pressure differentially regulate expression of hypertrophic markers in primary chondrocytes. *Bone* 2003;33:685-693.

Chapter 15

# EMF Regulates Growth Factor Synthesis by Osteoblasts

*Barbara D. Boyan, PhD*
*Bruce J. Simon, PhD*
*Jean C. Gan, PhD*
*Mary J. MacDougall, PhD*
*Christoph H. Lohmann, MD*
*Zvi Schwartz, DMD, PhD*

## Introduction

Although biophysical signals are used to promote bone healing, relatively little is known about the underlying mechanisms involved. To better understand these mechanisms, we have focused on the effects of electromagnetic fields (EMFs) on cells in the osteoblast lineage. More than 300 published studies using in vitro and in vivo models have investigated the effects of electric stimulation on bone-related cellular responses. With respect to osteoblasts and osteoprogenitor cells, a consistent theme has emerged indicating that electrophysical stimuli induce osteoblasts and osteoprogenitor cells to produce local regulatory factors. These studies are summarized here.

## Growth Factor Stimulation: An Intermediary Mechanism of Action

To determine if osteoblasts are sensitive to EMF stimulation, an in vitro model was used to examine cell response as a function of exposure time.[1] Confluent cultures were placed between Helmholtz coils and exposed to a 15-Hz pulsed electromagnetic signal for 8 hours per day for 1, 2, or 4 days. Controls were cultured under identical conditions, but no signal was applied. Treated and control cultures were alternated between two comparable incubators. Measurement of the temperature of the incubators and the culture medium indicated that application of the signal did not generate heat above the level found in the control incubator or culture medium.

Initial studies using human MG63 osteoblast-like cells suggested that pulsed electromagnetic fields (PEMF) promote osteogenic differentiation.[1] PEMF caused decreased proliferation and increased alkaline phosphatase-specific activity, osteocalcin synthesis, and collagen production. In addition, the levels of cytokines and growth factors present in the conditioned media of the cells were sensitive to PEMF treatment. Prostaglandin $E_2$ ($PGE_2$) was reduced at 1 and 2 days of PEMF treatment, whereas TGF-$\beta_1$ was increased. These effects were time dependent, and at 4 days of treatment, the levels of both local factors were similar to those in the controls.

Studies in our lab[1] and others[2-4] indicate that the response of osteoblasts to biophysical regulatory factors varies considerably with their maturation state in the osteoblast lineage, potentially explaining the disparity of observations among investigators with respect to EMF. To test this hypothesis, we examined the effects of the PEMF treatment regimen described above on terminally differentiated osteoblasts—osteocytes.[5] For these experiments, mouse osteocyte-like MLO-Y4 cells were cultured until they achieved contact and exposed to active PEMF or inactive devices. The cells were harvested at various time points, and cell number, alkaline phosphatase activity, and levels of osteocalcin, connexin 43, $PGE_2$, and $TGF-\beta_1$ were determined. PEMF treatment increased $TGF-\beta_1$ levels in the conditioned media, as noted for the MG63 cells. Unlike MG63 cells, PEMF also caused a time-dependent increase in $PGE_2$ in the MLO-Y4 cells.

This finding supports the hypothesis that growth factor production in response to the PEMF stimulus used in our experimental model is cell specific. Moreover, it also suggests that an increase in $TGF-\beta_1$ may be a common response, because other studies also reported an increase in this growth factor following EMF treatment.[6-8] To test whether this is the case for human cells—particularly cells targeted for clinical response to PEMF, we examined the effects of PEMF on human nonunion cells.[9] Cells were cultured from hypertrophic and atrophic nonunion tissues harvested from humans undergoing surgical revisions for nonunions. The cells were exposed to either active PEMF or inactive devices as noted above. PEMF treatment increased $TGF-\beta_1$ levels in the conditioned medium of the human nonunion cells. This effect was seen in cells from both hypertrophic and atrophic nonunions, although the magnitude of the response was greater and occurred at an earlier time point in the hypertrophic nonunion cell cultures. In contrast to the stimulation of $TGF-\beta_1$, PEMF decreased $PGE_2$ levels in the nonunion cells.

The culture media were replaced every 48 hours; therefore, the effect of PEMF treatment on $TGF-\beta_1$ or $PGE_2$ levels described above represents the cumulative change in the conditioned media over a minimum of 1 day and a maximum of 2 days. In addition, some responses required exposure to PEMF for 8 hours per day for 48 hours. This finding suggests that EMF elicits a time-dependent cascade of events, and in vivo experiments support this hypothesis. Studies using an L4-L5 posterolateral intertransverse fusion process in rabbits as the experimental model show that direct current (DC) stimulation caused time- and location-dependent increases in expression of BMP-2, -4, -6, and -7.[10]

Biophysical stimuli also elicit rapid changes in release of growth and differentiation factors from osteoblasts. Prostanoid production occurs within 30 minutes.[11,12] More recently Bodamyali and associates[2] showed that treatment of neonatal rat calvarial cells with active PEMF devices increased the number and size of bone-like nodules, and upregulated the levels of BMP-2 and BMP-4 mRNA. The effect on BMP expression occurred within 15 minutes.

To determine if PEMF modulates expression of BMPs in human cells, we assessed the effects of PEMF on mRNA levels in cells that were derived from resected human chronic nonunions characterized as hypertrophic. Of the three patients, one was female and two were males, with an average age

**Table 1 Effect of PEMF Stimulation on mRNA Expression in Cells Derived from Human Hypertrophic Chronic Nonunions**

Messenger RNA levels were determined by RT-PCR and normalized to GAPDH. Arrow denotes the direction of change in expression in cells treated with PEMF for 8 hours per day for 4 days compared with control cultures grown under identical conditions but using inactive coils. Symbols used are as follows: ↑, increase; ↑↑, large increase; ↓, decrease; (↑), small increase; —, no change.

|  | Change in mRNA Levels in Hypertrophic Nonunion Cells | | |
|---|---|---|---|
|  | Donor 1 | Donor 2 | Donor 3 |
| Osteonectin | ↑ | ↑ | ↓ |
| ALK-2 | — | ↑ | ↓ |
| ALK-3 | ↑ | ↑ | ↑ |
| Osteocalcin | ↓ | ↑↑ | ↑ |
| Osteopontin | ↑ | ↑ | — |
| BMP-2A | — | — | ↑ |
| BSP | ↑ | ↑↑ | — |
| Collagen I | ↑↑ | ↑↑ | — |
| Collagen II | — | (↑) | ↑ |

of 35.3 years. Cells were expanded in culture and confluent fourth passage cultures were treated for 8 hours per day for 4 days. RNA was extracted and examined by reverse transcription polymerase chain reaction (RT-PCR) for the presence of mRNAs for a number of extracellular matrix proteins associated with endochondral ossification, BMP-2, the BMP type Ia receptor ALK-3, and the BMP type I receptor ALK-2. Results were normalized to GAPDH mRNA and compared to mRNA levels in nonunion cells cultured under identical conditions in the absence of PEMF.

As shown in Table 1, there was interdonor variability, which may contribute to the variability in patient response to PEMF treatment. The sample size was too small to determine if this variability was due to the age or sex of the donor. Overall, however, trends were identified showing upregulation of osteoblast markers such as osteonectin (2/3), osteocalcin (2/3), osteopontin (2/3), bone sialoprotein (2/3), and collagen I (2/3). Most important, BMP-2 was upregulated in one patient's cells and the BMP-2 type Ia receptor ALK-3 was upregulated in all three sets of cells. This latter observation suggests that PEMF may act in part by sensitizing nonunion cells to osteoinductive factors such as BMP-2. Interestingly, these data correlated with those found in the human osteoblast-like MG63 cells cultured under identical conditions (Table 2). Messenger RNA levels for osteocalcin, osteopontin, bone sialoprotein, and collagen I were upregulated, as was mRNA for ALK-3.

# Mechanisms Mediating Biophysical Regulation of Growth Factors

Although the results described above show that cytokine and growth factor levels are modulated by biophysical signals, they do not demonstrate mech-

## Table 2 Effect of PEMF Stimulation on mRNA Expression in Human Osteoblast-like MG63 Cells

Messenger RNA levels were determined by RT-PCR and normalized to GAPDH. Arrow denotes the direction of change in expression in cells treated with PEMF for 8 hours per day for 4 days compared to control cultures grown under identical conditions but using inactive coils. Symbols used are as follows: ↑, increase; ↑↑, large increase; ↓, decrease; (↑), small increase; —, no change.

|              | + PEMF |
| ------------ | ------ |
| Osteonectin  | —      |
| ALK-2        | —      |
| ALK-3        | ↑      |
| Osteocalcin  | ↑↑     |
| Osteopontin  | ↑      |
| BMP-2A       | —      |
| BSP          | ↑      |
| Collagen I   | ↑↑     |
| Collagen II  | —      |

anisms to account for these time-dependent fluxes in amount, nor do they link changes in local regulators with altered osteoblast physiology. We used the osteocyte model to determine how the change in TGF-$\beta_1$ was modulated.[5] Previous work identified PGE$_2$ as a mediator of cell response to EMF,[11,12] and an interrelationship between prostaglandin production and TGF-$\beta_1$ synthesis has been reported.[13] These observations suggest that prostaglandin production might also play a role in the PEMF-dependent increase in TGF-$\beta_1$ observed in osteocytes. For these experiments, MLO-Y4 cells were treated for 24 hours or 4 days with PEMF (8 hours per day) in the presence and absence of cyclooxygenase (COX) inhibitors.[5] The general COX inhibitor indomethacin was used to block total prostaglandin production; resveratrol was used to block constitutively expressed COX-1; NS-398 was used to block inducible COX-2. The results showed that at least part of the effect of PEMF on TGF-$\beta_1$ levels in the conditioned media of the osteocytes was mediated by COX-1 but not by COX-2. Indomethacin blocked PEMF-dependent TGF-$\beta_1$ increases, and resveratrol caused a significant reduction, but NS-398 had no effect. The results were comparable at day 1 and at day 4.[5]

COX-1 is constitutively expressed; thus any change in reaction product requires a change in substrate availability, indicating that the regulatory effect of PEMF is upstream. The most likely contender is phospholipase A$_2$ (PLA$_2$), which catalyzes the release of arachidonic acid, the substrate for COX action. PLA$_2$ is a Ca$^{++}$ sensitive enzyme, and lysophospholipids produced as a consequence of arachidonic acid release have been shown to activate phospholipase C,[14] which has been linked to the mechanism by which mechanical stimuli modulate osteoblasts.[15]

The biochemical pathway mediating bone cell response to EMF also involves the release of calcium ions from intracellular stores, subsequent increases in cytosolic calcium ions, and increases in activated calmodulin, ultimately leading to cell proliferation in some osteoblastic populations. Thus the change in levels of local regulatory factors may be secondary to the change in the intracellular Ca$^{++}$ ion elicited by PEMF stimulation. Studies using MC3T3-E1 bone cells as the model showed that inhibition of Ca$^{++}$-sensitive signaling pathways blocked the stimulatory effect of PEMF on cell response.[16] Both TGF-$\beta_1$ and PGE$_2$ are regulated by Ca$^{++}$-dependent pathways[16,17] as are their effects on their target cells.[8] Similarly, stimulation of MC3T3-E1 osteoblast-like cells[8] and rat calvarial cells[12] via capacitive coupling, another type of electric stimulation, has been found to activate transmembrane calcium translocation via voltage-gated calcium channels, subsequently activating calmodulin and increasing PGE$_2$ as well as enhancing growth factor synthesis.

## Summary

The studies described here indicate that the effectiveness of EMF stimulation of osteoblasts may be mediated by growth factors. EMF upregulates expression of TGF-$\beta_1$, BMP-2, and BMP-4. Appropriately configured, EMF also stimulates synthesis of other osteogenic cytokines, such as insulin-like growth factor, BMP-5, and BMP-7. These growth factors in turn modulate bone cell proliferation, differentiation, and extracellular matrix synthesis. At least in the case of TGF-$\beta_1$, prostaglandin is required. The observation that COX-1 mediates this effect implicates PLA$_2$ in the mechanism. Our results also indicate that PEMF regulates the ability of cells to respond to local growth factors by modulating the availability of appropriate receptors.

DC electric stimulation also enhances bone growth by providing an osteogenic environment for bone formation.[18,19] At the cathode, the electric field and the faradic products from the electrochemical reaction both together and separately promote bone healing. The electrochemical reaction consumes oxygen and produces hydroxyl ions, thus reducing oxygen concentration and increasing tissue pH. A reduction in oxygen concentration stimulates osteoblastic activity, while an increase in pH decreases osteoclastic activity and thus bone resorption but increases osteoblastic activity.[20] Hydrogen peroxide, another faradic product, accelerates bone remodeling by stimulating osteoclasts to resorb bone, thus priming the bone surface for osteoblasts to then lay down new bone. In addition, hydrogen peroxide stimulates macrophages to release vascular endothelial growth factor,[21] which is an angiogenic factor that is crucial for fracture healing. Whether this occurs in the presence of DC is not yet known. DC stimulation also upregulates the gene expression of growth factors such as BMP-2, -4, -6, and -7, suggesting that growth factor stimulation may mediate the effectiveness of DC stimulation on bone healing.[10]

The effectiveness of capacitive coupling electric stimulation has been observed in bone healing, chondrogenesis, and osteoporosis. The mechanism of action of capacitive coupling stimulation involves transmembrane calcium translocation via voltage-gated calcium channels, subsequent activation of calmodulin and increases in $PGE_2$, and enhancement of growth factor (such as TGF-$\beta_1$) synthesis.

## Acknowledgments

Research in the Boyan laboratory was supported by grants from EBI, LP (Parsippany, NJ), the Center for the Enhancement of the Biology/Biomaterials Interface at the University of Texas Health Science Center at San Antonio (San Antonio, TX), and the Georgia Tech/Emory Center for the Engineering of Living Tissues at the Georgia Institute of Technology (Atlanta, GA). The authors acknowledge the support of the Georgia Research Alliance (Atlanta, GA), the Price Gilbert, Jr. Foundation, and the Institute of Bioengineering and Biosciences at Georgia Tech. Drs. Simon and Gan are employees of EBI, LP.

## References

1. Lohmann CH, Schwartz Z, Liu Y, et al: Pulsed electromagnetic field stimulation of MG63 osteoblast-like cells affects differentiation and local factor production. *J Orthop Res* 2000;18:637-646.

2. Bodamyali T, Bhatt B, Hughes FJ, et al: Pulsed electromagnetic fields simultaneously induce osteogenesis and upregulate transcription of bone morphogenetic proteins 2 and 4 in rat osteoblasts in vitro. *Biochem Biophys Res Comm* 1998;250:458-461.

3. Ciombor DM, Aaron RK: Influence of electromagnetic fields on endochondral bone formation. *J Cell Biochem* 1993;52:37-41.

4. Fitzsimmons R, Ryaby J, Magee F, Baylink D: IGF-II receptor number is increased in TE-85 osteosarcoma cells by combined magnetic fields. *J Bone Miner Res* 1995;10:812-819.

5. Lohmann CH, Schwartz Z, Liu Y, et al: Pulsed electromagnetic fields affect phenotype and connexin 43 protein expression in MLO-Y4 osteocyte-like cells and ROS 17/2.8 osteoblast-like cells. *J Orthop Res* 2003;21:326-334.

6. Aaron RK, Ciombor DM, Keeping H, Wang S, Capuano A, Polk C: Power frequency fields promote cell differentiation coincident with an increase in transforming growth factor-beta(1) expression. *Bioelectromagnetics* 1999;20:453-458.

7. Aaron RK, Wang S, Ciombor DM: Upregulation of basal TGFbeta1 levels by EMF coincident with chondrogenesis: Implications for skeletal repair and tissue engineering. *J Orthop Res* 2002;20:233-240.

8. Zhuang H, Wang W, Seldes RM, Tahernia AD, Fan H, Brighton CT: Electrical stimulation induces the level of TGF-$\beta$1 mRNA in osteoblastic cells by a mechanism involving calcium/calmodulin pathway. *Biochem Biophys Res Comm* 1997;237:225-229.

9. Guerkov HH, Lohmann CH, Liu Y, et al: Pulsed electromagnetic fields increase growth factor release by nonunion cells. *Clin Orthop* 2001;384:265-279.

10. Petersen EB, Fredericks DC, Bobst JA, Nepola JV, Simon BJ: Effects of direct current electrical stimulation on expression of BMP 2, 4, 6, 7, bFGF, VEGF, ALK 2, and ALK 3 in a rabbit posterolateral spine fusion model. *The Spine Journal* 2003;3:67S-171S.

11. Davidovitch Z, Shanfeld JL, Montgomery PC, et al: Biochemical mediators of the effects of mechanical forces and electric currents on mineralized tissues. *Calcif Tissue Int* 1984;36:S86-S97.

12. Lorich DG, Brighton CT, Gupta R, et al: Biochemical pathway mediating the response of bone cells to capacitive coupling. *Clin Orthop* 1998;350:246-256.

13. Klein-Nulend J, Semeins CM, Burger EH: Prostaglandin-mediated modulation of transforming growth factor-beta metabolism in primary mouse osteoblastic cells in vitro. *J Cell Physiol* 1996;168:1-7.

14. Schwartz Z, Shaked D, Hardin RR, et al: 1α,25(OH)2D3 causes a rapid increase in phosphatidylinositol-specific PLC-β activity via phospholipase A2 dependent production of lysophosphlipid. *Steroids* 2003;68:423-437.

15. Ajubi NE, Klein-Nulend J, Alblas MJ, Burger EH, Nijweide PJ: Signal transduction pathways involved in fluid flow-induced PGE2 production by cultured osteocytes. *Am J Physiol* 1999;276:E171-E178.

16. Brighton CT, Wang W, Seldes R, Zhang G, Pollack SR: Signal transduction in electrically stimulated bone cells. *J Bone Joint Surg Am* 2001;83:1514-1523.

17. Zonta M, Sebelin A, Gobbo S, Fellin T, Pozzan T, Carmignoto G: Glutamate-mediated cytosolic calcium oscillations regulate a pulsatile prostaglandin release from cultured rat astrocytes. *J Physiol* 2003;553:407-414.

18. Bassett CA, Herrmann I: Influence of oxygen concentration and mechanical factors on differentiation of connective tissues in vitro. *Nature* 1961;190:460-461.

19. Hellewell AB, Beljan JR: The effect of a constant direct current on the repair of an experimental osseous defect. *Clin Orthop* 1979;142:219-222.

20. Yamaguchi DT, Ma D: Mechanism of pH regulation of connexin 43 expression in MC3T3-E1 cells. *Biochem Biophys Res Commun* 2003;304:736-739.

21. Cho M, Hunt TK, Hussain MZ: Hydrogen peroxide stimulates macrophage vascular endothelial growth factor release. *Am J Physiol Heart Circ Physiol* 2001;280:H2357-H2363.

Chapter 16

# The Role of Genetics in Skeletal Mechanotransduction

*Charles H. Turner, PhD*

Osteoporosis is a complex disorder resulting from the influence of both genetic and environmental factors. Twin and family studies have consistently reported a substantial genetic contribution to bone mineral density (BMD).[1-3] Important factors contributing to osteoporosis include low BMD,[4,5] poor bone structure,[6,7] and impaired bone biomechanics.[8] Both BMD[9] and bone structure[10] have been shown to be highly heritable. Genetic polymorphisms affecting bone structure may follow a Mendelian pattern of inheritance in the case of a single gene effect, or a complex pattern of inheritance if several genes are acting on bone structure. An example of Mendelian inheritance is the autosomal dominant high bone mass (HBM) phenotype.[11] Individuals with HBM have areal BMD values that are four to five standard deviations above normal. The cause of HBM is a mutation in the extracellular domain of the low-density lipoprotein receptor-related protein-5 (LRP-5) gene;[12] LRP-5 mutations also cause the autosomal recessive disorder osteoporosis-pseudoglioma syndrome.[13] These findings illustrate the importance of the LRP-5 signaling pathway for development of bone structure and BMD. However, bone structure is a complex trait regulated by many genes besides LRP-5, and identification of additional polymorphic genes that are responsible for stronger (or weaker) bones will lead to discovery of other cellular pathways involved in bone biology.

One useful strategy for uncovering the genes contributing to complex traits like bone fragility uses inbred strains of mice that differ in BMD or bone strength. Mice within an inbred strain are identical "twins," and their environments can be closely controlled. Planned matings between mice from two inbred strains allow the segregation of genetic alleles important for bone structure or strength. Statistical models can be used to assess the cosegregation of a genetic region with a quantitative trait such as BMD. During the past decade, mouse models of osteoporosis have been used as a complementary means to identify genes contributing to osteoporosis susceptibility. A series of studies in recombinant inbred lines, as well as a variety of inbred second filial (F2) crosses, revealed several chromosomal regions consistently linked to quantitative trait loci (QTL) for BMD.[8,14-22] Additional mouse studies led to the identification of QTL that contribute uniquely to femoral structure[19-21] and to bone biomechanical properties.[20-22]

Several studies have shown that the long bones of C57BL/6J (B6) mice are more responsive to mechanical loading and are larger in cross-section than are bones from C3H/HeJ (C3H) mice.[23-27] Consequently, these two groups of mice may provide a means for mapping QTL associated with

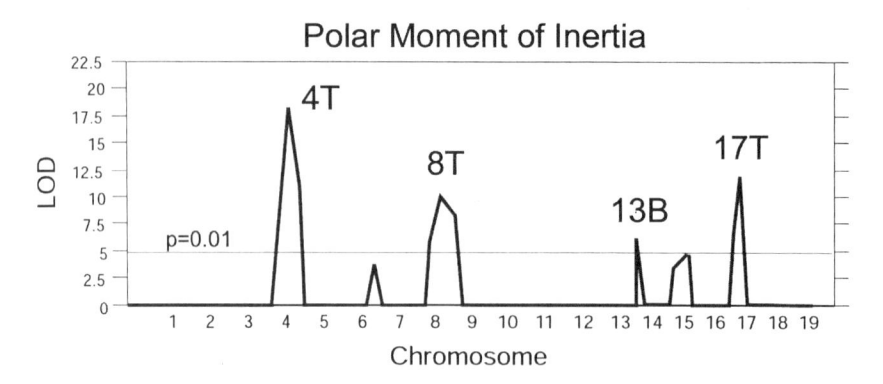

Section Four    Biophysical Regulation of Growth Factor Synthesis

**Figure 1** Genome-wide screen for an F2 population of mice from C3H and B6 parents. A QTL map was created for the phenotype of femoral cross-sectional size, represented by Ip. Four QTL achieved statistical significance at the $P = 0.01$ level. These QTL are located on chromosomes 4 (4T), 8 (8T), 13 (13B), and 17 (17T).

skeletal mechanotransduction. Genetic mapping of F2 offspring from B6 and C3H mice produced a QTL map for femoral cross-sectional size represented by the polar moment of inertia (Ip). Four QTL located on chromosomes 4, 8, 13, and 17 were statistically significant (Fig. 1). These QTL are linked to long bone cross-sectional size and shape and therefore may also affect the responsiveness of the bone to mechanical loads. To study this possibility further, the QTL were isolated onto separate congenic mouse lines.

Congenic mice were created using a backcross breeding strategy.[28,29] The C3H mice were first intercrossed with B6 mice and the offspring backcrossed with B6 mice for approximately 10 generations. Through each generation, the mice were genotyped at the QTL to identify carriers of C3H DNA within the QTL. The resulting congenic line is over 99% B6 with only a small region of C3H DNA at the QTL. Numerous congenic mouse lines have been developed for studying skeletal phenotypes by Wesley Beamer, PhD, of the Jackson Laboratory (Bar Harbor, Maine). The congenic lines derived from C3H and B6 mice are denoted B6.C3H-X in which B6 is the recipient strain, C3H is the donor strain, and X indicates the chromosomal location of the QTL. The congenic lines investigated here are B6.C3H-4T, B6.C3H-8T, B6.C3H-13B, and B6.C3H-17T. The femoral midshafts from these mice were scanned using microcomputed tomography (Scanco uCT 20, Scanco Medical AG, Bassersdorf, Switzerland) and the Ip was calculated using Scion software (Scion Image 4.0.2 for Windows, Scion Corporation, Frederick, MD).

After the effects of individual QTL were isolated in congenic mouse lines, it was possible to evaluate the biologic effects of each QTL. The gross effects of each QTL on femoral size (Ip) are shown in Figure 2. C3H mice have smaller Ip for the femoral midshaft compared with B6 mice. Consequently, we expected that the C3H QTL sequestered in the congenic mouse lines would contribute to smaller femoral size, and indeed, congenic lines

## Femoral Size in Congenic Mice

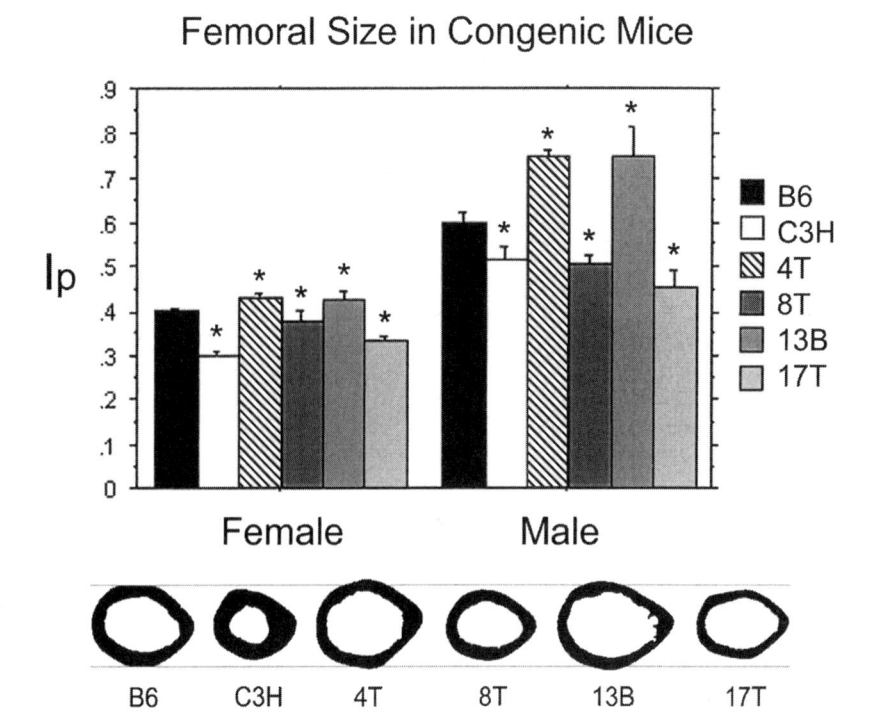

**Figure 2** Ip measured at the femoral midshaft for adult mice. Mouse strains include B6 and C3H as well as B6.C3H-4T (4T), B6.C3H-8T (8T), B6.C3H-13B (13B), and B6.C3H-17T (17T) congenic lines. Example femoral cross-sections are shown below the bar chart. Asterisks represent statistically significant ($P < 0.05$) differences from B6 mice.

B6.C3H-8T (8T) and B6.C3H-17T (17T) had smaller femoral size and significantly lower Ip compared with the B6 strain. However, the congenic lines B6.C3H-4T (4T) and B6.C3H-13B (13B) had significantly larger femoral cross-sections (Ip) compared with B6. These results suggest that the genetic influences on femoral Ip in C3H mice are complicated, involving genes on chromosomes 8 and 17 that suppress bone formation at the periosteum and genes on chromosomes 4 and 13 that promote periosteal growth. Interestingly, a striking feature of C3H mice—the thick femoral cortex—was not passed on to any of the congenic lines. Therefore, it appears that the genes that regulate cortical thickness are different from those that regulate cross-sectional size.

It has been speculated that the lower Ip in C3H mice is due mainly to impaired mechanotransduction causing reduced periosteal expansion during growth. In addition, it is reasonable to expect that differences in long bone cross-sectional size observed in congenic mouse strains are due to differences in the responsiveness of the bone to mechanical loading. The femoral cross-sectional Ip is significantly larger in 4T and 13B mice; therefore, their

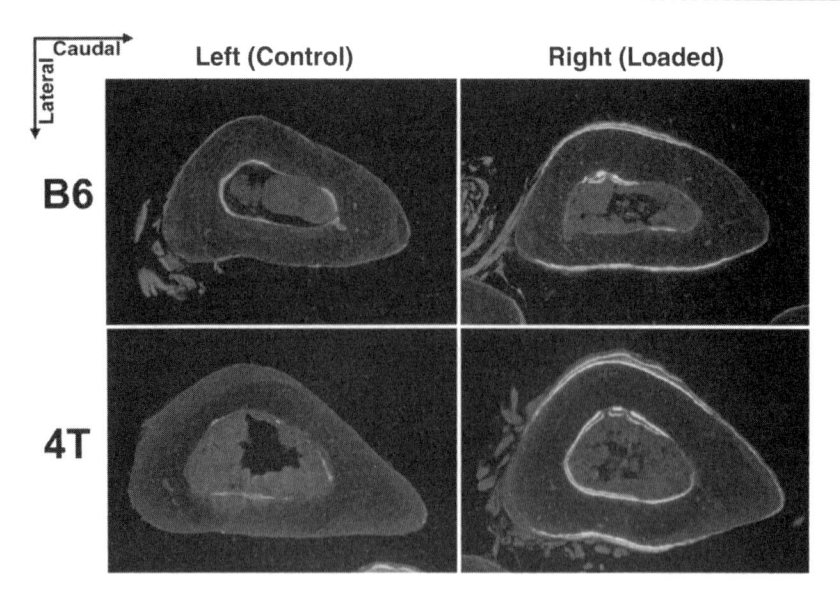

Section Four  Biophysical Regulation of Growth Factor Synthesis

**Figure 3** Fluorochrome labeling (white bands) on the periosteal surface of the ulnae from B6 or 4T mice. Loading induced almost twice as much bone formation in the 4T mice (as indicated by broader separation of the labels) than in B6 control mice. These findings indicate that ulnae from the 4T mice are more sensitive to mechanical loading than those from the B6 mice, suggesting that the QTL on chromosome 4 influences mechanotransduction in the skeleton. *(Adapted with permission from Robling AG, Li J, Shultz KL, Beamer WG, Turner CH: Evidence for a skeletal mechanosensitivity gene on mouse chromosome 4. FASEB J 2003;17:324-326.)*

femora are stouter and more resistant to bending than those of B6 control mice, even though the three groups have the same body weights. Thus, it would appear that 4T or 13B mice have skeletons that are hyperresponsive when exposed to similar loading conditions. The greater responsiveness to load would result in more periosteal bone formation during growth and broader, stiffer bones in adulthood. According to this proposition, bones from 4T or 13B mice should be more responsive to mechanical loading, causing increased periosteal apposition compared with B6 or C3H mice. This hypothesis was tested using the mouse ulna loading model. Mechanical responsiveness of the ulna was measured in 4T mice and compared with B6 or C3H mice.

Adult female mice from the different strains were subjected to mechanical loading of the ulna as described by Robling and associates.[30] Low-, medium-, or high-magnitude in vivo loading was applied under anesthesia to the right forearm of each mouse for 30 seconds per day for 3 consecutive days using a 2-Hz haversine waveform. An electromagnetic actuator was used for in vivo loading. The left forearms were not loaded and served as an internal control for loading effects. All mice were allowed normal cage activity between loading bouts. Intraperitoneal injections of calcein (42 mg/kg body

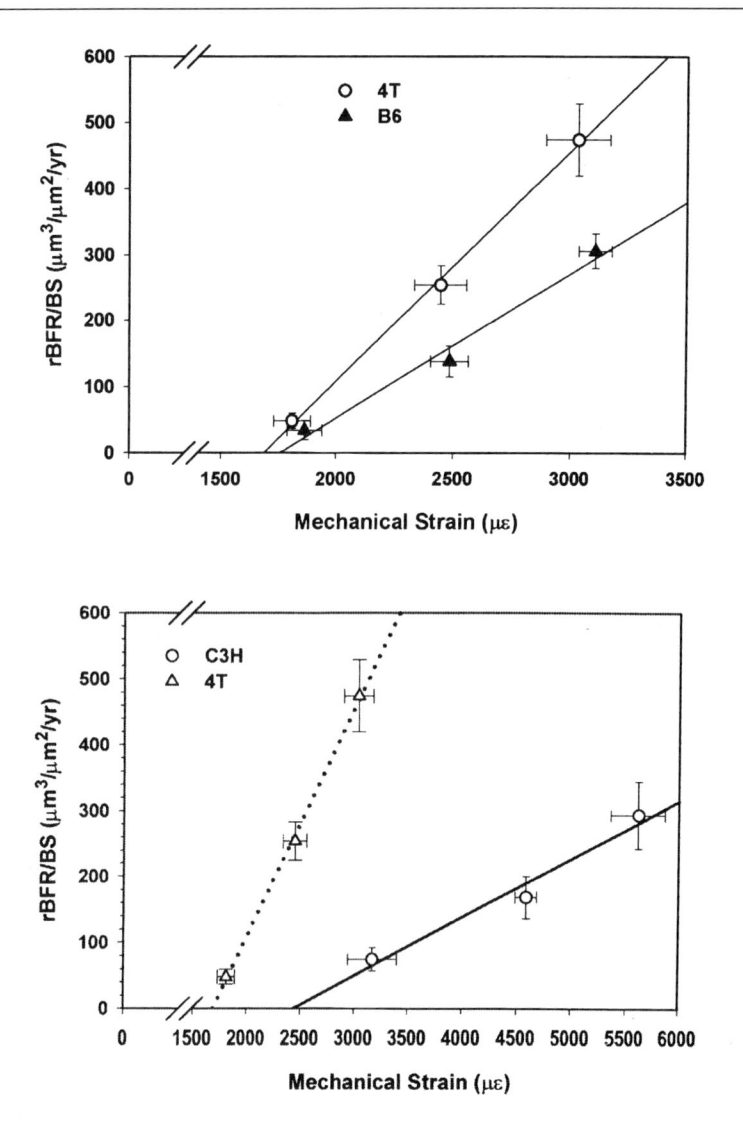

**Figure 4** Bone formation rate (rBFR/BS) of the ulna for 4T compared with either B6 or C3H mice. At about 3,000 $\mu\varepsilon$, the 4T ulna had almost twofold more bone formation than B6 and over sevenfold more bone formation than C3H.

mass; Sigma Chemical Co, St Louis, MO) were administered 4 and 8 days after the first load day. All animals were sacrificed 18 days after the first load day. Fluorochrome bone labels for B6 and 4T mice are shown in Figure 3. Ulnae from 4T mice were more responsive to loading than either B6 or C3H mice (Fig. 4). For instance, at about 3,000 $\mu\varepsilon$, the 4T ulna had almost twofold more bone formation than B6 and over sevenfold more bone formation than C3H.

The interesting aspect of the 4T congenic mice is that the donated chromosomal region from C3H made the long bones larger and more mechanically responsive even though the C3H mice themselves have smaller, less mechanically responsive long bones. This finding suggests that C3H mice contain QTL that have a dominant suppressive effect on periosteal apposition and mechanical responsiveness. Once these QTL are removed, their suppressive effect disappears, as in the 4T congenic mice. Our data suggest that the suppressive C3H QTL reside on chromosomes 8 and 17. Consequently, we expect that 8T and 17T congenic mice will have reduced long bone responsiveness to mechanical loading, similar to C3H mice.

The ultimate goal of these studies is to identify the specific genes that influence bone mechanotransduction. Identification of the important genetic polymorphisms within each QTL requires further work. New databases and technologies are becoming available to aid in the identification of polymorphisms. These include single nucleotide polymorphism (SNP) and expressed sequence tag (EST) databases. The largest mouse SNP database was developed by Celera and includes 3.4 million SNPs from five different inbred mouse strains. About 40% of Celera's mouse SNPs are within gene coding regions, giving an average density of 40 SNPs per gene. SNP databases for additional inbred mouse strains are under development at the Whitehead Institute and Roche. These SNP databases include both the B6 and C3H mouse strains. As these databases continue to grow, SNP genotyping will become increasingly precise. Soon it will be possible to fine-map a QTL region using SNPs. With improved SNP databases, candidate genes can be prioritized based on the number of SNPs within their coding sequence and where the SNPs are. Genes with more SNPs or genes with SNPs in highly conserved genomic regions are more likely candidates.

Over the past few years, considerable progress has been made toward developing a characterization of the mouse transcriptome, or a catalog of all RNAs synthesized by the mouse. These include protein coding, nonprotein coding, alternatively spliced, alternatively polyadenylated, alternatively initiated, sense, antisense, and RNA-edited transcripts. The transcriptome catalog is based largely on sequences from large-scale EST databases. There are considerably more transcripts than there are genes, due in part to alternative splicing of genes. As much as a third of mouse mRNAs result from alternative splicing;[31] as a result, the transcriptome is much more complex than the genome.[32] In addition, there are new technologies for connecting the transcriptome to the proteome. Antibodies are generated against peptides derived from ESTs that, in turn, are used to identify the full-length proteins.[33] These technologies allow more extensive evaluation of the functional outcomes caused by genetic polymorphisms. Therefore, gene expression derived from congenic mice may soon be more useful for identifying the altered genetic pathways that result in the observed phenotype.

# References

1. Seeman E, Tsalamandris C, Formica C, Hopper JL, McKay J: Reduced femoral neck bone density in the daughters of women with hip fractures: The role of low peak bone density in the pathogenesis of osteoporosis. *J Bone Miner Res* 1994;9:739-743.

2. Smith DM, Nance WE, Kang KW, Christian JC, Johnston CC Jr: Genetic factors in determining bone mass. *J Clin Invest* 1973;52:2800-2808.

3. Arden NK, Baker J, Hogg C, Baan K, Spector TD: The heritability of bone mineral density, ultrasound of the calcaneus and hip axis length: A study of postmenopausal twins. *J Bone Miner Res* 1996;11:530-534.

4. Melton LJ III, Atkinson EJ, O'Fallon WM, Wahner HW, Riggs BL: Long-term fracture prediction by bone mineral assessed at different skeletal sites. *J Bone Miner Res* 1993;8:1227-1233.

5. Marshall D, Johnell O, Wedel H: Meta-analysis of how well measures of bone mineral density predict occurrence of osteoporotic fractures. *Br Med J* 1996;312:1254-1259.

6. Peacock M, Turner CH, Liu G, Manatunga AK, Timmerman L, Johnston CC Jr: Better discrimination of hip fracture using bone density, geometry and architecture. *Osteoporos Int* 1995;5:167-173.

7. Faulkner KG, Cummings SR, Nevitt MC, Pressman A, Jergas M, Genant HK: Hip axis length and osteoporotic fractures: Study of Osteoporotic Fractures Research Group. *J Bone Miner Res* 1995;10:506-508.

8. Peacock M, Turner CH, Econs MJ, Foroud T: Genetics of osteoporosis. *Endocr Rev* 2002;23:303-326.

9. Koller DL, Econs MJ, Morin PA, et al: Genome screen for QTLs contributing to normal variation in bone mineral density and osteoporosis. *J Clin Endocrinol Metab* 2000;85:3116-3120.

10. Koller DL, Liu G, Econs MJ, et al: Genome screen for quantitative trait loci underlying normal variation in femoral structure. *J Bone Miner Res* 2001;16:985-991.

11. Johnson ML, Gong G, Kimberling W, Recker SM, Kimmel DB, Recker RR: Linkage of a gene causing high bone mass to human chromosome 11 (11q12-13). *Am J Hum Genet* 1997;60:1326-1332.

12. Little RD, Carulli JP, Del Mastro RG, et al: A mutation in the LDL receptor-related protein 5 results in the autosomal dominant high-bone-mass trait. *Am J Hum Genet* 2002;70:11-19.

13. Gong Y, Slee RB, Fukai N, et al: LDL receptor-related protein 5 (LRP5) affects bone accrual and eye development. *Cell* 2001;16:513-523.

14. Beamer WG, Shultz KL, Churchill GA, et al: Quantitative trait loci for bone density in C57BL/6J and CAST/EiJ inbred mice. *Mamm Genome* 1999;10:1043-1049.

15. Beamer WG, Shultz KL, Donahue LR, et al: Quantitative trait loci for femoral and lumbar vertebral bone mineral density in C57BL/6J and C3H/HeJ inbred strains of mice. *J Bone Miner Res* 2001;16:1195-1206.

16. Klein RF, Carlos AS, Vartanian KA, et al: Confirmation and fine mapping of chromosomal regions influencing peak bone mass in mice. *J Bone Miner Res* 2001;16:1953-1961.

17. Klein RF, Mitchell SR, Phillips TJ, Belknap JK, Orwoll ES: Quantitative trait loci affecting peak bone mineral density in mice. *J Bone Miner Res* 1998;13:1648-1656.

18. Benes H, Weinstein RS, Zheng W, et al: Chromosomal mapping of osteopenia-associated quantitative trait loci using closely related mouse strains. *J Bone Miner Res* 2000;15:626-633.

19. Klein RF, Turner RJ, Skinner LD, et al: Mapping quantitative trait loci that influence femoral cross-sectional area in mice. *J Bone Miner Res* 2002;17:1752-1760.

20. Turner CH, Sun Q, Schriefer J, et al: Genetic influences on bone density and geometry affect femoral bone strength. *Trans Orthop Res Soc* 2002;27:114.

21. Li X, Masinde G, Gu W, Wergedal J, Mohan S, Baylink DJ: Genetic dissection of femur breaking strength in a large population (MRL/MpJ x SJL/J) of F2 mice: Single QTL effects, epistasis, and pleiotropy. *Genomics* 2002;79:734-740.

22. Li X, Masinde G, Gu W, et al: Chromosomal regions harboring genes for the work to femur failure in mice. *Funct Integr Genomics* 2002;1:367-374.

23. Beamer WG, Donahue LR, Rosen CJ, Baylink DJ: Genetic variability in adult bone density among inbred strains of mice. *Bone* 1996;18:397-403.

24. Akhter MP, Cullen DM, Pedersen EA, Kimmel DB, Recker RR: Bone response to in vivo mechanical loading in two breeds of mice. *Calcif Tissue Int* 1998;63:442-449.

25. Kodama Y, Umemura Y, Nagasawa S, et al: Exercise and mechanical loading increase periosteal bone formation and whole bone strength in C57BL/6J mice but not in C3H/Hej mice. *Calcif Tissue Int* 2000;66:298-306.

26. Judex S, Donahue LR, Rubin C: Genetic predisposition to low bone mass is paralleled by an enhanced sensitivity to signals anabolic to the skeleton. *FASEB J* 2002;16:1280-1282.

27. Robling AG, Turner CH: Mechanotransduction in bone: Genetic effects on mechanosensitivity in mice. *Bone* 2002;31:562-569.

28. Silver LM: *Mouse Genetics: Concepts and Applications.* New York, NY, Oxford University Press, 1995.

29. Shultz KL, Donahue LR, Bouxsein ML, Baylink DJ, Rosen CJ, Beamer WG: Congenic strains of mice for verification and genetic decomposition of quantitative trait loci for femoral bone mineral density. *J Bone Miner Res* 2003;18:175-85.

30. Robling AG, Li J, Shultz KL, Beamer WG, Turner CH: Evidence for a skeletal mechanosensitivity gene on mouse chromosome 4. *FASEB J* 2003;17:324-326.

31. Brett D, Pospisil H, Valcarcel J, Reich J, Bork P: Alternative splicing and genome complexity. *Nat Genet* 2002;30:29-30.

32. FANTOM Consortium and the RIKEN Genome Exploration Research Group Phase I & II Team: Analysis of the mouse transcriptome based on functional annotation of 60,770 full-length cDNAs. *Nature* 2002;420:563-573.

33. Frisch C, Brocks B, Ostendorp R, Hoess A, von Ruden T, Kretzschmar T: From EST to IHC: Human antibody pipeline for target research. *J Immunol Methods* 2003;275:203-212.

## Consensus Panel 4

# Evaluation of Biophysical Regulation of Growth Factor Synthesis

**Dr. Hari Reddi:** There are two ways of thinking about physical signals. First, physical signals may influence extracellular growth factors. They can directly affect cells by way of physical—some people call them mechanical—receptors. Second, the chondrocyte is exposed to not one factor at a time but at least four families of factors.

**Dr. Mark Bolander:** I think we had a very exciting series of talks looking at a number of growth factors. I think a lot of the work has centered on TGF-β—the net effect of Anita Roberts' generous willingness to distribute reagents to everyone around the world was to make TGF-β seem, for a while, like it was the center of the universe. It certainly is important, but we are learning that it is not the center of the universe and there are other things that are involved. Clearly, one of the issues that we face is to find those significant soluble mediators and learn about how they are regulated. There is another issue that may be equally important. If there is a very variable spectrum of mechanical forces, we have to consider the possibility that there also is going to be a spectrum of growth factors that is changing in some way that may influence signaling.

With that introduction, a far cry from what I tried to prepare for you this morning, I'd like to begin our discussion. I'd like to begin with Regis.

**Dr. Regis O'Keefe:** I think that Hari Reddi has given a really outstanding summary to start this session. And I would emphasize, as he has, that we are aware that not only growth factor secretion but also probably the activators of growth factors are important. As we look at growth factors and gene expression of the growth factor, what is important are the matrices that they attach to and the things that can activate them. I think we need to use in vitro systems to define targets and then creatively think about ways to move in vivo to validate that this has a very important role in the biophysical responses and bone healing responses that we are interested in.

**Dr. Mark Bolander:** I think Charles Turner's presentation was quite unique and added something very important. Charles pointed out that LRP-5 was not something that would have been a candidate gene. Regis just referred to a paper in which MMP-9, which we think of as a matrix-degrading enzyme, actually activates growth factors. The first time I saw that was in a paper by Lynn Matrisian in which she was looking at the degradation of the spinal cord, and she also showed that MMP-9 activated a growth factor and that it had no effect at all on matrix degradation. What do these observations suggest about our assumptions regarding the functions of these different growth factors?

**Speaker:** I think we have learned from trying to analyze the signaling pathways about the complexity of the growth factor receptors. Although I talked about IL-6, I didn't talk about the IL-6 receptor and the fact that it is a complex multimeric receptor that requires GP130 versus another protein to actually be assembled in the presence of the receptor. And I talked a little bit about the fact that, if the receptor is not occupied, then there are downregulation and/or signaling pathways that get triggered by the absence of occupancy. I think Hari Reddi's point, that the models are too simple, is clear; as he has already pointed out, we think in terms of soluble factors.

**Speaker:** Beyond the growth factors, I think that there are some key transcription factors that are critical regulators. I think that one of the ways we can understand growth factors is that there are critical downstream signals inducing a plethora of effects that drive a cell in certain directions. One of the things that is very interesting, though, is if you look at BMPs and TGF-$\beta$, BMPs and the BMP-related SMADs drive maturation and differentiation of cartilage, whereas TGF-$\beta$ has completely the opposite effect. It is an inhibitor. So in regard to understanding some of the growth factors, we can understand their roles better in a context of what biophysical signals are mediating a cell. I think this morning Jim referred to that as well, that different signals have the same response if that downstream signal is the same.

**Dr. Mark Bolander:** The other thing you said, if I understand you correctly, is that the complexity that is obvious in the growth factor signaling can be simplified somewhat by using the transcription factors as surrogates because they were activating multiple genes and modulating a phenotype.

**Speaker:** I agree that TGF-$\beta$ definitely has a role in biophysical signaling. There are temporal growth factor responses, and there is differential expression of receptors. So, for example, I can tell you that some work that we are doing now suggests that during chondrogenesis a response to prostaglandins involves EP (E-prostanoid) receptors 1 through 4. That is probably the cell's ability to respond, and different growth factors need to be there at different times. It is a very, very complex process. The cell has to then integrate all the various signals through its machinery. It is amazing that you can put in a growth factor like BMP, as we are doing clinically, and it works.

**Dr. Deborah Ciombor:** One other level of complexity that I don't think we have approached is the concentration of TGF-$\beta$ protein or the level of gene expression. TGF-$\beta$ is often called the master regulator for a very good reason. It synergizes with other growth factors in ways that we still don't understand. And if you go all the way back to the fertilized ovum in embryology, the synergy of TGF-$\beta_1$ and FGF-1 is critical. And the upregulation of one gene and protein as TGF-$\beta$ is descending, or vice versa, is critical, as are the relative concentrations. We did choose TGF-$\beta$ because it was the most upregulated. But do you ignore the fact that there were slight upregulations of BMP-7 and there were slight upregulations of FGF? IGF-1 didn't change. IGF-2 went down a little bit. There is information there that we have not looked at. It is a very difficult thing to look at, not only because, as Jim points out, the animal model is extremely complex, but the matrix that you would have to evolve and the number of experiments that would have to be done to look at that would be enormous.

**Dr. Mark Bolander:** We have not talked about Charles Turner's work, and I would very much like to. This represents something that to those of us in orthopaedics is distinctly new and different and consequently a little confusing but I think has an obvious power. I have heard the work described as actually a family study where you have two grandparents, four parents, and 17,000 children. There are a very large number of mice that go into this work.

**Dr. Charles Turner:** This all came out of a population of 1,000 mice. The mice have been bred for IGF-1 levels, bone mass, bone size, trabecular bone, and cortical bone. That is the level of complexity we are talking about here. It is site specific, as you have different regulating genes for the trabecular bone in the vertebrae as opposed to trabecular bone in the distal femur, for instance.

**Dr. Mark Bolander:** You presented data about qualitative traits that control bone density in the femur. There are different sets of qualitative traits. As an aside, qualitative trait or QTL locus is probably something that people here are not familiar with. It just means a region of the gene.

**Dr. Charles Turner:** It means a region of a chromosome. It can contain 20 or maybe several hundred genes. It is just that the technique is not precise enough to pick out a single gene. It picks out a neighborhood.

**Dr. Hari Reddi:** If we want to study physical regulation of skeletal repair, we definitely have to choose some model for mechanistic studies, and that has to be the mouse. This point has been made three times by Dr. Mone Zaidi. Having said that, what is the point about it? Every problem, including physical regulation, can be done at the tissue level. You can study the cartilage, the growth plate, or articular cartilage. Of course one can study bone; not only just bone but the osteocyte network. The steady state of bone is the balance between the anabolic response of osteocytes and osteoblasts and degradation. This steady state homeostasis is indirectly influenced by such nonmusculoskeletal systems as the vascular system, which brings in both the precursor cells—the metabolic precursor cells for osteoblasts—and of course the pericytes. But from a mechanistic point of view, from the human genome studies, we know that we have about 32,000 genes, and mice are not too far off. So I am now putting the context for what our friend Charles Turner from Indiana has done. He has essentially taken two mice, one of which has dense bones, the other does not. For the purposes of this discussion, there might be about 1,000 genes for both, just like there might be 1,000 genes for your heart or 1,000 genes for your kidney. So he is studying a group of genes that are involved in bone mass. But bone mass does not come in one step. There is a cascade of 99 steps that cannot be described by map analysis. And these morphogenetic proteins at the cellular level are like these four families. I liken these four families to a chamber orchestra that has a string quartet with two violins, one cello, and a viola. If you take the same four instruments, you can have a chamber orchestra. The Indianapolis orchestra with a hundred instruments is giving you the whole organism, whereas the chamber orchestra gives you bone or kidney or brain. So that is a simple analogy. You have to analyze this problem of biophysical stimulation at the tissue level, but if you want to understand the mechanisms, you have to go to the cell. At the cell level, the cast of characters is different. Precursor cells are going to give rise to cartilage. As the differentiation proceeds, there is an intermediate stage in which there can be both growth plate and articular cartilage. Constellations of genes are turned on and off, the most important of which are transcription factors. I like to think, at least for purposes of this discussion, that there is nothing like free-floating growth factors, they are only sparingly soluble signals. They have a context and the context is their expression in the matrix. And for these purposes, I would say that the musculoskeletal system is an example par excellence for the study of this biologic problem. The growth factor complexes travel on predefined routes: SMAD-1 through -5 and their complexes have a route. SMAD-2 and -3 and their complexes have a route. And then of course there are intermediate points; the hedgehogs may crossregulate BMPs. Above all this, the pattern is a set of 34 to 39 genes called hox genes or homeobox genes that determine shape.

**Dr. Mark Bolander:** I think when Charles Turner gives his presentation, it will be clear that he does not have the gene now, but I'm sure that will happen relatively soon. Charles, do you expect this type of work to influence how we do our experiments or how we interpret the data from our experiments?

**Dr. Charles Turner:** I don't know if it necessarily changes the way experiments are done. The way I view a genetic screen is to open doors, to point toward genes that you never would have guessed before. Now maybe they are pattern genes, maybe Hari Reddi is right. Maybe it is a gene that has to do with parathyroid function, that is not even in the bone at all. This is not something you can know. You are pulling out the polymorphisms in the genome from two different strains of mice now. If you took two other strains of mice, some of the polymorphisms would be the same, some of them would be different. The value of the work is that it tells us something that is new and leads us in a direction we never would have gone if we had not had that clue. That is where I see the value. I think the LRP-5 story is a great story. I can tell you that probably two of the biggest discoveries in the last 10 years in bone biology were the RANKL signaling pathway and the cbfa1 or runx2 signaling pathway in osteoblasts. Both of those pathways came from molecular genetics approaches. I think there is a lot of value in the approach.

**Dr. Mone Zaidi:** I think what Charles Turner is looking at has to have a phenotype, for example, low bone mass and high bone mass. And then to try and trace back the gene or set of genes that might be responsible for that, that is a very logical approach. But that approach has yielded very little new information about new genes. If you have a clear-cut disease state, a more useful approach is to go forward. The parallel approach, however, would be to establish gene functionality by doing the more traditional arrays—for example to look at the physiologic regulation of a gene and then to knock it out.

**Dr. Joseph Lane:** Listening to this discussion, it seems to me that there are four things that we need to do as a very pragmatic approach. The first thing that I think we need to do is describe the initiator of the process, for whatever these biophysical techniques are. What is the initial signal that starts the pathway through this process? Because if we knew what that initiator is, we could then perfect the signal to that initiator. So that is one set of research. The second set of experiments needs to describe the obligatory steps, where there is no alternative pathway in the body, but the signal has to go through that step. Because if we knew an obligatory step, we could then point our therapies toward it. The third thing is if we could identify those components that are actually facilitators of the process. And TGFs may be a great facilitator. So then we could aim our therapy at making sure the facilitator achieves a high level. And the fourth one is to identify inhibitors like noggins. If you knew that there was an inhibitor, an alternative approach would be to knock out the inhibitor. So I think as we go through all these processes, we want the physiology, we want the cascades. But then we want to pick these kinds of targets.

**Dr. Mone Zaidi:** I think Joseph Lane has made a very, very important point, and we are trying to explore that in the bone area. If you look at my recent review in JBMR, we have called it obligatory and facilitatory. If you knock out an obligatory molecule to get a phenotype, that's potentially a drug target. If you knock out, for example, IL-6 in a mouse that was once thought to be obligatory, you don't get a phenotype. And that is because of redundancy of other genes going up and down. So I think that concept is a very important concept, and I have not actually seen that coming up in cartilage biology.

**Dr. Joseph Lane:** There has been a long-standing dilemma with respect to mesenchymal stem cells and populations of mesenchymal stem cells. The question is, could a hemopoietic stem cell actually do other things? For a long time there were two camps, one saying that there was a general mesenchymal stem cell that could go in a lot of directions other than just hemopoiesis. And in fact, the hemopoietic stem cell now has been shown to be able to go in a different direction but only under conditions in which it is a stressed tissue. One of the things that we do with some of the stimuli that have been talked about for the last 2 days obviously is in stressed tissue—nonunions.

**Dr. Solomon Pollack:** I just wanted to follow up a little bit on the previous comment. When I look at this picture that Hari Reddi drew and the level of complexity that underlies what you drew, I add to it what must be other dimensions of complexity with phenotype and cell phase and all the other factors that modulate this. And then on another easel, one might imagine the complexity of all the biophysical signals that one could apply to a system, whether it is through a cell system or through a tissue or an animal or the human system. And you look at the two complexities. In effect what you are doing is taking one or more of the stimuli and applying to this complex system. And you are looking for some outcome, but obviously there are countless outcomes. And so it's a complexity on top of a complexity. It might be helpful if there was some time for a discussion of all the things that could be done. What are the best things to do? And I will tell you, I thought I was a player in this field until I see this degree of complexity staring me in the face. It is hard to know what the next step is. Where are the most exciting basic science questions and why are they the most exciting and how would we even approach those questions?

## Future Directions

- Signaling in response to biophysical agents involves soluble growth factors and their membrane receptors. Downstream signaling, especially transcription factors, may present more specificity.

- Opportunities for studying mechanisms of physical regulation are offered by specific cell responses that may be particular to the cell type. Morphogenetic responses to biophysical signals are best studied at a higher order of integration, at the tissue level.

- Analysis of candidate genes responding to biophysical agents needs to be done in the context of the phenotype.

- Obligatory steps in signal transduction pathways and their inhibitors are important to identify and then target therapeutically.

# Section Five
Transduction of Biophysical Signals

# Chapter 17
# Transduction of Physical Signals in Articular Cartilage

*Farshid Guilak, PhD*
*Lori A. Setton, PhD*

## Introduction

Articular cartilage provides a low-friction surface for the transmission and distribution of joint loads, exhibiting little or no wear over decades of use.[1] These unique properties of cartilage are determined by the structure and composition of the extracellular matrix, which consists mostly of water with dissolved electrolytes, fibrillar collagens (mainly type II), and polyanionic glycosaminoglycans that are covalently attached to a core protein to form the proteoglycan aggrecan.[2-4] The remainder of the solid matrix consists of smaller, lesser amounts of other proteoglycans, collagens, and noncollagenous proteins. Under normal physiologic conditions, the components of the extracellular matrix are in a state of slow turnover, regulated by the catabolic and anabolic activities of a single cell type, the chondrocytes. These activities are controlled through the processing of both genetic and environmental information, such as the action of soluble mediators (eg, growth factors and cytokines), cell-matrix interactions (eg, matrix composition and integrin-mediated attachment), and physical factors such as mechanical stress.

The physical mechanisms involved in the regulation of cell activities involve various mechanical, chemical, and electric signals.[5] Deformation of the cartilage extracellular matrix due to joint loading is associated with changes in the mechanical environment of the cell, including a complex set of spatially-varying tensile, compressive, and shear stresses and strains; fluid flows; and hydrostatic and osmotic pressures.[6] Furthermore, the high density of negatively charged proteoglycans in the solid matrix (ie, fixed charge density) gives rise to coupled mechanical deformations with electric and chemical phenomena, such as streaming potentials and electro-osmosis effects, during joint loading.[7-9] The ability of the chondrocytes to alter their metabolic biologic activity in response to the mechanical, electric, or physicochemical signals engendered in their environment provides a means by which articular cartilage can modulate its composition, and possibly structure, in response to the physical demands of the joint.

A variety of approaches ranging from in vivo clinical or animal studies to in vitro experiments at the cellular and molecular levels have been used to elucidate the role of different physical stimuli on chondrocyte activity.[5,10-12] The objective of this chapter is to review those studies that describe the potential mechanisms by which physical forces may regulate chondrocyte metabolism at the molecular, cellular, tissue, and organ levels.

Section Five    Transduction of Biophysical Signals

# In Vivo Evidence of the Effects of Mechanical Stress on Cartilage

In vivo studies based on simulating physiologically relevant changes in joint loading provide a means to study long-term (ie, weeks to years) influences on joint tissues that are involved in the processes of growth, remodeling, degeneration, or aging.[13,14] Clinical and animal studies of altered joint loading provide strong evidence that abnormal loads lead to alterations in the composition, structure, metabolism, and mechanical properties of articular cartilage, with some of these changes involved in the etiopathogenesis of osteoarthritis (Fig. 1). For example, disuse of the joint achieved through casting or immobilization results in a resorption of cartilage matrix and proteoglycans that is associated with decreases in cartilage compressive stiffness and thickness.[15,16] Many of these changes seem to be partially reversible with remobilization. Long-term exercise may cause site-specific changes in proteoglycan content and cartilage stiffness, although these changes are not believed to be deleterious[17] and may potentially have a beneficial effect in the normal joint.[18,19] In contrast, obesity may be associated with chronic increases in joint loads and is strongly associated with osteoarthritis.[20] Indeed, a decrease of five kilograms of body weight has been shown to decrease the risk of osteoarthritis by over 50%.[21]

Altered joint loading due to injury of the soft-tissue stabilizers of the joint is now well known to be a significant risk factor for the onset and progression of osteoarthritis.[22-24] Joint instability induced by ligament transection[25,26] or meniscectomy[27,28] may also lead to joint degeneration. These processes result in profound and repeatable changes in joint tissues that mimic changes that occur in early human osteoarthritis, including increased hydration, collagen disruption, and matrix turnover accompanied by decreased tissue stiffness in tension, compression, and shear.[29-37] Articular cartilage and synovial fluid from these models of osteoarthritis show significant increases in various biomarkers[38] that are correlated with histologic damage in the joint.[39] Inflammatory mediators and cytokines seem to play an important role in these "altered loading" models of osteoarthritis, although the precise relationships between biomechanical factors and inflammation are not fully understood. Similarly, impact loads cause significant damage to the articular cartilage, including fissuring of the extracellular matrix, increased cellular activity, increased tissue hydration, and remodeling of the subchondral bone.[40] These characteristics are generally consistent with the early stages of osteoarthritis, suggesting that hyperphysiologic stresses may be an important factor in the etiopathogenesis of this disease.

These in vivo studies indicate an important relationship between mechanical loading and the health of the joint. Taken together, they suggest that a critical magnitude, and perhaps frequency, of joint loading is necessary to maintain the normal homeostatic balance of cartilage anabolism and catabolism. Conversely, progressive joint degenerative changes are largely initiated by hyperphysiologic magnitudes of loading or by alterations in the normal loading pattern on the joint surfaces (eg, loading of normally unloaded regions of cartilage).

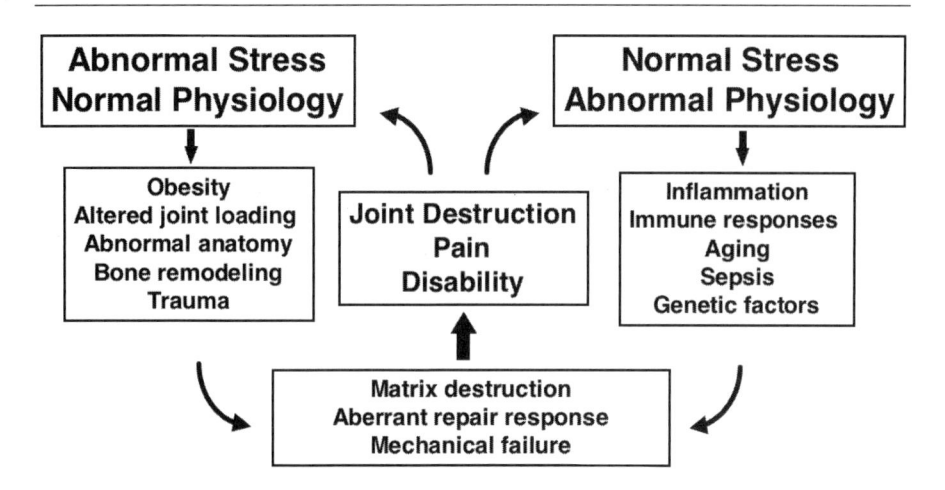

**Figure 1** Potential roles of mechanical stress in the etiopathogenesis of osteoarthritis.

## In Vitro Studies of the Effects of Physical Stimuli on Cartilage Metabolism

Considerable research has been directed toward understanding the processes by which biophysical signals are converted to a biochemical signal by chondrocytes. In vitro explant models of cartilage mechanical loading have been widely used in these studies, because the biomechanical and biochemical environments of the chondrocytes can be controlled while in situ interactions between the cells and the extracellular matrix are maintained. Given the central importance of compressive loading in the joint, most of these studies have focused on cellular responses to compressive stimuli. The general consensus of these studies is that static compression suppresses matrix biosynthesis, whereas cyclic and intermittent loading stimulate chondrocyte metabolism.[41-47] Such responses have been reported over a wide range of loading magnitudes and exhibit a dependency on the magnitude of stress or strain.[10] Excessive loading (eg, high magnitude or prolonged durations of loading) appear to have a deleterious effect, resulting in suppression of biosynthetic activity, cell death, and tissue disruption.[43,48-50] Injurious compression at hyperphysiologic magnitudes (7 to 12 MPa) can induce degradation of the collagen fibril network with a resultant increase in tissue swelling that inhibits the tissues' ability to recover homeostasis.[49]

In other studies, static or intermittent mechanical compression has increased the synthesis of nitric oxide (NO) and prostaglandin $E_2$ with significant interaction between the NO synthase and cyclooxygenase pathways.[51,52] However, altered osmotic stress in the absence of changes in tissue deformation did not affect NO production,[51] suggesting that the observed effects probably are not the result of changes in matrix fixed-charge density or cell volume secondary to altered osmolarity.

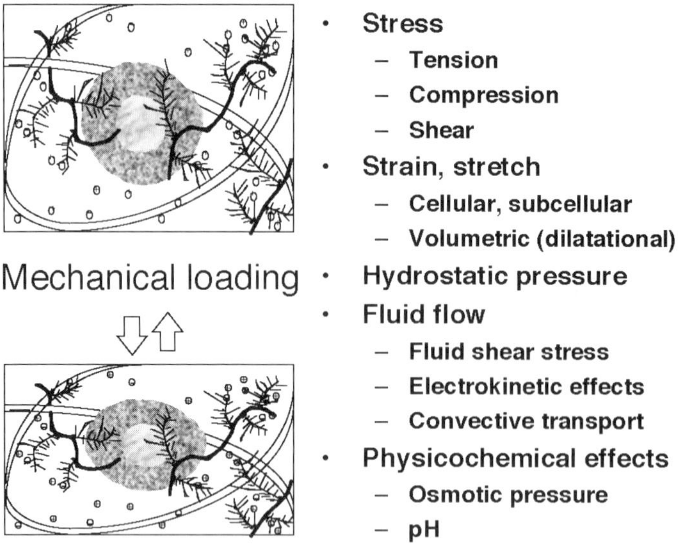

Section Five   Transduction of Biophysical Signals

- **Stress**
  - Tension
  - Compression
  - Shear
- **Strain, stretch**
  - Cellular, subcellular
  - Volumetric (dilatational)
- **Hydrostatic pressure**
- **Fluid flow**
  - Fluid shear stress
  - Electrokinetic effects
  - Convective transport
- **Physicochemical effects**
  - Osmotic pressure
  - pH

Mechanical loading

**Figure 2** At the cellular level, mechanical compression of articular cartilage induces a complex biomechanical microenvironment consisting of spatially varying tensile, compressive, and shear stresses and strains. Furthermore, the large fixed-charge density in the hydrophilic extracellular matrix couples mechanical, electric, and chemical phenomena that occur with tissue loading.

## Physical Signals at the Cellular and Subcellular Levels

Although in vivo and in vitro studies illustrate that mechanical stress may modulate the physiology of the chondrocyte, the identity of the specific biologic and physical pathways involved in the transduction of physical stimuli to an intracellular response is still unclear. A major complexity in examining the effects of specific biophysical phenomena on chondrocyte activity is the fact that many of these phenomena are intrinsically coupled within the cartilage extracellular matrix, and even simple compression of cartilage can change the stress-strain, fluid flow, fluid pressure, physicochemical, and electric environment of the chondrocytes (Fig. 2).

For example, the physicochemical environment within articular cartilage is determined by properties such as matrix hydration, fixed-charge density, interstitial ion concentrations, and activity coefficients for specific ions within the matrix.[9] Because of the coupling of tissue hydration and fixed charge density to tissue dilatation, compression of a cartilage explant by 20% can increase the negative fixed charge density by 15% to 20%.[8,53] The associated changes in local ionic environment with compression give rise to increased intratissue osmotic pressure and decreased pH, which may modify cell behavior.[42,54]

Chondrocytes may also perceive changes in their physical environment through cellular deformation (ie, changes in shape and volume). During

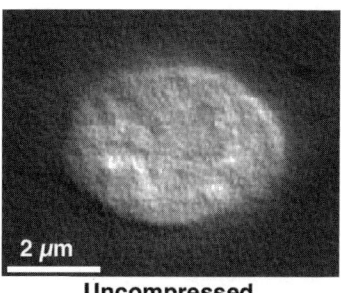

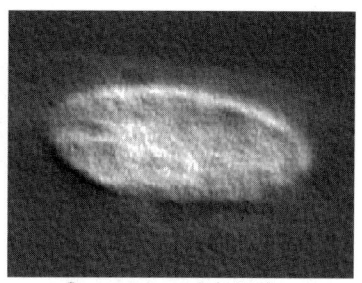

**Uncompressed**      **Compressed (15%)**

**Figure 3** Digitally enhanced confocal laser scanning microscopy images showing deformation of the chondrocyte nucleus in cartilage explants. Fluoresence images show the same nucleus from the cartilage middle zone prior to compression (left), and at equilibrium following a 15% surface-to-surface displacement of the tissue (right). Chondrocyte nuclei deformed in a coordinated manner with the cell and extracellular matrix during compression. *(Reproduced with permission from Guilak F, Sah RL, Setton LA: Physical regulation of cartilage metabolism, in Mow VC, Hayes WC (eds):* Basic Orthopaedic Biomechanics, *ed 2. Philadelphia, PA, Lippincott-Raven, 1997, pp 179-207.)*

physiologic levels of matrix compression, chondrocytes undergo significant shape changes, and cellular and nuclear volume in situ can be altered by as much as ~15% to 20%[55-57] (Fig. 3). The mechanisms resulting in chondrocyte volumetric decrease appear to involve both mechanical and osmotic effects associated with matrix compression[58] (Fig. 4). In many cell types, changes in cell volume are associated with biologic signaling via the transport of ions and organic compounds.[59-61] Alterations in the osmotic environment of isolated chondrocytes induce changes in cell volume and activate cell signaling pathways, such as the mobilization of calcium ion ($Ca^{2+}$) from intracellular stores.[62]

The water in cartilage may constitute as much as 80% of the cartilage extracellular matrix and is considered to be incompressible at physiologic pressures. Thus, hydrostatic fluid pressurization of cartilage does not cause measurable deformation of the extracellular matrix[63] or cells[64] but does appear to have a strong biologic effect on chondrocytes. The stimulatory effects of hydrostatic pressure on aggrecan biosynthesis may be regulated through membrane-mediated pathways by the alteration of membrane fluidity or changes in the transport of cations, amino acids, and macromolecules.[65] There is also evidence that hydrostatic pressure has a direct effect on the transmembrane potential of chondrocytes, which is hypothesized to occur due to altered intracellular $K^+$ concentrations via effects on the $Na^+/K^+$ pump.[66] Hydrostatic pressure can alter the structure of the chondrocyte cytoskeleton and intracellular organelles. For example, high hydrostatic pressures (30 MPa) can alter the organization of stress fibers, microtubules, and the Golgi apparatus in isolated chondrocytes.[67,68]

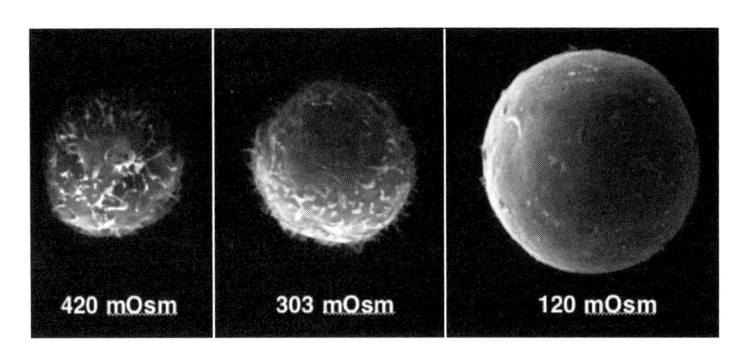

Section Five　　Transduction of Biophysical Signals

**Figure 4** Scanning electron microscopy of the effects of osmotic stress on chondrocyte morphology. Hyperosmotic medium (420 mOsm) causes a decrease in cell volume with an apparent increase in membrane ruffling. In iso-osmotic medium (300 to 350 mOsm), chondrocytes exhibited numerous membrane ruffles and microvilli, which represents an apparent "excess" membrane area of ~230% of the surface area of the cell. In hypo-osmotic medium (120 to 150 mOsm), chondrocytes swelled significantly, exhibiting a relatively smooth plasma membrane. Scale bar = 10 µm. *(Reproduced with permission from Guilak F, Erickson GR, Ting-Beall HP: The effects of osmotic stress on the viscoelastic and physical properties of articular chondrocytes. Biophys J 2002;82:720-727.)*

Because of the large proportion of water in the extracellular matrix, cyclic compression of cartilage produces hydrostatic fluid pressure gradients that can increase the convective transport of the interstitial fluid. Physiologic frequencies of compression (~1 Hz) can generate interstitial flow velocities greater than 1 µm/s,[44] which are predicted to be 1 to 2 orders of magnitude higher during physiologic joint contact.[69,70] The effects of fluid flow on chondrocytes may be due to a combination of physical effects, such as fluid-induced shear stresses on the cell surface, or to increased transport of solutes and metabolites to and from the cells.[41,71] Shear stress-induced cellular signal transduction has been studied extensively in other cell types;[72,73] in chondrocytes, fluid-induced shear stress influences aggrecan synthesis, cellular alignment, metalloproteinase expression, and NO production.[74-78] Mechanically induced fluid flow is also associated with increased convective transport, which appears to preferentially enhance the transport of larger molecules (eg, growth factors, cytokines, or enzymes).[41,71,79]

An additional interaction of fluid movement in cartilage with the proteoglycan-associated negative charges is the generation of electrokinetic phenomena, such as streaming potentials and streaming currents, that arise from motions of mobile cations in the interstitial fluid (eg, $K^+$, $Na^+$, $Ca^{2+}$).[7,8,80] The physiologic magnitude of streaming potentials in cartilage is estimated to be approximately ~15 mV, with corresponding field strengths of up to 1,500 V/m and current densities of ~100 mA/cm² during loading, although typical in vivo current densities may be 1 to 2 orders of magnitude lower.[81-83] Several studies have shown that such low-level electric fields can modulate chondrocyte activity,[84-89] suggesting that cellular response to mechanical loading, and possibly to interstitial fluid flow, may also involve electrokinetic phenomena. The mechanisms by which such electric potentials influence chondrocyte activity remain to be elucidated but may involve the gating of voltage-dependent ion channels and transient changes in chondrocyte membrane potential.

## Intracellular Signaling Pathways

To influence chondrocyte physiology, these physical signals must be transduced to an intracellular biochemical signal. Intracellular signaling in response to mechanical and other physical factors appears to involve many of the traditional second messenger and transmembrane cell signaling pathways, such as the adenylate cyclase system, the inositol trisphosphate system, and cytosolic $Ca^{2+}$ signaling.[11,62,78,90-94] In particular, increased concentrations of intracellular $Ca^{2+}$ appear to be an early response to various mechanical stimuli (eg, stretch, osmotic stress, fluid flow), and changes in $Ca^{2+}$ can influence a large number of cellular functions.[95] Intracellular transduction of physical stimuli also appears to involve the mitogen-activated protein kinase (MAPK) family of signaling molecules. Studies have shown that the suppression of aggrecan gene expression by fluid shear stress[75] and the increased proliferative response following chondrocyte stretch[96] are mediated in part by extracellular signal-regulated kinase 1/2 (ERK 1 and ERK 2) regulation.

Cellular deformation may be transduced to biologic responses through an effect on the cell membrane that is potentially regulated by mechanically sensitive, or "stretch-activated," ion channels.[60,92,93,97-99] Recent studies also demonstrate the presence in chondrocytes of members of the transient receptor potential vanilloid (TRPV) family of cation channels[100] that may serve as transducers of mechanical and osmotic signals, as they do in a variety of organisms.[101-103] As chondrocytes appear to express receptors and ion channels common to many other cell types, their involvement in the transduction of physical stimuli may provide important avenues of future study.

Mechanical signaling may be regulated by interactions between the extracellular matrix and the cells that control cellular attachment, cytoskeleton, and morphology and that potentially contribute to signaling cross-talk. For example, chondrocyte attachment to fibronectin through specific membrane-spanning integrin subunits regulates protein kinase C and MAPK signaling downstream of fibronectin adhesion and alters chondrocyte response to interleukin 1 and other cytokines.[104-109] Some studies suggest that these same integrin-mediated cell-matrix interactions are capable of transducing mechanical signals to the cytosol directly, through transmembrane pathways that bypass traditional second messenger cascades.[110] Indeed, numerous studies have shown that integrin-mediated connections directly modulate cytoskeletal organization and the proteins of the adhesion plaque (eg, α-actinin, vinculin, talin) that may regulate organization of cell trafficking pathways and the nucleus.[55,56,111-114] In chondrocytes, the adhesion of fibronectin to integrin subunits has been shown to phosphorylate proteins of the adhesion plaque that can be expected to modify cytoskeletal organization. Recent studies have shown that the amount of expressed integrin subunits is directly affected by exposure to compressive stimuli,[115] so it is clear that cell-matrix interactions are modulated by physical stimuli. It is likely that more complex interactions between traditional receptor-mediated and second messenger pathways, as well as cytoskeletal-mediated signaling mechanisms, contribute to the mechanisms by which cell-matrix interactions affect chondrocyte homeostasis.

## Conclusions

The process of physical signal transduction in cartilage involves a complex and interacting array of physical and biochemical processes. In vivo studies show that the mechanical environment of the chondrocytes plays an important role in the health and function of the diarthrodial joint, and that significant deviations from the normal pattern of joint loading may lead to deleterious and usually irreversible changes in the articular cartilage and joint tissues. Under normal conditions, the chondrocyte population is exposed to dynamic changes in the mechanical and electrochemical environment within the tissue extracellular matrix, including spatial and temporal variations in a variety of physical factors such as stress, strain, fluid flow, fluid pressure, osmotic pressure, fixed charge density, pH, and electric field effects.

A number of different model systems have been used to show that each of these physical phenomena has the potential to activate multiple cellular signaling pathways. Furthermore, it appears that a variety of physical and biochemical transduction pathways function together to orchestrate the overall cell response to mechanical loading. These findings suggest that physical stimuli applied exogenously or pharmacologic agents that mediate physical stimuli-induced signaling have potential as clinical modalities for preventing age- or disease-related changes in articular cartilage, or enhancing cartilage repair or regeneration.

## Acknowledgments

Supported by National Institutes of Health grants AR50245, AR48182, AG15768, EB02263, and AR47442. The authors thank Drs. Robert Sah and Clark Hung for many insightful and important discussions on this topic.

## References

1. Mow VC, Ratcliffe A, Poole AR: Cartilage and diarthrodial joints as paradigms for hierarchical materials and structures. *Biomaterials* 1992;13:67-97.

2. Eyre DR: The collagens of articular cartilage. *Semin Arthritis Rheum* 1991;21:2-11.

3. Mankin HJ, Brandt KD: Biochemistry and metabolism of articular cartilage in osteoarthritis, in Moskowitz RW, Howell DS, Goldberg VM, Mankin HJ (eds): *Osteoarthritis: Diagnosis and Medical/Surgical Management.* Philadelphia, PA, WB Saunders, 1992, pp 109-154.

4. Muir H, Hardingham TE: Structure of proteoglycans, in Whelan WJ (ed): *MTP International Review of Science: Biochemistry of Carbohydrates.* Baltimore, MD, Butterworth/University Park Press, 1975, pp 152-222.

5. Helminen HJ, Jurvelin J, Kiviranta I, Paukkonen K, Säämänen AM, Tammi M: Joint loading effects on articular cartilage: A historical review, in Helminen HJ, Kiviranta I, Tammi M, Säämänen AM, Paukkonen K, Jurvelin J (eds): *Joint Loading: Biology and Health of Articular Structures.* Bristol, England, Wright and Sons, 1987, pp 1-46.

6. Guilak F, Mow VC: The mechanical environment of the chondrocyte: A biphasic finite element model of cell-matrix interactions in articular cartilage. *J Biomech* 2000;33:1663-1673.

7. Frank EH, Grodzinsky AJ: Cartilage electromechanics: I. Electrokinetic transduction and the effects of electrolyte pH and ionic strength. *J Biomech* 1987;20:615-627.

8. Lai WM, Hou JS, Mow VC: A triphasic theory for the swelling and deformation behaviors of articular cartilage. *J Biomech Eng* 1991;113:245-258.

9. Maroudas A: Physicochemical properties of articular cartilage, in Freeman M (ed): *Adult Articular Cartilage.* Tunbridge Wells, England, Pitman Medical, 1979, pp 215-290.

10. Guilak F, Sah RL, Setton LA: Physical regulation of cartilage metabolism, in Mow VC, Hayes WC (eds): *Basic Orthopaedic Biomechanics,* ed 2. Philadelphia, PA, Lippincott-Raven, 1997, pp 179-207.

11. Stockwell RA: Structure and function of the chondrocyte under mechanical stress, in Helminen HJ, Kiviranta I, Tammi M, Säämänen AM, Paukkonen K, Jurvelin J (eds): *Joint Loading: Biology and Health of Articular Structures.* Bristol, England, Wright and Sons, 1987, pp 126-148.

12. van Campen GPJ, van de Stadt RJ: Cartilage and chondrocytes responses to mechanical loading in vitro, in Helminen HJ, Kiviranta I, Tammi M, Säämänen AM, Paukkonen K, Jurvelin J (eds): *Joint Loading: Biology and Health of Articular Structures.* Bristol, England, Wright and Sons, 1987, pp 112-125.

13. Moskowitz RW: Experimental models of osteoarthritis, in Moskowitz RW, Howell DS, Goldberg VM, Mankin HJ (eds): *Osteoarthritis: Diagnosis and Medical/Surgical Management,* ed 2. Philadelphia, PA, WB Saunders, 1992, pp 213-232.

14. Pritzker KPH: Animal models for osteoarthritis: Processes, problems and prospects. *Ann Rheum Dis* 1994;53:406-420.

15. Akeson WH, Amiel D, Abel MF, Garfin SR, Woo SL: Effects of immobilization on joints. *Clin Orthop* 1987;219:28-37.

16. Palmoski MJ, Perricone E, Brandt KD: Development and reversal of a proteoglycan aggregation defect in normal canine knee cartilage after immobilization. *Arthritis Rheum* 1979;22:508-517.

17. Lammi MJ, Hakkinen TP, Parkkinen JJ, et al: Adaptation of canine femoral head articular cartilage to long distance running exercise in young beagles. *Ann Rheum Dis* 1993;52:369-377.

18. Kraus VB: Pathogenesis and treatment of osteoarthritis. *Med Clin North Am* 1997;81:85-112.

19. Lane NE, Bloch DA, Jones HH, Marshall WH Jr, Wood PD, Fries JF: Long-distance running, bone density, and osteoarthritis. *JAMA* 1986;255:1147-1151.

20. Oliveria SA, Felson DT, Cirillo PA, Reed JI, Walker AM: Body weight, body mass index, and incident symptomatic osteoarthritis of the hand, hip, and knee. *Epidemiology* 1999;10:161-166.

21. Felson DT, Zhang Y, Anthony JM, Naimark A, Anderson JJ: Weight loss reduces the risk for symptomatic knee osteoarthritis in women: The Framingham Study. *Ann Intern Med* 1992;116:535-539.

22. Buckwalter JA: Osteoarthritis and articular cartilage use, disuse, and abuse: Experimental studies. *J Rheumatol* 1995;43:13-15.

23. Howell DS, Treadwell BV, Trippel SB: Etiopathogenesis of osteoarthritis, in Moskowitz RW, Howell DS, Goldberg VM, Mankin HJ (eds): *Osteoarthritis, Diagnosis and Medical/Surgical Management,* ed 2. Philadelphia, PA, WB Saunders, 1992, pp 233-252.

24. Lane JM, Chisena E, Black J: Experimental knee instability: Early mechanical property changes in articular cartilage in a rabbit model. *Clin Orthop* 1979;140:262-265.

25. Gilbertson EMM: Development of periarticular osteophytes in experimentally induced osteoarthrosis in the dog. *Ann Rheum Dis* 1975;34:12-25.

26. Pond MJ, Nuki G: Experimentally induced osteoarthritis in the dog. *Ann Rheum Dis* 1973;32:387-388.

27. Hoch DH, Grodzinsky AJ, Koob TJ, Albert ML, Eyre DR: Early changes in material properties of rabbit articular cartilage after meniscectomy. *J Orthop Res* 1983;1:4-12.

28. Moskowitz RW, Davis W, Sammarco J: Experimentally induced degenerative joint lesions following partial meniscectomy in the rabbit. *Arthritis Rheum* 1973;16:397-405.

29. Altman RD, Tenenbaum J, Latta L, Riskin W, Blanco LN, Howell DS: Biomechanical and biochemical properties of dog cartilage in experimentally induced osteoarthritis. *Ann Rheum Dis* 1984;43:83-90.

30. Carney SL, Billingham ME, Muir H, Sandy JD: Demonstration of increased proteoglycan turnover in cartilage explants from dogs with experimental osteoarthritis. *J Orthop Res* 1984;2:201-206.

31. Elliott DM, Guilak F, Vail TP, Wang JY, Setton LA: Tensile properties of articular cartilage are altered by meniscectomy in a canine model of osteoarthritis. *J Orthop Res* 1999;17:503-508.

32. Eyre DR, McDevitt CA, Billingham ME, Muir H: Biosynthesis of collagen and other matrix proteins by articular cartilage in experimental osteoarthrosis. *Biochem J* 1980;188:823-837.

33. Guilak F, Ratcliffe A, Lane N, Rosenwasser MP, Mow VC: Mechanical and biochemical changes in the superficial zone of articular cartilage in canine experimental osteoarthritis. *J Orthop Res* 1994;12:474-484.

34. McDevitt CA, Muir H: Biochemical changes in the cartilage of the knee in experimental and natural osteoarthritis in the dog. *J Bone Joint Surg Am* 1976;58:94-101.

35. Ratcliffe A, Billingham ME, Saed-Nejad F, Muir H, Hardingham TE: Increased release of matrix components from articular cartilage in experimental canine osteoarthritis. *J Orthop Res* 1992;10:350-358.

36. Sandy JD, Adams ME, Billingham ME, Plaas A, Muir H: In vivo and in vitro stimulation of chondrocyte biosynthetic activity in early experimental osteoarthritis. *Arthritis Rheum* 1984;27:388-397.

37. Setton LA, Mow VC, Muller FJ, Pita JC, Howell DS: Mechanical properties of canine articular cartilage are significantly altered following transection of the anterior cruciate ligament. *J Orthop Res* 1994;12:451-463.

38. Lindhorst E, Vail TP, Guilak F, et al: Longitudinal characterization of synovial fluid biomarkers in the canine meniscectomy model of osteoarthritis. *J Orthop Res* 2000;18:269-280.

39. Carlson CS, Kraus VB, Vail TP, Setton LA, Gardin JF, Guilak F: Articular cartilage damage following medial meniscectomy in dogs is predicted by synovial fluid biomarker levels. *Trans Orthop Res Soc* 1999;24:194.

40. Radin EL, Martin RB, Burr DB, Caterson B, Boyd RD, Goodwin C: Effects of mechanical loading on the tissues of the rabbit knee. *J Orthop Res* 1984;2:221-234.

41. Bonassar LJ, Grodzinsky AJ, Srinivasan A, Davila SG, Trippel SB: Mechanical and physicochemical regulation of the action of insulin-like growth factor-I on articular cartilage. *Arch Biochem Biophys* 2000;379:57-63.

42. Gray ML, Pizzanelli AM, Grodzinsky AJ, Lee RC: Mechanical and physiochemical determinants of the chondrocyte biosynthetic response. J Orthop Res 1988;6:777-792.

43. Guilak F, Meyer BC, Ratcliffe A, Mow VC: The effects of matrix compression on proteoglycan metabolism in articular cartilage explants. *Osteoarthritis Cartilage* 1994;2:91-101.

44. Kim YJ, Bonassar LJ, Grodzinsky AJ: The role of cartilage streaming potential, fluid flow and pressure in the stimulation of chondrocyte biosynthesis during dynamic compression. *J Biomech* 1995;28:1055-1066.

45. Palmoski MJ, Brandt KD: Effects of static and cyclic compressive loading on articular cartilage plugs in vitro. *Arthritis Rheum* 1984;27:675-681.

46. Sah RL, Kim YJ, Doong JY, Grodzinsky AJ, Plaas AH, Sandy JD: Biosynthetic response of cartilage explants to dynamic compression. *J Orthop Res* 1989;7:619-636.

47. Torzilli PA, Grigiene R: Continuous cyclic load reduces proteoglycan release from articular cartilage. *Osteoarthritis Cartilage* 1998;6:260-268.

48. Chen CT, Burton-Wurster N, Borden C, Hueffer K, Bloom SE, Lust G: Chondrocyte necrosis and apoptosis in impact damaged articular cartilage. *J Orthop Res* 2001;19:703-711.

49. Loening AM, James IE, Levenston ME, et al: Injurious mechanical compression of bovine articular cartilage induces chondrocyte apoptosis. *Arch Biochem Biophys* 2000;381:205-212.

50. Quinn TM, Grodzinsky AJ, Hunziker EB, Sandy JD: Effects of injurious compression on matrix turnover around individual cells in calf articular cartilage explants. *J Orthop Res* 1998;16:490-499.

51. Fermor B, Weinberg JB, Pisetsky DS, Misukonis MA, Banes AJ, Guilak F: The effects of static and intermittent compression on nitric oxide production in articular cartilage explants. *J Orthop Res* 2001;19:729-737.

52. Fermor B, Weinberg JB, Pisetsky DS, Misukonis MA, Fink C, Guilak F: Induction of cyclooxygenase-2 by mechanical stress through a nitric oxide-regulated pathway. *Osteoarthritis & Cartilage* 2002;10:792-798.

53. Lai WM, Setton LA, Mow VC: Conditional equivalence of chemical and mechanical loading on articular cartilage. *ASME Adv Bioeng BED* 1991;18:481-484.

54. Urban JP, Bayliss MT: Regulation of proteoglycan synthesis rate in cartilage in vitro: Influence of extracellular ionic composition. *Biochim Biophys Acta* 1989;992:59-65.

55. Buschmann MD, Hunziker EB, Kim YJ, Grodzinsky AJ: Altered aggrecan synthesis correlates with cell and nucleus structure in statically compressed cartilage. *J Cell Sci* 1996;109:499-508.

56. Guilak F: Compression-induced changes in the shape and volume of the chondrocyte nucleus. *J Biomech* 1995;28:1529-1542.

57. Guilak F, Ratcliffe A, Mow VC: Chondrocyte deformation and local tissue strain in articular cartilage: A confocal microscopy study. *J Orthop Res* 1995;13:410-421.

58. Guilak F, Erickson GR, Ting-Beall HP: The effects of osmotic stress on the viscoelastic and physical properties of articular chondrocytes. *Biophys J* 2002;82:720-727.

59. Christensen O: Mediation of cell volume by Ca2+ influx through stretch-activated channels. *Nature* 1987;330:66-68.

60. Sachs F: Mechanical transduction by membrane ion channels: A mini review. *Mol Cell Biochem* 1991;104:57-60.

61. Sarkadi B, Parker JC: Activation of ion transport pathways by changes in cell volume. *Biochem Biophys Acta* 1991;1071:407-427.

62. Erickson GR, Alexopoulos LG, Guilak F: Hyper-osmotic stress induces volume change and calcium transients in chondrocytes by transmembrane, phospholipid, and G-protein pathways. *J Biomech* 2001;34:1527-1535.

63. Bachrach NM, Mow VC, Guilak F: Incompressibility of the solid matrix of articular cartilage under high hydrostatic pressures. *J Biomech* 1998;31:445-451.

64. Wilkes R, Athanasiou KA: The intrinsic incompressibility of osteoblast-like cells. *Tissue Eng* 1996;2:167-181.

65. Urban JPG, Hall AC: The effects of hydrostatic and osmotic pressures on chondrocyte metabolism, in Mow VC, Guilak F, Tran-Son-Tay R, Hochmuth RM (eds): *Cell Mechanics and Cellular Engineering.* New York, NY, Springer Verlag, 1994, pp 398-419.

66. Wright MO, Stockwell RA, Nuki G: Response of plasma membrane to applied hydrostatic pressure in chondrocytes and fibroblasts. *Connect Tissue Res* 1992;28:49-70.

67. Parkkinen JJ, Lammi MJ, Inkinen R, et al: Influence of short-term hydrostatic pressure on organization of stress fibers in cultured chondrocytes. *J Orthop Res* 1995;13:495-502.

68. Parkkinen JJ, Lammi MJ, Pelttari A, Helminen HJ, Tammi M, Virtanen I: Altered Golgi apparatus in hydrostatically loaded articular cartilage chondrocytes. *Ann Rheum Dis* 1993;52:192-198.

69. Ateshian GA: A theoretical formulation for boundary friction in articular cartilage. *J Biomech Eng* 1997;119:81-86.

70. Ateshian GA, Wang H: Rolling resistance of articular cartilage due to interstitial fluid flow. Proc Inst Mech Eng Part H: *J Eng Med* 1997;211:419-424.

71. Garcia AM, Lark MW, Trippel SB, Grodzinsky AJ: Transport of tissue inhibitor of metalloproteinases-1 through cartilage: contributions of fluid flow and electrical migration. *J Orthop Res* 1998;16:734-742.

72. Davies PF: Flow-mediated endothelial mechanotransduction. *Physiol Rev* 1995;75:519-560.

73. Nerem RM, Harrison DG, Taylor WR, Alexander RW: Hemodynamics and vascular endothelial biology. *J Cardiovasc Pharmacol* 1993;21:S6-S10.

74. Das P, Schurman DJ, Smith RL: Nitric oxide and G proteins mediate the response of bovine articular chondrocytes to fluid-induced shear. *J Orthop Res* 1997;15:87-93.

75. Hung C, Henshaw D, Wang C, et al: Mitogen-activated protein kinase signaling in bovine articular chondrocytes in response to fluid flow does not require calcium mobilization. *J Biomechanics* 2000;33:73-80.

76. Lee MS, Trindade MCD, Ikenoue T, Schurman DJ, Goodman SB, Smith RL: Effects of shear stress on nitric oxide and matrix protein gene expression in human osteoarthritic chondrocytes in vitro. *J Orthop Res* 2002;20:556-561.

77. Smith RL, Trindade MC, Ikenoue T, et al: Effects of shear stress on articular chondrocyte metabolism. *Biorheology* 2000;37:95-107.

78. Yellowley CE, Jacobs CR, Li Z, Zhou Z, Donahue HJ: Effects of fluid flow on intracellular calcium in bovine articular chondrocytes. *Am J Physiol* 1997;273:C30-C36.

79. O'Hara BP, Urban JP, Maroudas A: Influence of cyclic loading on the nutrition of articular cartilage. *Ann Rheum Dis* 1990;49:536-539.

80. Gu WY, Lai WM, Mow VC: Transport of fluid and ions through a porous-permeable charged-hydrated tissue, and streaming potential data on normal bovine articular cartilage. *J Biomech* 1993;26:709-723.

81. Chen AC, Nguyen TT, Sah RL: Streaming potentials during the confined compression creep test of normal and proteoglycan-depleted cartilage. *Ann Biomed Eng* 1997;25:269-277.

82. Frank E, Grodzinsky A, Phillips S, Grimshaw P: Physicochemical and bioelectrical determinants of cartilage material properties, in Mow VC, Ratcliffe A, Woo SLY (eds): *Biomechanics of Diarthrodial Joints.* New York, NY, Springer Verlag, 1990, pp 261-282.

83. Gu WY, Rabin J, Lai WM, Mow VC: Measurement of streaming potential of bovine articular and nasal cartilage in 1-D permeation experiments. *ASME Adv Bioeng BED* 1995;31:49-50.

84. Aaron RK, Boyan BD, Ciombor DM, Schwartz Z, Simon BJ: Stimulation of growth factor synthesis by electric and electromagnetic fields. *Clin Orthop* 2004;419:30-37.

85. Aaron RK, Wang S, Ciombor DM: Upregulation of basal TGFbeta1 levels by EMF coincident with chondrogenesis: Implications for skeletal repair and tissue engineering. *J Orthop Res* 2002;20:233-240.

86. Chao P-HG, Roy R, Mauck RL, Liu W, Valhmu WB, Hung CT: Chondrocyte translocation response to direct current electric fields. *J Biomech Eng* 2000;122:261-267.

87. Ciombor DM, Aaron RK, Wang S, Simon B: Modification of osteoarthritis by pulsed electromagnetic field: A morphological study. *Osteoarthritis Cartilage* 2003;11:455-462.

88. Ciombor DM, Lester G, Aaron RK, Neame P, Caterson B: Low frequency EMF regulates chondrocyte differentiation and expression of matrix proteins. *J Orthop Res* 2002;20:40-50.

89. MacGinitie LA, Gluzband YA, Grodzinsky AJ: Electric field stimulation can increase protein synthesis in articular cartilage explants. *J Orthop Res* 1994;12:151-160.

90. Edlich M, Yellowley CE, Jacobs CR, Donahue HJ: Oscillating fluid flow regulates cytosolic calcium concentration in bovine articular chondrocytes. *J Biomech* 2001;34:59-65.

91. Erickson GR, Northrup DL, Guilak F: Hypo-osmotic stress induces calcium-dependent actin reorganization in articular chondrocytes. *Osteoarthritis Cartilage* 2003;11:187-197.

92. Guilak F, Zell RA, Erickson GR, et al: Mechanically induced calcium waves in articular chondrocytes are inhibited by gadolinium and amiloride. *J Orthop Res* 1999;17:421-429.

93. Mobasheri A, Mobasheri R, Francis MJO, Trujillo E, Delarosa DA, Martinvasallo P: Ion transport in chondrocytes: Membrane transporters involved in intracellular ion homeostasis and the regulation of cell volume, free [Ca2+] and pH. *Histol Histopathol* 1998;13:893-910.

94. Roberts SR, Knight MM, Lee DA, Bader DL: Mechanical compression influences intracellular Ca2+ signaling in chondrocytes seeded in agarose constructs. *J Appl Physiol* 2001;90:1385-1391.

95. Rasmussen H: The calcium messenger system. *N Engl J Med* 1986;17:1094-1170.

96. Chen Q, Zhen X, Wu QQ, Zhang Y: Activation of extracellular signal-regulated kinase and P38 MAP kinase is required for mechanical stimulation of chondrocyte proliferation. *Trans Orthop Res Soc* 1999;45:7.

97. Millward-Sadler SJ, Wright MO, Davies LW, Nuki G, Salter DM: Mechanotransduction via integrins and interleukin-4 results in altered aggrecan and matrix metalloproteinase 3 gene expression in normal, but not osteoarthritic, human articular chondrocytes. *Arthritis Rheum* 2000;43:209-219.

98. Morris CE: Mechanosensitive ion channels. *J Membr Biol* 1990;113:93-107.

99. Wright M, Jobanputra P, Bavington C, Salter D, Nuki G: Evidence for stretch-activated ion channels in human chondrocytes. *Bone Miner* 1994;1:S37.

100. Alford AI, Votta B, Nuttall ME, Kumar S, Lark M, Guilak F: Functional characterization of vanilloid receptor 4 in porcine articular chondrocytes. *Trans Orthop Res Soc* 2003;28:251.

101. Liedtke W, Choe Y, Marti-Renom MA, et al: Vanilloid receptor-related osmotically activated channel (VR-OAC), a candidate vertebrate osmoreceptor. *Cell* 2000;103:525-535.

102. Liedtke W, Friedman JM: Abnormal osmotic regulation in trpv4-/- mice. *Proc Natl Acad Sci USA* 2003;100:13698-13703.

103. Nilius B, Vriens J, Prenen J, Droogmans G, Voets T: TRPV4 calcium entry channel: A paradigm for gating diversity. *Am J Physiol Cell Physiol* 2004;286:C195-C205.

104. Attur MG, Dave MN, Clancy RM, Patel IR, Abramson SB, Amin AR: Functional genomic analysis in arthritis-affected cartilage: Yin-yang regulation of inflammatory mediators by alpha 5 beta 1 and alpha V beta 3 integrins. *J Immunol* 2000;164:2684-2691.

105. Forsyth CB, Pulai J, Loeser RF: Fibronectin fragments and blocking antibodies to alpha2beta1 and alpha5beta1 integrins stimulate mitogen-activated protein kinase signaling and increase collagenase 3 (matrix metalloproteinase 13) production by human articular chondrocytes. *Arthritis Rheum* 2002;46:2368-2376.

106. Gemba T, Valbracht J, Alsalameh S, Lotz M: Focal adhesion kinase and mitogen-activated protein kinases are involved in chondrocyte activation by the 29-kDa amino-terminal fibronectin fragment. *J Biol Chem* 2002;277:907-911.

107. Lee HS, Millward-Sadler SJ, Wright MO, Nuki G, Salter DM: Integrin and mechanosensitive ion channel-dependent tyrosine phosphorylation of focal adhesion proteins and beta-catenin in human articular chondrocytes after mechanical stimulation. *J Bone Miner Res* 2000;15:1501-1509.

108. Loeser RF: Integrins and cell signaling in chondrocytes. *Biorheology* 2002;39:119-124.

109. Salter DM, Millward-Sadler SJ, Nuki G, Wright MO: Integrin-interleukin-4 mechanotransduction pathways in human chondrocytes. *Clin Orthop* 2001;391:S49-S60.

110. Ingber DE, Folkman J: Mechanochemical switching between growth and differentiation during fibroblast growth factor-stimulated angiogenesis in vitro: Role of extracellular matrix. *J Cell Biol* 1989;109:317-330.

111. Hynes RO: Integrins: A family of cell surface receptors. *Cell* 1987;48:549-554.

112. Ingber D: Integrins as mechanochemical transducers. *Curr Opin Cell Biol* 1991;3:841-848.

113. Knight MM, Lee DA, Bolton JF, Bader DL: Cell and nucleus deformation in compressed chondrocyte-agarose constructs: Implications for mechanotransduction. *Trans Orthop Res Soc* 1999;24:710.

114. Pavalko FM, Otey CA, Simon KO, Burridge K: Alpha-actinin: A direct link between actin and integrins. *Biochem Soc Trans* 1991;19:1065-1069.

115. Lucchinetti E, Bhargava MM, Torzilli PA: The effect of mechanical load on integrin subunits alpha5 and beta1 in chondrocytes from mature and immature cartilage explants. *Cell Tissue Res* 2003;315:385-391.

Chapter 18

# Common Cellular Signaling Mechanisms for Mechanotransduction

*Jameel Iqbal, BS*
*Mone Zaidi, MD, PhD, FRCP*

Hughes-Fulford[1] states that "mechanotransduction is the process of translating mechanical force on a cell into a biological response." A "process of converting physical forces into biochemical signals and integrating these signals into [a] cellular response,"[2] mechanotransduction involves a series of discrete but common steps in which the general objective is growth.

Mechanical stimulation of the skeleton by exercise leads to increases in osteoblast proliferation and matrix deposition.[1] Exercise also stimulates chondrocyte proliferation and increases cartilage synthesis.[3] In tissues such as the gastrointestinal tract, shear stimulation following feeding enhances proliferation of the gut mucosa.[4] In the heart, an increase in mechanical pressure results in compensatory fibroblast proliferation and cardiomyocyte hypertrophy.[5] In most mechanosensitive tissues, the absence of mechanical stimulation leads to tissue degradation. Immobilization or microgravity causes acute, rapid, and severe bone loss in humans and animals.[6] Similarly, disuse of a limb leads selectively to bone degradation in that limb[7] due to a lack of stimulation of the key mechanosensitive cell, the osteocyte. Likewise, strict total parenteral nutrition without oral consumption of food results in gastrointestinal mucosal atrophy.[8] Mechanotransduction thus imparts an essential mitogenic stimulus to mechanosensitive tissues. In this chapter we will review the essential common steps—and variations on those steps—used by mechanosensitive cells for transducing the effects of mechanical stimulation into cellular responses, including effects on gene transcription.

Mechanical stimulation often leads to similar outcomes in many different tissue types; therefore, it is not surprising that common signaling mechanisms are involved. Specifically, it appears that all mechanical stimuli lead to activation of the MAP kinase ERK 1/2, whether it is cardiac, bone, or gastrointestinal tissue.[1-5,9] Phosphorylated ERK 1/2 can, in turn, upregulate and activate progrowth transcription factors such as c-fos as well as some cytoskeletal components like $\alpha$-actinin[5] (Fig. 1). Whereas several converging signals activate ERK 1/2, integrins specifically appear to be involved upstream for mechanotransduction, regardless of the mechanosensitive tissue involved. In both cartilage and intestinal epithelial cells, integrin $\beta_1$ is

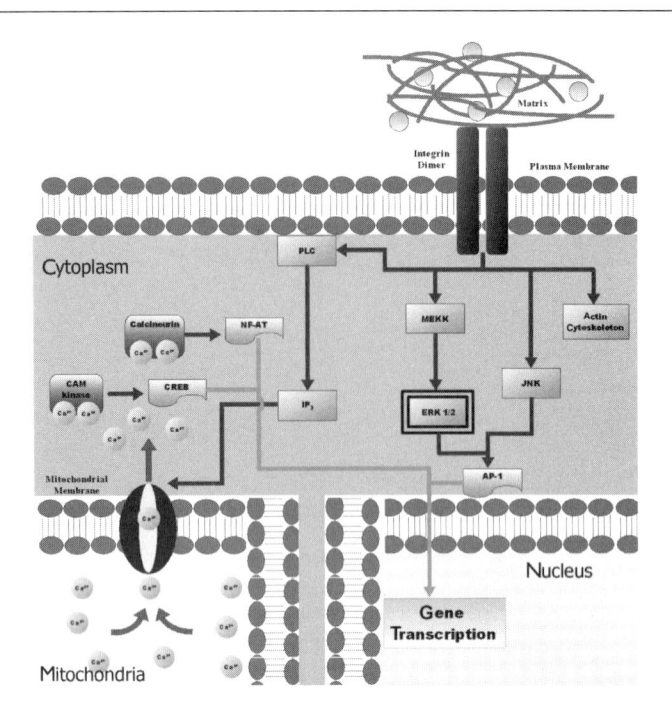

**Figure 1** The cellular mechanisms of mechanotransduction. A mechanical stress activates integrin receptors that are bound to the extracellular matrix. These receptors recruit adaptors to cause three main changes: (1) the phosphorylation and activation of MAP kinase signaling pathways (denoted by MEKK and JNK) that lead to ERK 1/2 phosphorylation, (2) the activation of PLC leading to $IP_3$ generation and elevation of intracellular $Ca^{2+}$ levels, and (3) alterations in the actin cytoskeleton network. Phosphorylated ERK 1/2 causes the activation of the AP-1 family of transcription factors, which are necessary for the progrowth response. Elevated $Ca^{2+}$ levels accentuate kinases (CAM kinase) and phosphatases (calcineurin) to activate the transcription factors CREB and NF-AT respectively. Alterations in the actin cytoskeleton serve to stabilize the cell against the applied forces.

essential for ERK 1/2 activation and other mitogenic signals in response to mechanical stimulation.[3,10,11]

Even though there appears to be a common mechanism whereby mechanical stimulation leads to integrin signaling, ERK 1/2 activation, and mitogenic responses, individual tissues display complex responses. Osteoblasts initially increase $IP_3$ production and intracellular $Ca^{2+}$ with the subsequent activation of protein kinase C (PKC) signaling pathways.[1] Increases in cAMP, and thus implied activation of PKA signaling pathways, follow later. It appears that integrin signaling leads to alterations in Rho stress fiber formation and phospholipase C (PLC) activation.[12] PLC serves to generate $IP_3$ and ultimately increases intracellular $Ca^{2+}$ levels. These signals in osteoblasts serve to activate MAP kinase signaling initially via MEKK and possibly p38 MAPK, ultimately culminating in ERK 1/2 phosphorylation.[12,13]

Another mechanism for ERK 1/2 activation involves focal adhesion kinase/c-Src-mediated recruitment of Grb2/sos, which in turn activates Ras and ultimately ERK 1/2.[5]

Signaling pathways exclusive of the MAP kinase cascades also play a role in adjusting the cellular response to mechanical stimulation. For example, signaling mechanisms responsible for generating elevated cAMP levels, delayed due to the time needed for COX-mediated prostaglandin production, serve to augment osteoblast c-fos production and proliferation.[14] Other signaling pathways involve an activation step by $Ca^{2+}$, probably through a PLC-mediated mechanism. For example, elevations in $Ca^{2+}$ activate a $Ca^{2+}$/calmodulin-dependent protein kinase to phosphorylate CREB and cause increased c-fos expression. As another example, calcineurin, a $Ca^{2+}$/calmodulin-activated phosphatase, dephosphorylates and activates the NF-AT family of transcription factors. Different NF-ATs, which are expressed in different cells including the heart, cartilage, and bone, serve as tissue-specific activators of cell growth and differentiation.[15-17]

Finally, different types of cells are best suited to respond to different types of stimuli. For example, a pulsed stimulus promotes cartilage growth, whereas a continuous stimulus leads to cartilage degradation and inflammation.[3] The frequency of the mechanical stimulus is also important. Strain at cycles of 60 to 90 per minute seems optimal in transducing mitogenic effects in vascular endothelial cells, whereas cycles of 6 per minute and 10 to 15 per minute are required for osteoblasts and intestinal epithelial cells, respectively.[4] Cells also appear to respond best to certain stimulus strengths. For example, the strength of the stimulus leads to differential gene transcription in cartilage tissue.[18] Thus, each cell type appears fine-tuned to respond largely to the mechanical stimuli most often encountered or relevant to its physiology. The eventual response of a given cell type to mechanical stimulation thus appears to arise from (1) the type of mechanical stimulation per se and (2) the types of signaling molecules and transcription factors that are expressed.

Focal adhesions of cells to the extracellular matrix contain integrins, which are critical in mediating the transduction of mechanical forces in most cells that have been studied. Integrins bind to paxillin, caveolin, and focal adhesion kinase, and through these binding partners recruit kinases to activate pathways leading ultimately to ERK 1/2 and possibly JNK phosphorylation.[11] This function of integrins serves to transmit the mitogenic or differentiation response.

Another function of integrins is to stabilize cell adhesion in response to mechanical stimulation, "a force-dependent stiffening response."[5] Specifically, integrins connect to the actin cytoskeleton through their binding partners tensin, $\alpha$-actinin, and filamin. It has been hypothesized that this arm of integrin signaling serves to modulate gene expression through the connections of the actin cytoskeleton with the nuclear envelope, laminin networks, and ultimately chromatin.[19]

Interestingly, the central importance of integrins in mechanotransduction has highlighted the role of their extracellular binding partners. In general, it appears that different matrices signal through different integrins and these integrins serve to transduce different signals—that is to say, the response to mechanical strain is matrix-dependent. For example, cardiac fibroblasts or intestinal epithelial cells, when cultured on collagen or laminin, demonstrate patterns of ERK 1/2 activation and a mitogenic response to mechanical stimulation. In contrast, when the same cells are cultured on fibronectin, the same stimulus inhibits mitogenesis.[5,20]

The differential activation of signaling using the same receptor in a matrix-dependent manner may have pathophysiologic implications. Under inflammatory conditions, some cells show an increased synthesis and deposition of acute phase reactant proteins, including fibronectin.[3] The secreted fibronectin, when incorporated into the matrix, alters the response of mechanosensitive cells that use this newly formed matrix. Thus, conditions that alter matrix properties, such as inflammation or cancer, influence a cell's response to mechanical stimulation.

Furthermore, although certain potent inflammatory cytokines inhibit the promitogenic effects of mechanical stimulation under pathologic conditions, other cytokines—such as interleukin-6 (IL-6)—that are produced through mechanical stimulation serve as paracrine transducers of promitogenic stimuli. For example, the cytokine IL-6 is produced in response to mechanical strain in intestinal epithelial cells.[21] Through its gp130 receptor, which causes ERK 1/2 phosphorylation, IL-6 may accentuate the response triggered by mechanical stimulation.[5] There is also evidence that mechanical stimulation of therapeutic intensity leads to resistance of NF-κB activation in response to the inflammatory cytokine IL-1β.[3] Thus, because signaling pathways triggered by inflammatory cytokines and mechanical stress converge, the two stimuli are cross-modulated in both healthy and inflamed tissue.

## Summary

In conclusion, there appears to be a common mechanism for mechanotransduction regardless of the cell type. Specifically, integrins interacting with their matrix or environment mediate the generation of a Ca2+ signal and the activation of MAP kinase cascades, leading ultimately to ERK 1/2 phosphorylation and a pro-growth signal. Each cell appears fine-tuned for the specific type of stimulus, with accessory mechanotransduction signaling pathways adjusting the outcome of signaling in each case.

## References

1. Hughes-Fulford M: Signal transduction and mechanical stress. *Sci STKE* 2004;249:RE12.

2. Huang H, Kamm RD, Lee RT: Cell mechanics and mechanotransduction: Pathways, probes, and physiology. *Am J Physiol Cell Physiol* 2004;287:C1-C11.

3. Deschner J, Hofman CR, Piesco NP, Agarwal S: Signal transduction by mechanical strain in chondrocytes. *Curr Opin Clin Nutr Metab Care* 2003;6:289-293.

4. Basson MD: Paradigms for mechanical signal transduction in the intestinal epithelium. *Digestion* 2003;68:217-225.

5. Ruwhof C, van der Laarse A: Mechanical stress-induced cardiac hypertrophy: Mechanisms and signal transduction pathways. *Cardiovasc Res* 2000;47:23-37.

6. Zerath E: Effects of microgravity on bone and calcium homeostasis. *Adv Space Res* 1998;21:1049-1058.

7. Semb H: Experimental limb disuse and bone blood flow. *Acta Orthop Scand* 1969;40:552-562.

8. Inoue Y, Espat NJ, Frohnapple DJ, Epstein H, Copeland EM, Souba WW: Effect of total parenteral nutrition on amino acid and glucose transport by the human small intestine. *Ann Surg* 1993;217:604-612.

9. Thamilselvan V, Basson MD: Pressure activates colon cancer cell adhesion by inside-out focal adhesion complex and actin cytoskeletal signaling. *Gastroenterology* 2004;126:8-18.

10. Han O, Li GD, Sumpio BE, Basson MD: Strain induces Caco-2 intestinal epithelial proliferation and differentiation via PKC and tyrosine kinase signals. *Am J Physiol* 1998;275:G534-G541.

11. MacKenna DA, Dolfi F, Vuori K, Ruoslahti E: Extracellular signal-regulated kinase and c-Jun NH2-terminal kinase activation by mechanical stretch is integrin-dependent and matrix-specific in rat cardiac fibroblasts. *J Clin Invest* 1998;101:301-310.

12. Chen NX, Ryder KD, Pavalko FM, et al: Ca2+ regulates fluid shear-induced cytoskeletal reorganization and gene expression in osteoblasts. *Am J Physiol Cell Physiol* 2000;278:C989-C997.

13. You J, Reilly G, Zhen X, et al: Osteopontin gene regulation by oscillatory fluid flow via intracellular calcium mobilization and activation of mitogen-activated protein kinase in MC3T3-E1 osteoblasts. *J Biol Chem* 2001;276:13365-13371.

14. Fitzgerald J, Hughes-Fulford M: Mechanically induced c-fos expression is mediated by cAMP in MC3T3-E1 osteoblasts. *FASEB J* 1999;13:553-557.

15. Matsuo K, Galson DL, Zhao C, et al: Nuclear factor of activated T-cells (NFAT) rescues osteoclastogenesis in precursors lacking c-Fos. *J Biol Chem* 2004;279:26475-26480.

16. Ranger AM, Gerstenfeld LC, Wang J, et al: The nuclear factor of activated T cells (NFAT) transcription factor NFATp (NFATc2) is a repressor of chondrogenesis. *J Exp Med* 2000;191:9-22.

17. Crabtree GR: Generic signals and specific outcomes: Signaling through Ca2+, calcineurin, and NF-AT. *Cell* 1999;96:611-614.

18. Long P, Gassner R, Agarwal S: Tumor necrosis factor alpha-dependent proinflammatory gene induction is inhibited by cyclic tensile strain in articular chondrocytes in vitro. *Arthritis Rheum* 2001;44:2311-2319.

19. Lelievre S, Weaver VM, Bissell MJ: Extracellular matrix signaling from the cellular membrane skeleton to the nuclear skeleton: A model of gene regulation. *Recent Prog Horm Res* 1996;51:417-432.

20. Zhang J, Li W, Sumpio BE, Basson MD: Fibronectin blocks p38 and jnk activation by cyclic strain in Caco-2 cells. *Biochem Biophys Res Commun* 2003;306:746-749.

21. Kishikawa H, Miura S, Yoshida H, et al: Transmural pressure induces IL-6 secretion by intestinal epithelial cells. *Clin Exp Immunol* 2002;129:86-91.

# Chapter 19
# Calcium Signaling in Osteoblasts in Response to Mechanical Stimulation

*Randall L. Duncan, PhD*
*Damian C. Genetos, PhD*

## Introduction

Bone mass and skeletal architecture are dependent on the mechanical environment encountered throughout our lifetimes. When met with a novel mechanical load, bone cells have the ability to perceive these vectorial changes and initiate a cascade of cellular events that result—via bone resorption and formation—in alterations in bone architecture to adapt to these new loads. In vivo studies have demonstrated that a single, brief loading bout can increase bone formation rates sixfold in rats.[1] Thus, the anabolic response to mechanical stimulation is greater than that of any other factor that affects bone formation. Study of the cellular mechanisms that initiate this response may lead to new methods of intervention capable of maintaining or improving bone mass.

At the cellular level, the process of mechanotransduction is divided into four distinct phases: (1) mechanocoupling, (2) biochemical coupling, (3) transmission of signal, and (4) effector cell response.[2] The first phase, mechanocoupling, refers to the transduction of the mechanical force applied to the bone into a local mechanical signal perceived by the cell. Bending of bone during locomotion undoubtedly produces strains on cells of the bone. Yet the movement of fluid within the canaliculi and Haversian canals of bone has been proposed as a significant mechanical signal.[3] It is unclear from either in vivo or in vitro studies which mechanical signal plays the leading role in mechanotransduction. In vitro studies have shown that fluid shear induces many second messengers and signaling molecules that may be important to the osteogenic response to mechanical loading.[3-7] Additionally, we have shown that expression of osteoblastic anabolic markers is more sensitive to fluid forces than to physiologic levels of strain.[8] Thus, fluid shear may be a dominant mechanical stimulus in bone.

## The Role of $[Ca^{2+}]_i$ in Mechanotransduction

The earliest measured response of osteoblasts to either mechanical strain or fluid shear is a rapid rise in the concentration of intracellular calcium ($[Ca^{2+}]_i$).[4,9] This increase in $[Ca^{2+}]_i$ is dependent on both the movement of $Ca^{2+}$ into the cell and the release of $Ca^{2+}$ from intracellular stores.[10] In-

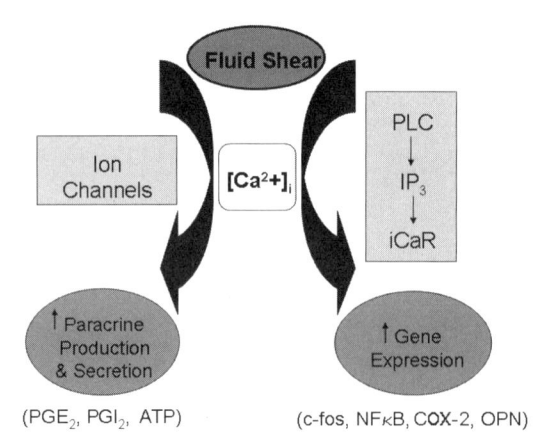

**Figure 1** Possible roles for subcellular $Ca^{2+}$ domains within the osteoblast in response to fluid shear. In this hypothesis, $Ca^{2+}$ entry through ion channels would promote release of factors that would stimulate surrounding cells to amplify the response. Conversely, activation of intracellular $Ca^{2+}$ release would mediate changes in gene expression associated with osteogenesis.

hibition of $Ca^{2+}$ entry with ion channel blockers significantly reduced this response, yet thapsigargin, an intracellular $Ca^{2+}$ release inhibitor, also abrogated the rise in $[Ca^{2+}]_i$ in response to shear.[10] Furthermore, inhibition of either of these sources of $Ca^{2+}$ decreased $PGE_2$ release from osteocytes in response to fluid shear[11] and prevented shear-induced increases in gene expression.[5] These observations indicate that both $Ca^{2+}$ entry through ion channels and intracellular $Ca^{2+}$ release are necessary for the response of osteoblasts to fluid shear and suggest a complex interaction of signaling from these two pools in response to fluid shear. Holda and associates[12] postulated that intracellular $Ca^{2+}$ can be increased within discrete domains of the cell to promote different functional responses based on the stimulation. We also hypothesize that activation of mechanisms involved in $Ca^{2+}$ entry and release increase $[Ca^{2+}]_i$ in discrete domains within the cell, but that both $Ca^{2+}$ pools are required for the complete shear response to osteoblasts. In this scenario, intracellular $Ca^{2+}$ release increases $[Ca^{2+}]_i$ levels throughout the interior of the cell, whereas rapid $Ca^{2+}$ entry via channels elevates the $Ca^{2+}$ concentration near the membrane where many membrane-bound enzymes and signaling molecules reside. Thus, release of $Ca^{2+}$ from intracellular stores is optimally placed for activating mechanisms associated with gene expression, whereas channel-mediated $Ca^{2+}$ entry activates a variety of membrane-bound kinases and other enzymes to release factors associated with signal amplification (Fig. 1). This hypothesis is strengthened by the observations that inhibition of intracellular $Ca^{2+}$ release abolishes cytoskeletal rearrangement and subsequent changes in gene expression in osteoblasts in response to fluid shear,[5] whereas inhibition of channel activation blocks release of $PGE_2$,[11] nitric oxide (NO),[13] and TGF-$\beta_1$.[14]

## Ca²⁺ Channels and Regulation of Bone Cell Function

A likely candidate for a mechanoreceptor that could initiate Ca$^{2+}$ entry is an ion channel that is responsive to membrane perturbation. Such a channel has been characterized in many diverse types of tissues[15] and has been found in UMR-106.01 cells,[16] MG63 osteosarcoma cell lines,[17] and MC3T3-E1 osteoblasts.[18] These channels are mechanosensitive, cation-selective (MSCC), and inhibited by gadolinium (Gd$^{3+}$). Patch clamp studies indicate that the kinetics of these channels are modulated by chronic, intermittent strain,[19] suggesting that chronic strain "primes" the channel for activation by additional mechanical stimulation. The importance of the MSCC in mechanotransduction has been demonstrated in studies showing that Gd$^{3+}$ blocks early, mechanically induced responses of the osteoblast and osteocyte. Gd$^{3+}$ significantly blocks the rise in [Ca$^{2+}$]$_i$ in response to fluid shear in osteoblasts[10] and inhibits NO release and glucose 6-phosphate dehydrogenase (G6PD) activity in osteocytes in response to mechanical strain.[13] Previous studies have shown that NO is released from osteoblasts in response to fluid shear[20] and has been implicated in the osteogenic response of bone to exogenous strain.[21] In addition, Gd$^{3+}$ significantly reduces the release of PGE$_2$ from osteocytes[11] and the production of TGF-$\beta_1$[14] in osteoblasts in response to shear. These data indicate that the MSCC plays a significant role in the response of osteogenic cells to mechanical loading.

In addition to MSCCs, L-type voltage-sensitive Ca$^{2+}$ channels (L-VSCC) have been identified using patch clamp techniques in primary osteoblasts[22] and osteosarcoma cell lines.[16,23-25] L-VSCCs are a ubiquitously expressed subfamily of voltage-sensitive Ca$^{2+}$ channels composed of heteromeric protein complexes and characterized by their sensitivity to dihydropyridines.[18] The $\alpha_1$ subunit forms the pore of the channel and contains the sequences for the dihydropyridine receptor and the voltage sensor. The L-VSCCs found in bone cells exhibit all of the kinetic characteristics of L-type Ca$^{2+}$ channels found in other tissues. These channels, extremely important in excitable tissues, are also important in bone physiology. When growing rabbits were given small doses of nifedipine twice daily for 10 weeks, epiphyseal growth plate thickness was reduced and the mineral apposition rate was severely compromised.[26] The morphology of the growth plate was also quite different from untreated controls. However, no toxic effects or differences in body weight were observed. In vitro studies demonstrate that pharmacologic block of these channels decreases both osteocalcin production[27] and proliferation in osteoblasts.[28] A significant reduction in Ca$^{2+}$ uptake[29] and production of extracellular matrix proteins[30] by mechanically stimulated osteosarcoma cells with inhibition of the L-VSCC, suggests a role for these channels in mechanoreception.

Conflicting reports have been published on the role of L-VSCCs in mechanotransduction in vivo. When rat tibiae are loaded for 12 weeks using the 4-point bending model in conjunction with inhibition of the L-VSCC with verapamil, periosteal bone formation increased significantly, leading the authors to conclude that L-VSCC inhibition had no effect on the response of bone to mechanical loading.[31] In contrast, we recently demonstrated that when rats or mice were injected with verapamil or nifedipine and subjected to a single bout of either tibial bending or ulnar loading at peak serum levels of inhibitor, endosteal bone formation rates decreased by 50% to 75%.[32,33] Although we were unable to decrease bone formation below 50%, this effect was most likely due to the fact that channels were only inhibited by approximately 50%. Higher doses of these inhibitors are lethal to the animal because of the role of the L-VSCC in the action potential of cardiac muscle.

We postulate that MSCCs and VSCCs can cooperate to produce an enhanced $[Ca^{2+}]_i$ response to shear. If shear activates the MSCC, the entry of $Ca^{2+}$ and $Na^+$ into the cell can depolarize the cell membrane, as we demonstrated previously with PTH activation of the MSCC.[34] This depolarization could then activate L-VSCCs, creating a large $Ca^{2+}$-conducting pathway. We observed similar cooperativity between these channels in osteoblasts stimulated with both 1,25 $(OH)_2$ vitamin $D_3$ and PTH.[35] Although 1,25 $(OH)_2$ vitamin $D_3$ alters L-VSCC kinetics to reduce the amount of depolarization required for activation of this channel,[25] addition of vitamin $D_3$ alone does not alter $[Ca^{2+}]_i$, and addition of PTH alone only elicits a small increase in $[Ca^{2+}]_i$. However, when MC3T3-E1 osteoblasts are pretreated with 1,25 $(OH)_2$ vitamin $D_3$, PTH addition produces a large increase in $[Ca^{2+}]_i$. Inhibition of L-VSCCs with nifedipine effectively blocked the vitamin $D_3$ enhancement of the rise in $[Ca^{2+}]_i$, and $Gd^{3+}$ inhibition of the MSCC totally blocked any changes in $[Ca^{2+}]_i$ during combined treatment, strengthening our hypothesis of cooperativity between these channels.

## Intracellular Calcium Release in Mechanotransduction

Although $Ca^{2+}$ entry pathways have proved to be important in the response of osteoblasts to mechanical loading in both in vivo and in vitro studies, $Ca^{2+}$ entry does not appear to be involved in changes in gene expression in osteoblasts in response to mechanical stimulation. When MC3T3-E1 osteoblasts were subjected to fluid shear (12 dynes/cm$^2$) in the presence of $Ca^{2+}$ channel inhibitors, neither shear-induced actin stress fiber formation nor the increase in c-fos and COX-2 was altered.[5] However, chelation of intracellular $Ca^{2+}$ with 1,2-Bis (2 aminophenoxy)ethane-N,N,N',N'-tetra-acetic acid (BAPTA) completely inhibited actin stress fiber formation and production of c-fos and COX-2 in sheared osteoblasts. Osteoblasts can also increase intracellular $Ca^{2+}$ levels via release of $Ca^{2+}$ from intracellular stores. Cellular studies have shown that intracellular $Ca^{2+}$ release is mediated through two receptors, the ryanodyne receptor and the $IP_3$ receptor. Although ryanodyne receptors have been reported in MC3T3-E1 osteoblasts,[36] we have yet to assign a functional role to these receptors in mechanotransduction. In the $IP_3$-mediated mechanism, membrane-bound phospholipase C (PLC) cleaves phosphatidylinositol 4,5 bisphosphate into diacylglycerol and D-*myo*-inositol 1,4,5-triphosphate ($IP_3$). $IP_3$ then binds to $IP_3$ receptors on the endoplasmic reticulum to release calcium stores and increase cytosolic $[Ca^{2+}]_i$ levels. Addition of thapsigargin, which empties intracellular $Ca^{2+}$ stores and prevents refilling of these stores, completely suppresses actin reorganization and production of c-fos and COX-2 in response to fluid shear.[5] When activation of PLC was inhibited with U73122, similar inhibition of fluid shear-induced responses was observed. We also demonstrated that the increase in COX-2 in response to shear results from the translocation of the transcription factor nuclear factor kappa B (NFκB).[37] Translocation of NFκB was also sensitive to IP$_3$-mediated intracellular Ca$^{2+}$ release, but not Ca$^{2+}$ entry. These observations suggest that IP$_3$-mediated intracellular Ca$^{2+}$ release and not Ca$^{2+}$ entry is necessary for changes in osteoblastic gene expression that accompany fluid shear stimulation. These results strengthen our hypothesis of differing functional roles of increased Ca$^{2+}$ concentrations within discrete domains of the cell (Fig. 1).

## ATP Release and Purinergic Receptors

The question of how fluid shear activates intracellular Ca$^{2+}$ release is still unknown; however, one likely mechanism is ATP activation of purinergic (P2) receptors. ATP, and probably other nucleotides, is constitutively released from cells in nanomolar concentrations with levels of ATP probably higher near the cell surface due to membrane trapping and unstirred layers.[38] It has been postulated that this constitutive release of ATP is a key determinant in setting the threshold of response for activation of signal transduction pathways.[39] Fluid shear and mechanical stimulation increase ATP release in numerous cell types,[40-42] including osteoblasts.[43]

Also known as P2 receptors, purinergic receptors are transmembrane proteins that bind extracellular nucleotides to initiate intracellular Ca$^{2+}$ signals. Based on their molecular structure and activated signaling pathways, P2 receptors are divided into two subclasses (Fig. 2): ionotropic or ligand-gated channels (P2X) or metabotropic or G-protein coupled receptors (P2Y).[44] In mammalian cells, six P2Y receptor isoforms (P2Y$_1$, P2Y$_2$, P2Y$_4$, P2Y$_6$, P2Y$_{11}$, and P2Y$_{12}$) and seven P2X isoforms (P2X$_{1-7}$) have been sequenced and pharmacologically characterized.[45] P2Y$_5$, P2Y$_7$, P2Y$_9$, and P2Y$_{10}$ have also been isolated; however, they primarily bind nonnucleotides. P2Y$_3$ and P2Y$_8$ are found in chick brain and *Xenopus* neural plate respectively.

P2Y receptors have seven membrane-spanning regions with the N-terminus exposed to the pericellular environment and the C-terminus on the cytosolic side of the membrane. ATP binding to these receptors activates several G-protein linked pathways. Most P2Y receptors stimulate phosphoinositide breakdown through activation of PLC-β via G$_{q/11}$.[46] P2Y$_1$, P2Y$_2$, and P2Y$_4$ have also been shown to activate G$_i$, which in turn inhibits adenylate cyclase.[46] P2Y$_4$ has also been reported to activate phospholipase D, although the mechanism for how this enzyme is activated is unclear.[47] Interestingly, P2Y$_{11}$ has been shown to activate both PLC through G$_{q/11}$ and adenylate cyclase via G$_s$.[45]

P2X receptors are ATP-gated channels that are ubiquitously expressed in mammalian tissues.[48-50] Typically, P2X channels are permeable to monovalent and divalent cations such as Na$^+$, K$^+$, and Ca$^{2+}$. However, the P2X$_7$ receptor, also known as a P2Z receptor, has been shown to be able to

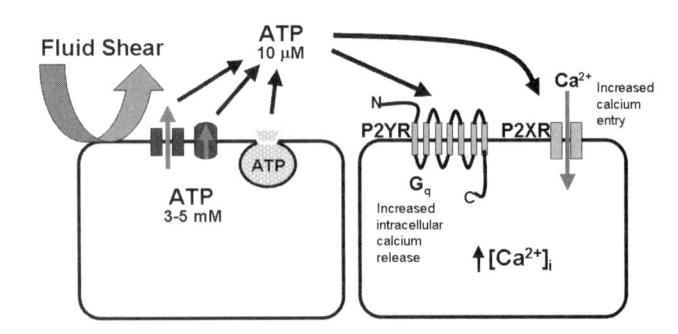

**Figure 2** ATP release and effects of binding to P2 receptors. ATP binds to both the P2Y receptor, inducing IP$_3$-mediated intracellular Ca$^{2+}$ release, and the P2X ligand-gated channel. *(Adapted with permission from Schwiebert EM, Morales MM, Devidas S, Egan ME, Guggino WB: Chloride channel and chloride conductance regulator domains of CFTR, the scystic fibrosis transmembrane conductance regulator.* Proc Natl Acad Sci *1998;95:2674-2679.)*

increase its pore size to act as a nonselective pore.[51-53] P2X receptors have two membrane-spanning regions with both the N- and C-terminus on the cytosolic side of the membrane.[45] It is postulated that these receptors form multimeric structures to create the pore of the channel.

Both osteoclasts and osteoblasts have multiple purinergic receptor types,[54] with osteoblasts expressing most of the isoforms of both P2X and P2Y. However, the expression of P2 receptors varies between primary osteoblasts and clonal cell lines, as well as between different cell lines.[55-57] Activation of P2 receptors in bone cells, like most other tissues, increases [Ca$^{2+}$]$_i$. Like the [Ca$^{2+}$]$_i$ response, activation of P2 receptors has been shown to modulate COX-2,[58] prostaglandin secretion[59,60] and c-fos expression[55] in osteoblasts and other cell types. A recent study demonstrated that knockout of the P2X$_7$ receptor significantly reduced total and cortical bone content and periosteal circumference in femurs, and increased bone resorption and reduced periosteal formation in the tibia,[61] suggesting a role for this receptor in normal bone development and growth. However, activation of P2 receptors has also been shown to inhibit bone formation,[62] and induce osteoclastogenesis, and bone resorption.[63]

We have recently shown that fluid shear applied to MC3T3-E1 osteoblasts produced a fivefold increase in ATP release, most of which was released during the first 5 minutes of shear.[64] Inhibition of Ca$^{2+}$ entry with the mechanosensitive channel blocker Gd$^{3+}$ or L-VSCC blockers nifedipine or verapamil significantly abrogated shear-induced ATP release but had no effect on basal ATP release in static cells. Inhibition of intracellular Ca$^{2+}$ release had no effect on ATP release. Since we demonstrated that fluid shear induced translocation of the transcription factor NFκB, which required activation of PLC/IP$_3$ to release calcium stores within the endoplasmic reticu-

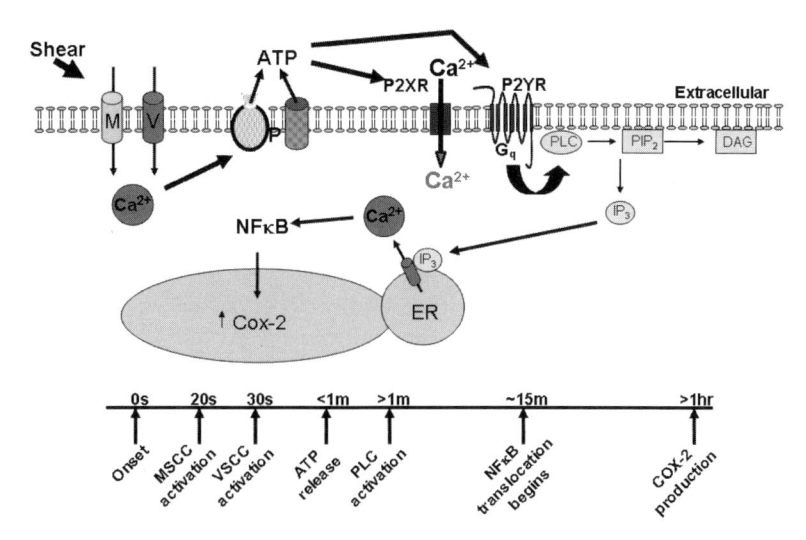

**Figure 3** Working model of $Ca^{2+}$ signaling in the osteoblasts in response to fluid shear.

lum, we used apyrase to degrade any extracellular nucleotides released in response to shear and examined the resultant NFκB translocation. Apyrase completely blocked NFκB translocation, indicating that release of nucleotides by osteoblasts in response to shear requires extracellular $Ca^{2+}$ entry and that this release is important in the activation of intracellular $Ca^{2+}$ release.

## Calcium Signaling in Mechanotransduction: A Working Model

These studies have led to a working model of $Ca^{2+}$ signaling in osteoblasts in response to mechanical stimulation presented in Figure 3. In this model, fluid shear activates the MSCC to allow $Ca^{2+}$ and $Na^+$ to enter the cell, producing a depolarization of the membrane. This depolarization activates the L-VSCC to further increase $Ca^{2+}$ entry. The submembrane increase in $[Ca^{2+}]_i$ enhances ATP or nucleotide release from the osteoblast. ATP then binds to a P2Y receptor to activate PLC via a G protein, thereby inducing intracellular $Ca^{2+}$ release via $IP_3$. However, this model has many limitations and unanswered questions. It is still unknown how membrane deformation activates the MSCC and whether there is a direct effect of this deformation on the L-VSCC. Furthermore, if $Ca^{2+}$ entry through either the MSCC or VSCC increases ATP release, which in turn activates intracellular $Ca^{2+}$ release, why doesn't channel inhibition block shear-induced gene expression? Although many questions remain, the role of $Ca^{2+}$ signaling in osteoblasts is essential to the response of bone to mechanical loading and may be the focal point for modulating bone formation in vivo.

## References

1. Forwood MR, Owan I, Takano Y, Turner CH: Increased bone formation in rat tibiae after a single short period of dynamic loading in vivo. *Am J Physiol Endocrinol Metab* 1996;270:E419-E423.

2. Duncan RL, Turner CH: Mechanotransduction and the functional response of bone to mechanical strain. *Calcif Tissue Int* 1995;57:344-358.

3. Weinbaum S, Cowin SC, Zeng Y: A model for the excitation of osteocytes by mechanical loading-induced bone fluid shear stresses. *J Biomechanics* 1994;27:339-360.

4. Jones DB, Bingmann D: How do osteoblasts respond to mechanical stimulation? *Cells Mater* 1991;1:329-340.

5. Chen NX, Ryder KD, Pavalko FM, et al: $Ca^{2+}$ regulates fluid shear-induced cytoskeletal reorganization and gene expression in osteoblasts. *Am J Physiol Cell Physiol* 2000;278:C989-C997.

6. Klein-Nulend J, Burger EH, Semeins CM, Raisz LG, Pilbeam CC: Pulsating fluid flow stimulates prostaglandin release and inducible prostaglandin G/H synthase mRNA expression in primary mouse bone cells. *J Bone Miner Res* 1997;12:45-51.

7. Reich KM, Frangos JA: Effect of flow on prostaglandin $E_2$ and inositol trisphosphate levels in osteoblasts. *Am J Physiol Cell Physiol* 1991;261:C428-C432.

8. Owan I, Burr DB, Turner CH, Qiu J, Duncan RL: Osteoblasts do not respond to physiological levels of mechanical strain, but are responsive to fluid effects. *Trans Orthop Res Soc* 1997;22:176.

9. Hung CT, Pollack SR, Reilly TM, Brighton CT: Real-time calcium response of cultured bone cells to fluid flow. *Clin Orthop* 1995;313:256-269.

10. Hung CT, Allen FD, Pollack SR, Brighton CT: Intracellular calcium stores and extracellular calcium are required in the real-time calcium response of bone cells experiencing fluid flow. *J Biomechanics* 1996;29:1411-1417.

11. Ajubi NE, Klein-Nulend J, Alblas MJ, Burger EH, Nijweide PJ: Signal transduction pathways involved in fluid flow-induced $PGE_2$ production by cultured osteocytes. *Am J Physiol Endocrinol Metab* 1999;276:E171-E178.

12. Holda JR, Klishin A, Sedova M, Huser J, Blatter LA: Capacitative calcium entry. *News Physiol Sci* 1998;13:157-166.

13. Rawlinson SC, Pitsillides AA, Lanyon LE: Involvement of different ion channels in osteoblasts' and osteocytes' early responses to mechanical strain. *Bone* 1996;19:609-614.

14. Sakai K, Mohtai M, Iwamoto Y: Fluid shear stress increases transforming growth factor β1 expression in human osteoblast-like cells: Modulation by cation channel blockades. *Calcif Tissue Int* 1998;63:515-520.

15. Morris CE: Mechanosensitive ion channels. *J Membrane Biol* 1990;113:93-107.

16. Duncan RL, Misler S: Voltage-activated and stretch-activated $Ba^{2+}$ conducting channels in an osteoblast-like cell line (UMR-106). *FEBS Lett* 1989;251:17-21.

17. Davidson RM, Tatakis DW, Auerbach AL: Multiple forms of mechanosensitive ion channels in osteoblast-like cells. *Pflugers Arch* 1990;416:646-651.

18. Duncan RL, Akanbi KA, Farach-Carson MC: Calcium signals and calcium channels in osteoblastic cells. *Semin Nephrol* 1998;18:178-190.

19. Duncan RL, Hruska KA: Chronic, intermittent loading alters mechanosensitive channel characteristics in osteoblast-like cells. *Am J Physiol* 1994;267:F909-F916.

20. Johnson DL, McAllister TN, Frangos JA: Fluid flow stimulates rapid and continuous release of nitric oxide in osteoblasts. *Am J Physiol Endocrinol Metab* 1996;271: E205-E208.

21. Turner CH, Takano Y, Owan I, Murrell GAC: Nitric oxide inhibitor L-NAME suppresses mechanically induced bone formation in rats. *Am J Physiol Endocrinol Metab* 1996;270:E634-E639.

22. Chesnoy-Marchais D, Fritsch J: Voltage-gated sodium and calcium currents in rat osteoblasts. *J Physiol* 1988;398:291-311.

23. Grygorczyk C, Grygorczyk R, Ferrier J: Osteoblastic cells have L-type calcium channels. *Bone Miner* 1989;7:137-148.

24. Guggino SE, Wagner JA, Snowman A, Hester L, Sacktor B, Snyder S: Phenylalkylamine-sensitive Ca channels in osteoblast-like osteosarcoma cells. *J Biol Chem* 1988;263: 10155-10161.

25. Caffrey JM, Farach-Carson MC: Vitamin $D_3$ metabolites modulate dihydropyridine-sensitive calcium current in clonal rat osteosarcoma cells. *J Biol Chem* 1989;264: 20265-20274.

26. Duriez J, Flautre B, Blary MC, Hardouin P: Effects of the calcium channel blocker nifedipine on epiphyseal growth plate and bone turnover: A study in rabbit. *Calcif Tissue Int* 1993;52:120-124.

27. Guggino SE, Lajeunesse D, Wagner JA, Snyder SH: Bone remodeling signaled by a dihydropyridine- and phenylalkylamine-sensitive calcium channel. *Proc Natl Acad Sci USA* 1989;86:2957-2960.

28. Loza JS, Stephan E, Dolce C, Dziak R, Simasko S: Calcium currents in osteoblastic cells: Dependence upon cellular growth stage. *Calcif Tissue Int* 1994;55:128-133.

29. Vadiakas GP, Banes AJ: Verapamil decreases cyclic load-induced calcium incorporation in ROS 17/2.8 osteosarcoma cell cultures. *Matrix* 1992;12:439-447.

30. Walker LM, Publicover SJ, Preston MR, Said Ahmed MA, El Haj AJ: Calcium-channel activation and matrix protein upregulation in bone cells in response to mechanical strain. *J Cell Biochem* 2000;79:648-661.

31. Samnegard E, Cullen DM, Akhter MP, Kimmel DB: No effect of verapamil on the local bone response to in vivo mechanical loading. *J Orthop Res* 2001;19:328-336.

32. Li J, Duncan RL, Burr DB, Turner CH: L-type calcium channels mediate mechanically induced bone formation in vivo. *J Bone Miner Res* 2002;17:1795-1800.

33. Li J, Duncan RL, Burr DB, Turner CH: Parathyroid hormone enhances mechanically induced bone formation, possibly involving L-type voltage-sensitive calcium channels. *Endocrinology* 2003;144:1226-1233.

34. Duncan RL, Hruska KA, Misler S: Parathyroid hormone activation of stretch-activated cation channels in osteosarcoma cells (UMR-106.01). *FEBS Lett* 1992;307:219-223.

35. Li W, Duncan RL, Karin NJ, Farach-Carson MC: $1,25(OH)_2D_3$ enhances parathyroid hormone-induced $Ca^{2+}$ transients in pre-osteoblasts by activating L-type $Ca^{2+}$ channels. *Am J Physiol Endocrinol Metab* 1997;273:E599-E605.

36. Adebanjo OA, Biswas G, Moonga BS, et al: Novel biochemical and functional insights into nuclear $Ca^{2+}$ transport through $IP_3Rs$ and RyRs in osteoblasts. *Am J Physiol Renal Physiol* 2000;278:F784-F791.

37. Chen NX, Geist DG, Genetos DC, Pavalko FM, Duncan RL: Fluid shear-induced NFκB translocation in osteoblasts is mediated by intracellular calcium release. *Bone* 2003;33:399-410.

38. Bowler WB, Tattersall JA, Hussein R, Dixon CJ, Cobbold PH, Gallagher JA: Real time measurement of ATP release from human osteoblasts. *J Bone Miner Res* 1998; 13:525-531.

39. Ostrom RS, Gregorian C, Insel PA: Cellular release of and response to ATP as key determinants of the set-point of signal transduction pathways. *J Biol Chem* 2000; 275:11735-11739.

40. Graff RD, Lazarowski ER, Banes AJ, Lee GM: ATP release by mechanically loaded porcine chondrons in pellet culture. *Arthritis Rheum* 2000;43:1571-1579.

41. Grierson JP, Meldolesi J: Shear stress-induced $[Ca^{2+}]_i$ transients and oscillations in mouse fibroblasts are mediated by endogenously released ATP. *J Biol Chem* 1995; 270:4451-4456.

42. Shen J, Luscinskas FW, Connolly A, Dewey CF Jr, Gimbrone MA Jr: Fluid shear stress modulates cytosolic free calcium in vascular endothelial cells. *Am J Physiol Cell Physiol* 1992;262:C384-C390.

43. Romanello M, Pani B, Bicego M, D'Andrea P: Mechanically induced ATP release from human osteoblastic cells. *Biochem Biophys Res Commun* 2001;289:1275-1281.

44. Abbracchio MP, Burnstock G: Purinoceptors: Are there families of P2X and P2Y purinoceptors? *Pharmacol Ther* 1994;64:445-475.

45. DiVirgilio F, Chiozzi P, Ferrari D, et al: Nucleotide receptors: An emerging family of regulatory molecules in blood cells. *Blood* 2001;97:587-600.

46. Ralevic V, Burnstock G: Receptors for purines and pyrimidines. *Pharmacol Rev* 1998; 50:413-492.

47. Purkiss JR, Boarder MR: Stimulation of phosphatidate synthesis in endothelial cells in response to P2-receptor activation: Evidence for phospholipase C and phospholipase D involvement, phosphatidate and diacylglycerol interconversion and the role of protein kinase C. *Biochem J* 1992;287:31-36.

48. Soto F, Garcia-Guzman M, Stuhmer W: Cloned ligand-gated channels activated by extracellular ATP (P2X receptors). *J Membr Biol* 1997;160:91-100.

49. Buell G, Collo G, Rassendren F: P2X receptors: An emerging channel family. *Eur J Neurosci* 1996;8:2221-2228.

50. Brake AJ, Wagenback MJ, Julius D: New structural motif for ligand-gated ion channels defined by an ionotropic ATP receptor. *Nature* 1994;371:519-523.

51. Surprenant A, Rassendren F, Kawashima E, North RA, Buell G: The cytolytic P2Z receptor for extracellular ATP identified as a P2X receptor ($P2X_7$). *Science* 1996;272:735-738.

52. DiVirgilio F, Falzoni S, Mutini C, Sanz JM, Chiozzi P: Purinergic $P2X_7$ receptor: A pivotal role in inflammation and immunosuppression. *Drug Dev Res* 1998;45:207-213.

53. Collo G, Neidhart S, Kawashima E, Kosco-Vilbois M, North RA, Buell G: Tissue distribution of the $P2X_7$ receptor. *Neuropharmacology* 1997;36:1277-1283.

54. Bowler WB, Buckley KA, Gartland A, Hipskind RA, Bilbe G, Gallagher JA: Extracellular nucleotide signaling: A mechanism for integrating local and systemic responses in the activation of bone remodeling. *Bone* 2001;28:507-512.

55. Bowler WB, Dixon CJ, Halleux C, et al: Signaling in human osteoblasts by extracellular nucleotides. *J Biol Chem* 1999;274:14315-14324.

56. Kumagi H, Sacktor B, Filburn CR: Purinergic regulation of cytosolic calcium and phosphoinositide metabolism in rat osteoblast-like osteosarcoma cells. *J Bone Miner Res* 1991;6:697-708.

57. Reimer CJ, Dixon SJ: Extracellular nucleotides elevate $Ca^{2+}$ in rat osteoblastic cells by interaction with two receptor subtypes. *Am J Physiol Cell Physiol* 1992;263:C1040-C1048.

58. Brambilla R, Abbracchio M: Modulation of cyclooxgenase-2 and brain reactive astrogliosis by purinergic P2 receptors. *Ann NY Acad Sci* 2001;939:54-62.

59. Koolpe M, Pearson D, Benton HP: Expression of both P1 and P2 purine receptor genes by human articular chondrocytes and profile of ligand-mediated prostaglandin $E_2$ release. *Arthritis Rheum* 1999;42:258-267.

60. Suzuki A, Kotoyori J, Oiso Y, Kozawa O: Prostaglandin $E_2$ is a potential mediator of extracellular ATP action in osteoblast-like cells. *Cell Adhes Commun* 1993;1:113-118.

61. Ke HZ, Qi H, Weidema AF, et al: Deletion of the $P2X_7$ nucleotide receptor reveals its regulatory roles in bone formation and resorption. *Mol Endocrinol* 2003;17:1356-1367.

62. Jones SJ, Gray C, Boyde A, Burnstock G: Purinergic transmitters inhibit bone formation by cultured osteoblasts. *Bone* 1997;21:393-399.

63. Morrison MS, Turin L, King BF, Burnstock G, Arnett TR: ATP is a potent stimulator of the activation and formation of rodent osteoclasts. *J Physiol* 1998;511:495-500.

64. Genetos DC, Geist DG, Liu D, Donahue HJ, Duncan RL: Fluid shear-induced ATP secretion mediates prostaglandin release in MC3T3-E1 osteoblasts. *J Bone Miner Res* 2005;20:41-49.

Chapter 20

# Effect of Low Frequency Electromagnetic Fields on $A_{2A}$ and $A_3$ Adenosine Receptors in Human Neutrophils

*Pier Andrea Borea, PhD*
*Katia Varani, PhD*
*Stefania Gessi, PhD*
*Stefania Merighi, PhD*
*Elena Cattabriga, PhD*
*Fabrizio Vincenzi, MSc*
*Annalisa Benini, MSc*
*Ruggero Cadossi, MD*

## Introduction

Adenosine, an endogenous modulator of a wide range of biologic functions, interacts with at least four cell surface subtypes classified as $A_1$, $A_{2A}$, $A_{2B}$, and $A_3$ receptors, which are coupled to G proteins.[1] The $A_1$ and $A_3$ subtypes, via Gi and Go proteins, mediate inhibition of adenylyl cyclase activity; in contrast, the $A_{2A}$ and $A_{2B}$ subtypes, coupled to Gs proteins, determine the stimulation of cAMP production.[2] Recently, a good correlation was found between cAMP accumulation data and inhibition of superoxide anion generation by typical adenosine receptor agonists, suggesting that cAMP may be involved in the anti-inflammatory actions of $A_{2A}$ and $A_3$ receptors linked to the inhibition of superoxide anion formation.[3] In particular, activation of $A_{2A}$ receptors appears to be associated with inhibition of tumor necrosis factor, interleukin (IL)-6, IL-8, and elastase by peripheral blood cells.[4] Of particular interest is that in human neutrophils, $A_3$ receptors exert their anti-inflammatory properties by inhibiting degranulation, chemotaxis, and superoxide anion production.[5]

Interest has grown concerning the use of pulsed electromagnetic fields (PEMFs) for therapeutic purposes.[6] The osteoinductive activity of PEMFs and their action on local inflammation,[7] osteogenesis, and the different phases of bone repair[8] is well established. A careful investigation of possible genotoxic effects of PEMFs has suggested that the exposure does not induce any chromosomal alteration such as breakages, translocations, or inversion.[9] Recently, the effects of prolonged exposure to PEMFs on chondrocyte proliferation and cell density have been investigated.[10] Several hypotheses have been proposed to explain the influence of PEMFs on the cell membrane and, in particular, on ligand binding with membrane receptors, which can also affect membrane protein distribution.[11]

This chapter describes the effect of PEMFs on $A_{2A}$ and $A_3$ adenosine receptors in human neutrophils. $A_{2A}$ and $A_3$ saturation binding experiments performed using high affinity radioligand antagonists [$^3$H]-ZM 241385 (4-(2-[7-amino-2 (2-furyl)-[1,2,4] triazolo [2,3-a]-[1,3,5]triazin-5-y-lamino]ethyl) phenol) and [$^3$H]-MRE 3008F20 (5N-(4-methoxyphenyl-carbamoyl) amino –8– propyl –2 -(2-furyl) pyrazolo-[4,3-e]1,2,4-triazolo[1,5-c]pyrimidine) respectively revealed a significant increase of the $A_{2A}$ and $A_3$ adenosine receptor density in neutrophils treated with PEMFs. The effect of PEMFs was specific for the $A_{2A}$ and $A_3$ adenosine receptors and dependent on both time and intensity. Competition of radioligand binding by the high affinity $A_{2A}$ receptor agonists NECA [5'N-ethylcarboxamidoadenosine] and HE-NECA [2hexynyl-5'N-ethyl carboxamidoadenosine] and by $A_3$ receptor agonists like Cl-IB-MECA [N$^6$-(3-iodo-benzyl)-2-chloro-adenosine-5'-N-methyluronamide] and IB-MECA [N$^6$-(3-iodo-benzyl)adenosine-5'-N-methyluronamide] in the absence and in the presence of PEMFs was performed. In functional assays, the effect of these typical $A_{2A}$ and $A_3$ adenosine agonists on the inhibition of adenylyl cyclase activity and of superoxide anion ($O_2^-$) production were evaluated. The results indicate significant alterations in $A_{2A}$ and $A_3$ adenosine receptor density and functionality in human neutrophils treated with PEMFs.

## Methods

### Preparation of Cell Suspensions
The cell preparations were isolated and prepared according to Varani and associates[3] from heparin-treated peripheral blood provided by the blood bank of the University Hospital of Ferrara. Blood (100 to 200 mL) was donated by healthy human volunteers after written informed consent to research was obtained.

### Field Characteristics
The neutrophils or neutrophil membranes were exposed to PEMFs generated by a pair of rectangular horizontal coils (14 × 23 cm), each made of 1,400 turns of copper wire; coils were powered by a pulse generator (IGEA, Carpi, Italy). The general characteristics of the field have been reported in previous work.[9] Briefly, the exposure system had three components: (1) the signal generator, which produced the input voltage of pulses at 75 Hz; (2) the amplifier, which produced the electric voltage output (200 V) supplying coils; and (3) the coils, which produced the magnetic field varying from 0.2 to 3.5 mTesla (mT) to evaluate the effect of intensity on binding parameters. The induced electric field in air was 0.04 mVcm$^{-1}$. The neutrophils or neutrophil membranes were PEMF treated or untreated for incubation times ranging from 30 to 240 minutes. The temperature, continuously monitored by a thermoresistor within the incubator, was constant throughout the exposure time and exactly maintained during the binding and functional experiments.

## Binding Assays in the Neutrophil Membranes
In saturation studies on $A_{2A}$ adenosine receptors, untreated or PEMF-treated neutrophil membranes were incubated with 8 to 10 different concentrations of [$^3$H]-ZM 241385 (specific activity 17 Ci/mmol) ranging from 0.05 to 10 nM.[12] In saturation studies on $A_3$ adenosine receptors, untreated or PEMF-treated neutrophil membranes were incubated with 8 to 10 different concentrations of [$^3$H]-MRE 3008F20 (specific activity 67 Ci/mmol) ranging from 0.2 to 20 nM.[13,14] Different incubation times were used (ranging from 30 to 240 minutes at 4°C) according to the results of previous time course experiments. Saturation experiments were also performed under magnetic fields ranging from 0.2 to 3.5 mT to evaluate the effect of intensity on binding parameters. In competition experiments carried out to determine the $IC_{50}$ values, 1 nM of [$^3$H]-ZM 241385, neutrophil membranes, and at least six to eight different concentrations of HE-NECA or NECA were incubated at 4°C for 60 minutes. In competition experiments carried out to determine the $K_i$ values, 2 nM of [$^3$H]-MRE 3008F20, neutrophil membranes, and at least six to eight different concentrations of Cl-IB-MECA or IB-MECA were incubated at 4°C for 120 minutes.

## Measurement of Cyclic AMP Levels in Human Neutrophils
PEMF-treated or untreated human neutrophils ($10^6$ cells/mL) were suspended and prepared for cAMP assays as described by Varani and associates.[3] Then forskolin, typical $A_{2A}$ adenosine agonists such as NECA or HE-NECA, or known $A_3$ adenosine agonists like Cl-IB-MECA or IB-MECA at different concentrations (1 nM to 10 µM) were added to the mixture, and the incubation continued for an additional 5 minutes. The effect of the selective $A_{2A}$ antagonist SCH 58261 (7-(2-phenylethyl)-2-(2-furyl)-pyrazolo[4,3-e]-1,2,4-triazolo-[1,5-c]pyrimidine) on NECA stimulation and of the $A_3$ antagonist MRE 3008F20 (1 µM) on Cl-IB-MECA (100 nM)-induced reduction of cyclic AMP levels was evaluated.

## Superoxide Anion Production in Human Neutrophils
$O_2^-$ production was measured by the superoxide dismutase–inhibitable (0.5 mg/mL) reduction of ferricytochrome c modified for microplate-based assays.[3] Inhibitory activity was determined by measuring the $A_{2A}$ and $A_3$ agonists' ability to inhibit $O_2^-$ production as activated by fMLF (N-formyl-L-methionyl-L-leucyl-L-phenylalanine). The percentage of activity was obtained by comparing the nmoles of $O_2^-$ in the absence (100%) and in the presence of typical $A_{2A}$ and $A_3$ adenosine agonists at different concentrations (1 nM to 1 µM).

## PEMF Response Specificity
Binding to $\alpha_2$ adrenergic receptors was carried out with [$^3$H]UK 14304 (0.2-10 nM) (specific activity 62 Ci/mmol) on human neutrophils in a 50 mM Tris HCl buffer pH 7.4 containing $MgCl_2$ 10 mM for 60 minutes at 25°C. Nonspecific binding was determined with 1 µM of UK 14304.[15] Binding to $\beta_2$ adrenergic receptors was carried out with [$^3$H]CGP 12177

(0.1-10 nM) (specific activity 43 Ci/mmol) on human neutrophils in a 50 mM Tris HCl buffer pH 7.4 containing MgCl$_2$ 10 mM for 60 minutes at 25°C. Nonspecific binding was determined with 10 μM of CGP 12177.[16] Binding to μ- and k-opioid receptors was performed on human neutrophils with [$^3$H]DAMGO (specific activity 65 Ci/mmol) and [$^3$H]U69593 (specific activity 44 Ci/mmol) in a 50 mM Tris HCl buffer pH 7.4 for 60 minutes at 25°C. Nonspecific binding was determined with 100 μM of bremazocine.[17]

## Data Analysis

Saturation and competition binding studies were analyzed with the program LIGAND.[18] The EC$_{50}$ and IC$_{50}$ values obtained in cyclic AMP and superoxide anion production assays were calculated by nonlinear regression analysis using the equation for a sigmoid concentration-response curve. All data were expressed as the arithmetic mean ± standard error of the mean. Analysis of data was performed with Student's $t$ test (unpaired analysis). Differences were considered significant at a value of $P < 0.01$.

## Results

### Binding Assays to A$_{2A}$ and A$_3$ Adenosine Receptors

The PEMF incubation times (ranging from 30 to 240 minutes) do not modify the A$_{2A}$ and A$_3$ affinity values of either PEMF-treated or untreated neutrophils. In contrast, the Bmax values of A$_{2A}$ and A$_3$ adenosine receptors present in human neutrophils are altered after 30 and 90 minutes of PEMF treatment respectively and remain at a steady value for the other incubation times. A series of experiments were carried out to evaluate the relationship between intensity of PEMFs (ranging from 0.2 to 5 mT) and changes in the A$_{2A}$ and A$_3$ binding parameters. No effect was observed under 0.5 mT, and the maximum effect on Bmax values of A$_{2A}$ and A$_3$ adenosine receptors appeared from 1 to 3.5 mT and then reached a stable plateau. Figure 1 presents the saturation curves of [$^3$H]-ZM 241385 binding to A$_{2A}$ adenosine receptors in untreated or PEMF-treated human neutrophils (A) respectively. The linearity of the Scatchard plot (B) indicates the presence of a single class of binding sites with a K$_D$ value of 1.06 ± 0.11 nM and a Bmax value of 126 ± 12 fmol/mg protein in untreated human neutrophils. Moreover, in human neutrophils treated with PEMFs, the K$_D$ value was 1.09 ± 0.13 nM and the Bmax value was 219 ± 18* fmol/mg protein (*$P < 0.01$ versus control). Figure 2 illustrates saturation curves of [$^3$H]-MRE 3008F20 binding to A$_3$ adenosine receptors in untreated or PEMF-treated human neutrophil (A) respectively. The Scatchard plot (B) reveals the presence of a single class of binding sites with a K$_D$ value of 2.32 ± 0.18 nM and Bmax value of 455 ± 22 fmol/mg protein in untreated human neutrophils. In human neutrophils treated with PEMFs, the K$_D$ value was 2.46 ± 0.17 nM and the Bmax value was 740 ± 26* fmol/mg protein (*$P < 0.01$ versus control).

The competition curves of typical A$_{2A}$ agonists HE-NECA and NECA revealed a Ki value of 9.6 ± 0.1 nM and 25 ± 3 nM respectively in untreated human neutrophils. In PEMF-treated human neutrophils, HE-NECA and

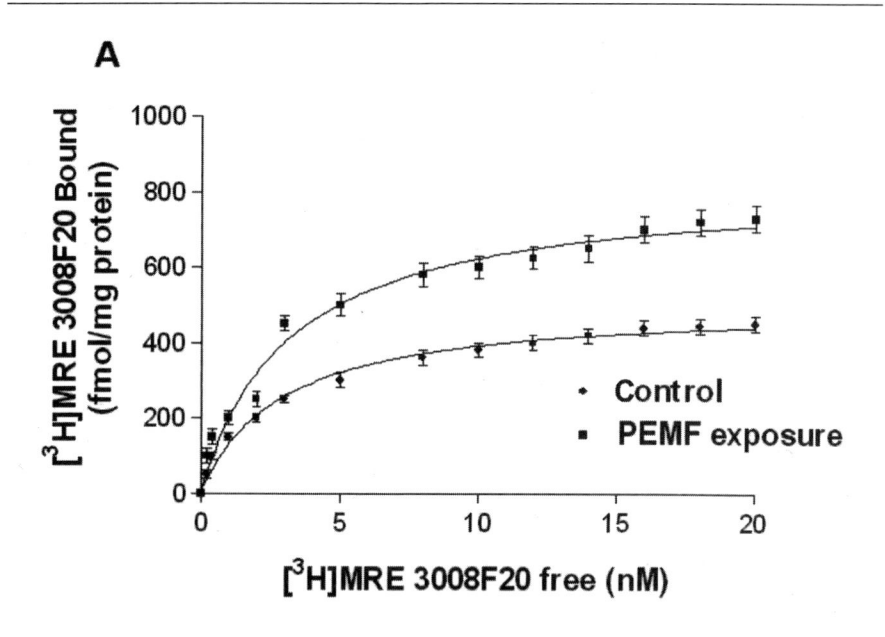

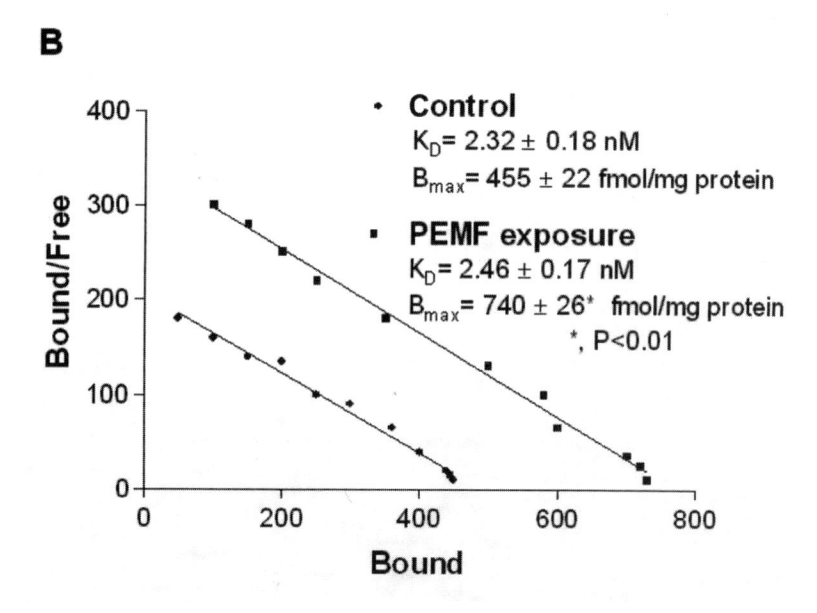

Effect of Low Frequency Electromagnetic Fields   Chapter 20

**Figure 1 A,** Saturation of [³H]ZM 241385 binding to $A_{2A}$ adenosine receptors on untreated and PEMF-treated human neutrophil membranes. **B,** Scatchard plot shows that the $K_D$ value was 1.06 ± 0.11 nM and the Bmax value was 126 ± 12 fmol/mg protein in control neutrophils. The $K_D$ value was 1.09 ± 0.13 nM and the Bmax value was 219 ± 18* fmol/mg protein in PEMF-treated neutrophils (*$P < 0.01$). Values are the means and vertical lines the standard error of the mean of three separate experiments.

Section Five  Transduction of Biophysical Signals

**A**

[graph: Saturation binding curve, $[^3H]$-ZM 241385 Bound (fmol/mg protein) vs $[^3H]$-ZM 241385 free (nM), with Control (●) and PEMF exposure (■)]

**B**

[Scatchard plot: Bound/Free vs Bound]

Control
$K_D = 1.06 \pm 0.11$ nM
$B_{max} = 126 \pm 12$ fmol/mg protein

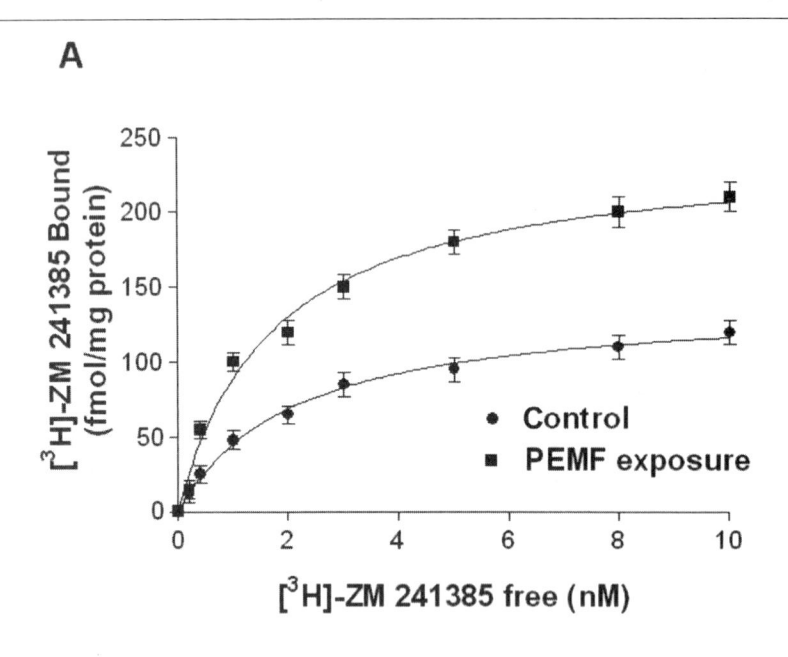

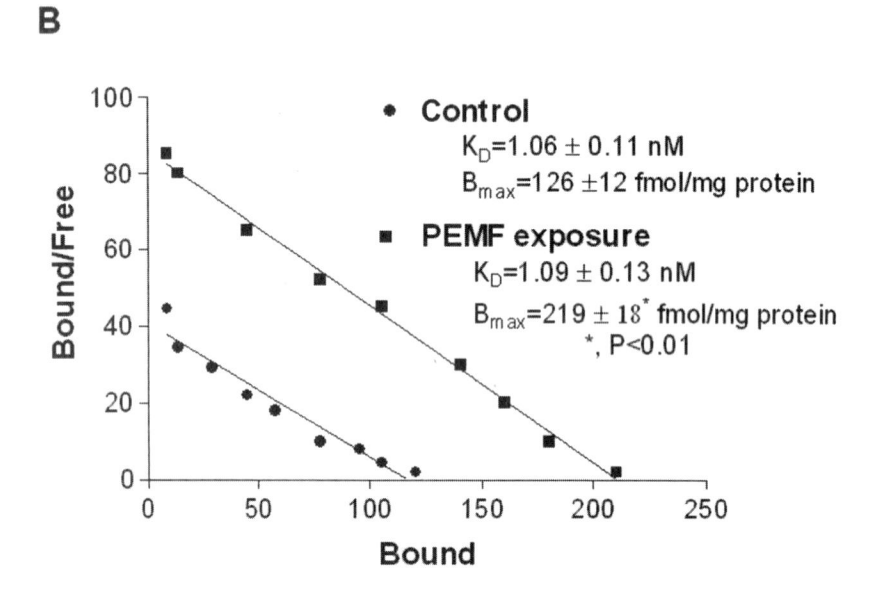

PEMF exposure
$K_D = 1.09 \pm 0.13$ nM
$B_{max} = 219 \pm 18^*$ fmol/mg protein
*, P<0.01

**Figure 2 A,** Saturation of [³H]MRE 3008F20 binding to $A_3$ adenosine receptors on untreated and PEMF-treated neutrophil membranes. **B,** Scatchard plot shows that the $K_D$ value was $2.32 \pm 0.18$ nM and the Bmax value was $455 \pm 22$ fmol/mg protein in control neutrophils. The $K_D$ value was $2.46 \pm 0.17$ nM and the Bmax value was $740 \pm 26^*$ fmol/mg protein in PEMF-treated neutrophils (*P < 0.01). Values are the means and vertical lines the standard error of the mean of three separate experiments.

NECA exhibited Ki values of 8.8 ± 0.9 nM and 23 ± 2 nM respectively. In parallel studies on untreated human neutrophils, Cl-IB-MECA, a typical $A_3$ agonist, showed a $K_H$ value of 0.68 ± 0.20 nM and a KL value of 89 ± 12 nM. In human neutrophils after PEMF treatment, Cl-IB-MECA has a $K_H$ value of 0.65 ± 0.14 nM and a $K_L$ value of 72 ± 10 nM. In untreated human neutrophils, IB-MECA showed a $K_H$ value of 1.83 ± 0.32 nM and a $K_L$ value of 102 ± 15 nM, whereas in PEMF-treated human neutrophils IB-MECA revealed a $K_H$ value of 1.64 ± 0.43 nM and a $K_L$ value of 98 ± 11 nM. The competition curves of both the agonists performed in the absence and in the presence of PEMFs exhibited Hill coefficients less than unity (0.54 and 0.62 for Cl-IB-MECA and 0.52 and 0.64 for IB-MECA, respectively) and were best described by the existence of one high-affinity ($K_H$) and one low-affinity ($K_L$) agonist-receptor binding state. Coupling of the $A_3$ receptors to G proteins was investigated in the presence of 100 µM GTP that is able to shift the competition binding curves of the agonist from a biphasic to a monophasic shape, suggesting that Ki values for Cl-IB-MECA were 93 ± 11 nM and 78 ± 9 nM and for IB-MECA were 122 ± 16 nM and 115 ± 13 nM in the absence and in the presence of PEMF treatment respectively.

## Functional Assays to $A_{2A}$ and $A_3$ Adenosine Receptors

Untreated or PEMF-treated neutrophils did not reveal changes of basal enzyme activity and of the response of adenylyl cyclase to the direct activator forskolin used in the absence or presence of the cAMP-dependent phosphodiesterase inhibitor, Ro 20-1724 (4-(3-butoxy-4-methoxybenzyl)-2-imidazolidinone. When the examined adenosine agonists were incubated with PEMF-treated or untreated neutrophils, an amplification of adenylyl cyclase response was detected, revealing a significant alteration of cAMP production in a concentration-dependent manner. HE-NECA determines an increase of stimulation of cAMP levels in untreated or PEMF-treated human neutrophils with EC50 values of 43 ± 4 nM and 10 ± 2* nM respectively (*$P$ < 0.01). NECA elicited a stimulation of cAMP levels in untreated or PEMF-treated human neutrophils with EC50 values of 255 ± 28 nM and 61 ± 10* nM respectively (*$P$ < 0.01). The selective $A_{2A}$ antagonist SCH 58261 (1 µM) totally inhibited the rise in cAMP levels induced by the examined agonists, suggesting that the stimulatory effect was essentially $A_{2A}$ mediated. We also evaluated the effect of the $A_3$ agonist Cl-IB-MECA that determines a decrease of cAMP levels in untreated or PEMF-treated human neutrophils with $IC_{50}$ values of 2.89 ± 0.14 and 1.18 ± 0.09* nM respectively (*$P$ < 0.01). Also, IB-MECA mediated a decrease of cAMP levels in untreated or PEMF-treated human neutrophils with $IC_{50}$ values of 5.84 ± 0.62 and 2.36 ± 0.38* nM respectively (*$P$ < 0.01). The selective $A_3$ antagonist MRE 3008F20 (1 µM) antagonized Cl-IB-MECA- or IB-MECA-mediated (100 nM) cAMP inhibition, suggesting that the inhibitory effect was essentially $A_3$ mediated. We also evaluated the effect of typical $A_{2A}$ (HE-NECA or NECA) and $A_3$ (Cl-IB-MECA or IB-MECA) adenosine agonists on $O_2^-$ generation by fMLF-stimulated neutrophils. In untreated neutrophils, these compounds were able to inhibit the generation of $O_2^-$ stimulated by fMLF (1 μM) in a dose-dependent manner. HE-NECA and NECA showed an $EC_{50}$ value of 3.61 ± 0.32 nM and 23 ± 2 nM respectively. Moreover, in PEMF-treated human neutrophils, HE-NECA and NECA revealed an $EC_{50}$ value of 1.62 ± 0.21* nM and 6.03 ± 0.58* nM respectively (*$P < 0.01$). HE-NECA and NECA (100 nM) mediated inhibitory effects, which were completely blocked by SCH 58261 (1 μM). Cl-IB-MECA showed an $IC_{50}$ value of 458 ± 35 nM and 263 ± 27* nM in control and PEMF-treated human neutrophils (*$P < 0.05$). IB-MECA showed an IC50 value of 930 ± 85 nM and 575 ± 65* nM in control and PEMF-treated human neutrophils (*$P < 0.05$). In untreated or PEMF-treated human neutrophils, the inhibitory capability of Cl-IB-MECA (1 μM) was blocked in a different way using selective adenosine antagonists such as SCH 58261 and MRE 3008F20 (100 nM), suggesting an involvement of the $A_{2A}$ and $A_3$ response.

## PEMF Response Specificity

To verify that the effect of PEMF was strictly correlated to the presence of the adenosine receptors, we studied other types of membrane receptors coupled to G proteins. The expression of $\alpha_2$ and $\beta_2$ adrenergic and μ and k opioid receptors in PEMF-treated and untreated human neutrophils was determined by performing saturation binding experiments using [$^3$H]UK14304, [$^3$H]CGP12177, [$^3$H]DAMGO, and [$^3$H]U69593 respectively. A single saturable binding site was detected for all types of receptors. Saturation of [$^3$H]UK14304 binding showed a $K_D$ value of 2.12 ± 0.24 nM and a Bmax value of 34 ± 4 fmol/mg$^{-1}$ protein. [$^3$H]CGP12177 exhibited high affinity for $\beta_2$ receptors with a $K_D$ value of 0.16 ± 0.04 nM and Bmax value of 9.0 ± 0.8 fmol/mg$^{-1}$ protein. [$^3$H]DAMGO and [$^3$H]U69593 labeled μ and k opioid receptors and revealed a $K_D$ value of 2.29 ± 0.12 and 0.80 ± 0.09 nM and a Bmax value of 4.7 ± 0.5 and 4.6 ± 0.6 fmol/mg$^{-1}$ protein respectively. None of these bindings was significantly affected by PEMF treatment at 2.5 mT, an intensity that promotes an upregulation of $A_{2A}$ and $A_3$ adenosine receptors.

## Discussion

The discovery of the detailed processes of inflammation has revealed a close relationship between inflammation and the presence of adenosine receptor subtypes. Studies demonstrating the presence of $A_{2A}$ and $A_3$ adenosine receptors in human neutrophils strongly suggest that adenosine could play an important role in inflammatory processes.[14] It has been shown that electric or magnetic fields can affect membrane functions and specialized molecules—such as receptors, enzymes, ion channels, and integrins—that are essential for many fundamental cell functions.[6] In the present study, we evaluated the effect of PEMFs on $A_{2A}$ and $A_3$ adenosine receptors in human neutrophils using a typical pharmacologic approach based on binding and functional characterization of these important receptor subtypes. A set of experiments was designed to study changes in the density and affinity of adenosine $A_{2A}$ and $A_3$ receptors treated with different incubation times. These studies showed that treatment of 30 to 90 minutes is able to induce an upregulation of $A_{2A}$ and $A_3$ adenosine receptors, respectively. In addition, treatment with different intensities of PEMFs revealed that magnetic intensity in the range of 1 to 3.5 mT produced a significant increase in adenosine $A_{2A}$ and $A_3$ density. These experimental conditions are similar to those used in other studies investigating the in vitro effect of PEMFs on human chondrocytes.[10] Moreover, the signal characteristics of PEMFs used in the present study are comparable with those used in orthopaedic and traumatologic treatments, even if the time of exposure is much longer (for 6 hours/day up to 90 days) than that used in in vitro experiments.[19,20]

Of particular interest is that saturation binding experiments with $A_{2A}$ and $A_3$ adenosine receptors revealed that the predominant effect of PEMFs was a significant increase of $A_{2A}$ and $A_3$ adenosine receptor density, suggesting that the upregulation cannot be ascribed to the synthesis of new receptors during the short time of PEMF treatment. On the contrary, the upregulation of adenosine receptors is most likely due to a translocation of this receptor subtype to the membrane surface. Moreover, it was demonstrated that PEMF treatment did not modify the binding parameters of $\alpha_2$ and $\beta_2$ adrenergic and $\mu$, and k opioid receptors, suggesting a specificity of PEMF treatment to adenosine receptors. Another aim of the present study was to investigate if PEMF treatment causes modulation of adenylyl cyclase activity. Our results do not show any change of basal and forskolin-stimulated enzyme activity after PEMF treatment. Interestingly, the potency of $A_{2A}$- and $A_3$-adenosine agonists in the PEMF-treated neutrophils was significantly increased compared with the untreated neutrophils. Finally, we investigated the effect of PEMFs on the inhibitory capability of $A_{2A}$- and $A_3$-adenosine agonists in oxidative burst. The capability of adenosine agonists to inhibit fMLF-stimulated superoxide anion production was statistically increased after PEMF treatment of human neutrophils. All these data provide evidence that PEMF treatment evokes an upregulation of the $A_{2A}$ and $A_3$ adenosine receptors and alters the response of these receptor subtypes in human neutrophils. It is of interest that PEMF treatment causes an alteration of functional responses such as adenylyl cyclase activity and superoxide anion production as a result of upregulation of the adenosine receptors located on the neutrophil surface. Moreover, the involvement of $A_{2A}$ and $A_3$ adenosine receptors in the inhibition of fMLF-stimulated superoxide anion production in neutrophils indicates relevant interaction between adenosine receptors and mechanisms strictly correlated with anti-inflammatory effects.

## References

1. Fredholm BB, Ijzerman AP, Jacobson KA, Klotz KN, Linden J: Nomenclature and classification of adenosine receptors. *Pharmacol Rev* 2001;53:527-552.

2. Fredholm BB, Arslan G, Halldner L, Kull B, Schulte G, Wassserman W: Structure and function of adenosine receptors and their genes. *Naunyn Schmiedeberg's Arch Pharmacol* 2002;362:364-374.

3. Varani K, Gessi S, Dionisotti S, Ongini E, Borea PA: [$^3$H]-SCH 58261 labelling of functional $A_{2A}$ adenosine receptors in human neutrophil membranes. *Br J Pharmacology* 1998;123:1723-1731.

4. Elenkov IJ, Chrousos GP, Wilder RL: Neuroendocrine regulation of IL-2 and TNF-alpha/IL-10 balance: Clinical implications. *Ann NY Acad Sci* 2000;917:94-105.

5. Ezeamuzie CI, Philips E: Adenosine $A_3$ receptors on human eosinophils mediate inhibition of degranulation and superoxide anion release. *Br J Pharmacol* 1999;127:188-194.

6. Bersani F, Marinelli F, Ognibene A, et al: Intramembrane protein distribution in cell cultures is affected by 50 Hz pulsed magnetic fields. *Bioelectromagnetics* 1997;18:463-469.

7. De Mattei M, Caruso A, Traina GC, Pezzetti F, Baroni T, Sollazzo V: Correlation between pulsed electromagnetic fields exposure time and cell proliferation increase in human osteosarcoma cell lines and human normal osteoblast cells in vitro. *Bioelectromagnetics* 1999;20:177-182.

8. Matsumoto H, Ochi M, Abiko Y, Hirose Y, Kaku T, Sakaguchi K: Pulsed electromagnetic fields promote bone formation around dental implants inserted into the femur of rabbits. *Clin Oral Implants Res* 2000;11:354-360.

9. Cadossi R, Bersani F, Cossarizza A, et al: Lymphocytes and low-frequency electromagnetic fields. *FASEB J* 1992;6:2667-2674.

10. De Mattei M, Caruso A, Pezzetti F, Pellati A, Stabellini G, Traina GC: Effects of pulsed electromagnetic fields on human articular chondrocyte proliferation. *Connect Tissue Res* 2001;42:269-279.

11. Chiabrera A, Bianco B, Moggia E, Kaufman JJ: Zeaman-Stark modeling of the RF EMF interaction with ligand binding. *Bioelectromagnetics* 2000;21:312-324.

12. Varani K, Gessi S, Merighi S, et al: Effect of low frequency electromagnetic fields on A2A adenosine receptors in human neutrophils. *Br J Pharmacology* 2002;36:57-66.

13. Varani K, Merighi S, Gessi S, et al: [$^3$H]-MRE 3008-F20: A novel antagonist radioligand for the pharmacological and biochemical characterization of human $A_3$ adenosine receptors. *Mol Pharmacol* 2000;57:968-975.

14. Gessi S, Varani K, Merighi S, et al: A3 adenosine receptors in human neutrophils and promyelocytic HL60 cells: A pharmacological and biochemical study. *Mol Pharmacol* 2002;61:415-424.

15. Zaccaria M, Borea PA, Opocher G, et al: Effects of high altitude chronic hypoxia on platelet $\alpha_2$ receptors in man. *Eur J Clin Invest* 1997;27:316-321.

16. Borea PA, Amerini S, Masini I, et al: $\beta_1$ and $\beta_2$ adrenoceptors in sheep cardiac ventricular muscle. *J Mol Cell Cardiol* 1992;24:753-764.

17. Varani K, Rizzi A, Calò G, et al: Pharmacology of [Tyr1]nociceptin analogs: Receptor binding and bioassay studies. *Naunyn Schmiedeberg's Arch Pharmacol* 1999;360:270-277.

18. Munson PJ, Rodbard D: Ligand: A versatile computerized approach for the characterization of ligand binding systems. *Anal Biochem* 1980;107:220-239.

19. Yonemori K, Matsunaga S, Ishidou Y, Maeda S, Yoshida H: Early effects of electrical stimulation on osteogenesis. *Bone* 1996;19:173-180.

20. Satter SA, Islam MS, Rabbani KS, Talukder MS: Pulsed electromagnetic fields for the treatment of bone fractures. *Bangladesh Med Res Counc Bull* 1999;25:6-10.

# Consensus Panel 5

# Evaluation of Transduction of Biophysical Signals

**Dr. Mone Zaidi:** What has been emerging throughout this meeting is that different biophysical signals seem to be activating fairly similar cellular responses. This morning, the presentations had to do with mitogen-activated protein kinase (MAPK) and extracellular regulated kinase (ERK), as well as with nuclear factor kappa B (NFκB) and a host of calcium signals. To elaborate on calcium signaling, there could be a variety of calcium signals, and what we have seen is that calcium goes up in these cells. What we need to start focusing on is, what are the mechanisms through which calcium goes up in these cells? The use of inhibitors to block certain processes is really not going to be specific enough, and I think we have to go more toward the cardiovascular than the musculoskeletal field, where they have been able to identify motifs within channels that can be modulated specifically. The mechanically sensitive calcium channel has never been cloned or sequenced. There are aspects of the cell membrane that could be potential targets for biophysical activation, and I think we need to look at that. And of course there are exchangers for calcium and sodium, and there are the intracellular calcium channels—for example, the IP-3 receptor. We also heard about the concept that the nucleus could be regulated specifically, and as I mentioned previously, we have some data showing that nuclear calcium can be regulated specifically. One of the other things that came up was molecules involved in cross-talk between cells, and we had some glimpses into some very interesting data regarding receptors, albeit in neutraphils, but it really opens up a new area of the relationship of biophysical information and the release of ADP from the cells. The other area that was highlighted was the connexin field, which we have not touched on at all. So these are the areas for future exploration. And before I move to the panel, I would just like to say that we have not heard a word about apoptosis. Apoptosis is a fundamentally important process for all living cells. Can physical stimuli actually change the life or the fate of these cells? We have been talking about cell proliferation and cell function, but I think we need to get into the big picture, the overall framework, and address issues about cell death and cell fate.

**Dr. Hari Reddi:** You laid the framework for this discussion very well. After listening this morning, I think there seems to be an important need for examining whether there is a common pathway between these mechanical, electric, magnetic, and ultrasound stimuli, and therefore I think it should be a very high priority to identify a mechanosensitivity.

**Dr. Lane Smith:** I have two issues to discuss. Farshid Guilak brought up a really interesting point with respect to cartilage when he pointed out that, in the absence of pain, people would never come to be treated. So in an avascular, aneural tissue, you could have a lot of damage. We have talked a lot at this meeting about cell, tissue, and organismal levels, and Regis O'Keefe and Joe Lane have stressed getting back to the organism at some point. So in the case of cartilage, I think for repair and regeneration, of course the cell is the target. But to have that tissue survive in a reasonable state, you have to work back to the total joint, and clearly the joint is a composite of synovial cells, cartilage cells, and these inflammatory mediators. Finally, our model systems have to start combining tissues to be able to approach the level of control that we are seeking.

**Dr. Mone Zaidi:** I'm going to ask Regis a specific question: could you elaborate a little more about the control of cell fate? What do you think would be the biophysical impact on a cell's lifespan?

**Dr. Regis O'Keefe:** The ability to alter receptors, as we heard, is really astounding and may have something to do with degradation of the receptors. It may involve other enzymes or some signaling pathways. It appears that one of the paradigms that is emerging is that calcium signaling is very, very important. And calcium can have huge effects because of its linkage to protein kinase C and then the MAP kinases, which can alter a number of the physiologic responses in the cell. I would again say that it has to be integrated with everything else that is happening in the matrix and cell environment. There is a lot of work to be done to organize and sort out how the cells at different stages of the differentiation process will interpret those signals, and how they will modulate the differentiation process. So, again, I think there should be a great emphasis on cell signaling. I think it's a very exciting time in this field.

**Dr. Mone Zaidi:** Janet, would you like to comment on how your signals— such as the MAPK signals that you see in the osteoclast in particular— would affect cell fate? Can you prolong the lifespan of cells with biophysical stimulus to a positive effect? Because if you are increasing ERK, that is clearly one signal that would actually enhance the lifespan.

**Dr. Janet Rubin:** I actually have killed a lot of cells by inhibiting MAPK. So if you make a dominant negative MAPK and you give it to cells, they will live for about 4 hours. They are not happy in culture.

**Speaker:** One of the things we started with the NFκB project was to look at protection against apoptosis. And that kind of went by the wayside when we found it affected cyclooxygenase-2. But when we were starving cells to induce apoptosis, we were able to protect the cells somewhat. The question is whether flow has a direct effect on the cell as a protection agent or whether you are simply refeeding the cell. One of the things you do in epithelial transport, which is where I come from originally, is that you have unstirred layers against the membrane that actually act as a defusion barrier. And whether you are reducing those unstirred layers with flow is something that still is unknown. But I think you are right, we do need to start looking at how mechanical stimulation, any kind of mechanical stimulation, can protect cells from apoptosis or maybe induce it in some cases.

**Dr. Hari Reddi:** There is a school of thought that says, so what if you kill one cell. There is a dynamic process through which cells are made and cells die. And we have to look at cell death as a function of cell birth to determine total cell numbers. So, although I have doubts about some of the glucocorticoid data as it stands, and I think a lot of people would go with me on that, I still think that, in particular, Brendan Boyce's work from your group has clearly demonstrated that apoptosis is fundamentally important to bone physiology, and whether that could be modulated in a positive way to affect the life of an osteocyte would be interesting.

**Speaker:** We think that apoptosis of osteocytes plays this crucial role in determining bone remodeling. And we have shown that isolated osteocytes, when subjected to fluid flow, are inhibited in their apoptosis. I would also like to mention that in human bone cells, apoptosis was inhibited by fluid shear. These data underscore the importance of apoptosis in bone remodeling in vivo.

**Dr. Lane Smith:** Actually, we have talked about disparate modalities here, from the electric field and upregulation of receptors to changes in the cell in response to compression. I wonder if I could ask Alan Grodzinsky and Farshid Guilak to put in perspective what compression may mean in the intact joint where we have basically confined compression. There is going to be some compression and deformation over time; what may that mean in terms of the extracellular matrix, taking into consideration the negative charge of the material, the counter ions, and then whether or not that brings deformation back together with electric effects? And those kinds of changes that we talk about in cartilage may also be present, although at much lower levels, in bone.

**Dr. Farshid Guilak:** I'm not sure I can exactly answer that. I think there are some commonalities, but I don't think anybody has done a real head-to-head comparison. Even some of the mechanisms that you proposed in your talk I think are potentially closely related—for example, hydrostatic pressure inhibiting interleukin effects, and having effects on nitric oxide and prostaglandins. We are applying dynamic compression, which has a hydrostatic pressure component, and there is a good possibility for linkage among these different mechanisms. I agree that we still have not been able to paint the whole picture of which signal relates to which outcome. It's possible that they overlap.

**Dr. Alan Grodzinsky:** I'm not sure I have too much to add, but as we have all seen from the literature, and we discussed it briefly here, the same kinds of compressive regimes induce local streaming potential. Sol Pollack has done a lot of work with that over many years in bone in particular. And, yes, those fields are there and the issue is that we always see a cell response. But can we peel apart the different stimuli, including the local fluid flow, pressure gradients, the actual electric field that is induced right near the cell, and the compaction of the proteoglycan-rich matrix, which would change the local charge density and therefore osmotic swelling pressure? All of that is occurring roughly at the same time rate of change or frequency of the loading. There are definitely some things that have been able to be done because you can look at explants and look at different regions of the tissue and, using quantitative autoradiography, look at particular regions in which there might be more fluid flow or more or less hydrostatic pressure. So some of that has been able to be parsed but certainly not all. In particular, I feel a bit frustrated that the issue of the streaming potential, which is always tagged to the fluid velocity, has not clearly been separated from the fluid velocity itself. Is it the mechanical or electric stimuli, I don't know.

**Dr. Solomon Pollack:** In bone, the streaming potentials have been measured very accurately within the osteonal geometry. The one way of separating the fluid flow from those potentials is that you can take the measured potentials and compute the gradients, which are the electric fields. You then apply the electric fields without deformation so that in the absence of fluid flow, you have the presence of the field. It turns out that, with the geometry of the osteon, the gradients reach values of the order of a volt per meter down to maybe two orders of magnitude lower than that. And that just happens to be the range of the electric field in several of the Food and Drug Administration-approved modalities. So one would argue that the amplitudes of the field are what is observed physiologically, although the frequencies are not. That does not begin to explain why there are frequency windows, but certainly you can replicate the amplitudes.

**Dr. Mone Zaidi:** Just to carry that point on in terms of the cellular signal, I believe that you probably need pulses because of cellular memory. There is a lot of memory in cellular transduction systems; what Howard Rasmussen said many years ago is still valid—that a single calcium signal can be memorized by the cell. And now it is quite clear that the amplitude, as well as the frequency of the calcium signals, could have differential effects even on gene expressions, as you pointed out earlier. So you could basically translate that biophysical signal, which is a much faster signal I understand, into changes in cell signaling. Let me pose a question. From Bob Sah's work, we saw that the cartilage had various compartments. And you presented data with one of the molecules, lubricin I think it was, which is selectively upregulated in the superficial zone and is downregulated in the deep zone. What other molecular events do you think would be preferentially regulated? And then I am going back to Dr. Borea to see if his findings are going to fit with yours.

**Dr. Robert Sah:** So the question is, how do these cells talk to each other in the different layers? Do they talk to each other in the different layers? It seems like the cells are different in the superficial and deeper zones, but they do not do exactly what you would expect from a straight mix, suggesting that there is some interaction between the two. As far as dissecting that out, I don't think people have really gotten too far. One of the things that we are working on is to direct cells into very defined geographic regions so you can start to look at cell-cell interactions, not just as they appear in the normal tissue.

**Dr. Mone Zaidi:** Dr. Borea, how do your findings with the adenosine receptors, assuming there are adenosine receptors on chondrocytes, relate to a ubiquitous second messenger for cross-talk? Would it be a mechanism through which PEMFs might modulate cell behavior?

**Dr. Pier Borea:** Normally receptors are more or less everywhere, with some exception obviously. And so why not in chondrocytes, why not in osteocytes? I have not seen a systematic study about this. I think that this cross-talking can exist, and I also think that this externalization of receptors can happen easily on these cells as you suggest.

**Speaker:** We've talked about proinflammatory factors, and Farshid Guilak brought up a lot of proinflammatory responses. I think that our end points between injury repair, fluid shear, whatever, are all similar responses. We may want to read the inflammatory literature a little bit more.

**Dr. Mone Zaidi:** I think you are absolutely right in the larger context. I think the inflammatory story that you brought out is extremely important because clearly there could be differences in responsiveness to physical stimulation in the presence and absence of inflammation near the tissue. I think we have to bear that in mind. So, could we now make three consensus statements? The first consensus statement, in general terms, would be that different biophysical signals produce really the same group of cellular signals. Are we all more or less in line with that? We have expanded on that, and I think Roy and Mark are going to write this up in the consensus statement. There appears to be a group of signals that are common to at least some of the biophysical responses that have been looked at. I think the second consensus statement that we could make is the fact that there are geometrically different areas within the cartilage and the interface with bone, they could perhaps be cross-talk, and they could contain molecules important for the cross-talk to occur. I think the third consensus statement should be that we really need to look at apoptosis. I think it is an important biologic process. It is clearly a black box as far as the biophysical signals are concerned, and of course there are the issues about inflammation.

**Speaker:** All of the speakers today were very much involved with the receptor or sets of receptors. There is an emerging hypothesis that there are specific receptors that then connect to classic pathways. That seemed to be a unifying sense from all of the speakers this morning that I thought was really very interesting.

**Dr. Mone Zaidi:** I think that is another important aspect to the consensus—that although we have not established a single receptor as being the biophysical receptor, there is clear evidence now from the talks that we have heard of different molecules serving that function. Notably there appears to be a unified function for a diverse set of molecules, as happened with the calcium-sensing receptor many years ago. There are different molecules that appear to be responsive to biophysical stimulation, and those could be called receptors for biomechanical stress. So, there is a unified function for a diverse set of molecules that appears to be evolving.

**Dr. Hari Reddi:** I think we really had a wonderful 3 days. Meetings like this don't happen spontaneously. They are the product of the efforts of people like Roy Aaron and Mark Bolander and a host of the excellent team from the American Academy of Orthopaedic Surgeons. Let's give them all a wonderful hand.

## Future Directions

- Calcium signaling appears to be a very important mediator of physical regulation. It needs to be integrated with other signaling events in the extracellular matrix.
- Dosimetry in terms of amplitude and frequency may be related to cell memory, especially of calcium signaling.
- Biophysical agents as a group produce a similar set of cellular signals. Specificity may be a function of zonal arrangement of signals and cross-talk among tissues.
- Activation of receptors and classic signaling pathways appears to be produced by biophysical agents, although no specific physical receptor(s) have been identified.

# Index

## A

Acoustic pressure waves, 62, 175–176
Acoustic streaming, 4
Actin, 132, 186, 250
Activator protein-1 (AP-1), 175, 180–181
ADAMTS-4, 127
Adenosine receptors
  binding assays, 262–265, *263, 264*
  functional assays, 265–266
  low-frequency electromagnetic fields and, 259–268
  PEMFs and, 260–265
  saturation assays, *263, 264*
Adenosine triphosphate (ATP), 251–253, *252*
Adenylate cyclase system, 231
Adhesion plaques, 231
Adriamycin, 55
Agarose gel cultures, 126, *127*
Age/aging, bone loss and, 69
Aggrecanase-1, 124
Aggrecans
  hydrostatic pressure and, 192, 193
  mRNA, 88, 189
  ramp-and-hold compression and, *123*
  static compression and, 124
  synthesis, 229
Alizarin complexone, 101
ALK-2, 203, *203, 204*
ALK-3, 203, *203, 204*
Alkaline phosphatase, 89, 91, 132, 177, 201
Angiogenesis, PEMF and, 179
Ankle arthroses, 12
Arthritis, 153, 159. *See also* Osteoarthritis
Arthropathies, noninflammatory, 152
Articular cartilage. *See also* Cartilage
  chemomechanical coupling, 151–161
  description of, 151
  hydrostatic pressure and, 192–193
  mechanical compression, *228*
  metabolism, 191–193
  signal transduction, 225–239
Attenuation coefficients, 86–87
Axial torsion tests, 100

## B

BAPTA-AM, 125
Bcl-2, 189
Bed rest, response to, 62
Bending stiffness, *79*
Binding assays, 261, 262–265, *263, 264*
Biolectron/EBI Spinalpak, *11*
Biomarkers, 53–57
Biomechanical factors, 173–175
Biomechanical testing, 100, 103, *104*
Biophysical signals, transduction of, 269–274
Bioquant System IV, 100
Biostim, waveforms, *45*
Body mass index (BMI), *71*
Bone
  calcium channels, 249–250
  degradation, 241
  formation rates, *213*
  functional environment and, 62
  gap junctions, 131
  healing, 17–26, 53–58, 111–116 (*See also* Bone repair)
  interstitial fluid flow in, 133–134
  lacunocanalicular network, 131
  lengthening, 190
  metabolism, 189–191
  mineral apposition rate, *40*
  modeling of, 17
  piezoelectric properties, 3
  quality, 30–31, *66*
  quantity, *66*
  response to low-level mechanical signals, 65
  turnover, 97–100
Bone formation rates/bone volume (BFR/BV), 68, 104
Bone loss
  aging and, 69
  body mass index and, *71*
  low-level mechanical signals and, 70–71
Bone marrow sinusoids, 136
Bone mineral density (BMD)
  genetic factors in, 209
  impact of PLIUS treatment, 31

Index

low-level mechanical signals and, 70–71
in osteoporosis, 108
quantitative trait loci (QTL), 209
skeletal loading and, 191
Bone morphogenetic proteins (BMPs), 175
BMP-2, 55, 176, 190, 202, *203, 204*
BMP-4, 190, 202, *204*
BMP-7, 190
cell metabolism and, 187
electromagnetic fields, 178
signaling by, 115
upregulation of, *174*
Bone multicellular units (BMUs), 135–139, *136, 137*
Bone remodeling, 62, 77
Bone repair. *See also* Bone, healing
decision tree, *48*
device-related modulation, 19
electric stimulation of, 39–51
endogenous, 47–48
imposed controlled mechanical stimulation and, 19–21
magnetic stimulation of, 39–51
mechanical factors in, *78*
mechanical modulation of, 18
mechanical regulation, 23, 77–84
prostaglandins in, 21
time-related regulation of, 22
Bone resorption, 144–146, 191, 252
Bone sialoprotein, 203, *203*
BSP, *203*

## C

C-fos, 22, 250, 251, 252
C-fos genes, 124, 174
C-jun, 22
C-jun genes, 124
C-jun N-terminal kinase (JNK), 126, 146, 193
Calcein, 212–213
Calcein blue, 100
Calcium
bone metabolism and, 191
callus mineralization, 90–91
in mechanotransduction, 247–248, *248*
release, 205
signaling, 125, 229, 231, 242, 247–257, *253*
Calcium channels, 249–250
Callus
area of, *79*
biomechanical function of, 78

estrogen receptors in, 22
formation, 28, 77, 79
interfragmentary displacements and, 19
longitudinal expansion, 190
measurement of, 100, *102*
mineralization, 90–91
Calmodulin, 205
Camptodactyly, 152
Camptodactyly-arthropathy-coxa vara-pericarditis syndrome, 152
Capacitively coupled electric fields (CCEF), 4
bone repair and, 39
efficacy trials, 8, *8*
European experience, 41
prospective, controlled studies, 5
in spinal fusion, 10, *11*
Cardiomyocyte hypertrophy, 241
Cartilage. *See also* Articular cartilage
culture, 154
culture methods, 154, *155*
degeneration, 188
degradation, 243
dynamic compression of, 120
dynamics, *153*
fluid movement in, 230
gene expression, 122–125
harvest, 154
mechanical stress on, 226–227
metabolism of, 227
synthesis, 241
Caveolin, 243
Cbfa1/Runx2, 93
CD44 receptors, 134
Cdx-1 genes, 89, *90*
Cell adhesion, 243
Charcot neuroarthropathy, 12
Charged coupled device cameras, 101
Chemomechanical coupling, 151–161
Chemotaxis, 259
Chondroblasts, recruitment, 77
Chondrocytes
agarose gel cultures, 126, *127*
anabolic activity, 225
attachment to fibronectin, 231
cellular deformation, 228–229
compression of, 120–122
electric stimulation of, 126–127
exercise and, 241
function, 79
gene expression, 122–125
hydrostatic pressure and, 125, 192
intermittent compression and, 193

278

loading, 193–194
metabolic activity, 151–152
nuclei, deformation, *229*
osmotic stress and, 125, *230*
osteoarthritic, 189
PRG4, 154–157, *155, 157*
regulation of, 151–161
response to ultrasound, 88–89
shear deformation, 121–122
superficial zone, 152
Chondrogenesis, 21, 106
CI-1B-MECA, 265–266
Collagens
in articular cartilage, 151, 225
biosynthesis of, 120
degradation, 227
synthesis, 122, 201
type I, *203*
type II
DC stimulation and, 178
hydrostatic pressure and, 192, 193
mechanical stimulation and, 188
PEMF and, *203, 204*
ramp-and-hold compression and, *123*
static compression and, 124
type X, 174
Colony forming units-macrophage (CFU-M), 144, 145
Combined magnetic fields (CMFs), 4
in Charcot neuroarthropathy, 12
prospective, controlled studies, 5
in spinal fusion, 10–11, *11*
tibial nonunion treatment, *6*
Compression
biosynthetic response to, 120–122
connective tissue loading and, 186
direct mechanical, 122–125
dynamic, 121
hydrostatic intermittent, 134
intermittent, 193
intermittent mechanical, 227
ramp-and-hold, 122, *123*
static, 124, 192, 227
Congenital pseudarthrosis, 42
Connective tissues, 185–200
Consensus panels
biophysical regulation of bone healing in animal models, 111–116
regulation of clinical bone healing, 53–58
regulation of growth factor synthesis, 217–222

regulation of skeletal cells and tissues, 163–169
transduction of biophysical signals, 269–274
Contact microradiographs, 101
Continuous wave ultrasound, 28
Contralateral limbs, 114–115
Cortical bone, *105*
Coxa vara deformity, 152
Culture media, 154
Cutting cones, *136, 137*
Cyclic adenosine monophosphate (cAMP), 261
Cyclooxygenase-1 (COX-1), 177–178, 191, 204
Cyclooxygenase-2 (COX-2), 93, 135, 176
blockade of, 204
effects of compression, 124
P2 receptor function and, 252
production of, 250, 251
Cytokines. *See also* specific cytokines
electromagnetic fields and, 205
mechanical stimulation and, 244
PEMF and, 201
response to joint injury, 153
shear stresses and, 188

# D

Decision trees, *48*
Deformation
cell morphology and, 125–126
cellular, 228–229
cellular function and, 225
chondrocyte nuclei, *229*
connective tissue loading and, 186–187
cyclical, 19
extracellular matrix, 120
mechanical, 3, 17
osteoblast proliferation and, 21
osteoclasts, 17
osteocytes, 17
shear, 121–122
stretch-induced, 174–175
Degranulation, 259
Delayed unions, 30, 34–36, 98
Demineralized bone matrix (DBM), 112
Developmental mechanics, 173
Developmental morphogenesis, 173
Digital image analysis, 100
Direct current (DC)
efficacy of, 40–41
implantable stimulators, 4, 9–10, 178

Index

Distraction osteogenesis, 190
Disuse osteopenia, 67–69
DNA synthesis, 126
Dorsiflexion, 81
DXC-151, 101
Dynamic fluid pressures, 21
Dynamic force plates, 99
Dynamic tissue shear, 121–122
Dynamization, 19

**E**

Early intermediate genes, *180*
Early response genes, 174
EBI, *11,* 98
Egr-1 genes, 174
Elastase, 259
Electrokinetic phenomena, 173
Electromagnetic fields (EMFs)
  cytokines and, 205
  dosimetric relationships, 111
  growth factors and, 176–179, *177,* 201–207
  low-frequency, 259–268
Electromagnetic induction devices, 4
Embryonic development, 126
Endochondrial ossification, 88
Endoplasmic reticulum, 125, 252–253
Endothelial cell nitric oxide synthase (eNOS), 138, 147
Endothelial cells, 146, 175
*Entwicklungsmechanik,* 173
Epidermal growth factor, 174
Epiphyseal growth plates, 249
Epiphyseal region, 31
Epithelial cells, 243
Estrogen receptors, 22
Exercise
  bone response to, 62
  mechanical stimulation via, 241
  site-specific changes, 226
  TGF-β and, 175
External fixation, 20–21
Extracellular matrix (ECM), 125
  composition, 225
  deformation of, 120
  effects of electrical stimulation, 126
  hydration, 228
  inhibition of, 153
  integrins and, 174
Extracellular signal-regulated kinases (ERK 1/2)
  activation, 146, 231, 241, 242
  mechanical stimulation and, 244
  phosphorylation of, 193, 241
  regulation of, 174
  signaling by, 126
  static compression and, 124
  ultrasound-induced activation of, 92, *93*

**F**

Faradic systems, 39, 40–41
Fat tissue, *87*
Femoral neck fractures, 47
Femurs
  nonunion, *87*
  osteotomies, 44
  size of, *211*
Fibroblast growth factors (FGFs), 174, 179, 188, 190
Fibroblasts, proliferation, 241
Fibronectin, 92, 186, 231, 244
Fibula, nonunion, *87*
Filamin, 243
Film, high-resolution, 101
Fimbrin, 132
Fixation devices, 19, 82
Flexcell devices, 145
Fluid flow, 62, 135, 173
Fluid shear, 146, 248, 249, 250–251
Fluorochrome labeling, *212*
Focal adhesion kinase (FAK), 92, 243
Focal adhesions, 243
Food and Drug Administration (FDA), 4, *7*
Fractures. See also Delayed unions; Nonunion
  callus formation, 77
  casted, 31
  delayed unions, 34–36
  FDA-approved treatments, 4
  flexible fixation, 82
  fresh, 5–9, 32–34, 44–47
  gap size, 78, *79*
  healing, 27–38, 77, *78,* 85–96 (*See also* Bone repair)
  intramedullary fixed, 9
  micromotion, 80
  nailed, 31
  nonunion, 34–36, 42–44, *44*
  repair mechanisms, 77–78

**G**

G protein-coupled channels, 251
G proteins, 94
Gadolinium, 249

# Index

Gap junctions, bone, 131
Gastrointestinal tract, 241
Glycosaminoglycan (GAG), 125, 126, 192, 225
Golgi apparatus, 124, 125, 229
Granulation, 77
Gravitational forces, 62
Grb2/sos, 243
Growth factors
  biomechanical factors and, 173–175
  biophysical regulation of, 203–205
  cell metabolism and, 187–188
  connective tissue metabolism and, 185–200
  consensus panel, 217–222
  distraction osteogenesis and, 190
  electromagnetic fields and, 176–179, *177*, 201–207
  PEMFs and, 201–203, *203*
  stimulation of, 3, 173–183, 201–203

## H

Haversian channels, 136
HE-NECA, 265–266
Healing end points, *29, 33*
Heart, mechanical pressures, 241
Helmholtz coils, 201
Hemiosteons, 136
High bone mass (HBM) phenotypes, 209
Histologic analyses, 100–101, 103–104
Histomorphometric analyses, 100–101, 103–104, 193
Histomorphometry
  dynamic, *66*
  static, *66*
Humeral fractures, *87*
Hydrostatic pressures
  aggrecan synthesis, 229
  articular cartilage and, 192–193
  cellular organization and, 229–230
  chondrocyte biosynthesis and, 125
  connective tissue loading and, 186–187
  growth factors and, 173
  intermittent compression, 134
  osteoclast formation and, 144–145
  stress, 79
  transcription factors and, 194
Hypertrophic chronic nonunions, *203*
Hypertrophic synovitis, 152

## I

IB-MECA, 265–266

IHA, 175
Immobilization, effects of, 241
Immunolocalization, 154–155, 156–158, *157*
Index of connectivity, 66
Indian Hedgehog (IHH), 174
Indomethacin, 21, 204
Inductive coupling techniques, 4
Inductive systems, 39, 41–47
Inflammation
  adenosine receptors and, 259, 266
  fracture healing and, 77
  mechanical stimulation and, 244
  strain and, 243
Inositol trisphosphate system, 231, 242, 250, 251
Insulin-like growth factor-1 (IGF-1), 121, 175, 176–177, 187–189
Integrins
  ECM and, 174
  fibronectin adhesion and, 231–232
  kinase recruitment and, 243
  mechanotransduction and, 125, 134, 241
  ultrasound signals and, 92–93
Interfragmentary displacements, 19, 78, 80–81
Interfragmentary strain hypothesis, 78–79, *79*
Interleukin-6 (IL-6), 188, 244, 259
Interleukin-8 (IL-8), 259
Interleukin-1α, 151–161
Interleukin-1β, 244
Intermittent hydrostatic compression, 134
Interstitial fluid flow, 133–134
Intracellular signaling. *See also* Signal transduction
  loading and, 193–194
  pathways, 231–232
Intramedullary nailing, 34
Ionotropic channels, 251
Iris Indigo Elan, 101

## J

Joint injuries. *See also* Inflammation
  cytokine response to, 153
  degeneration and, 226

## K

Ketamine, 100

## L

L-N(5)-(1-iminoethyl) ornithine, 189

281

# Index

L-NAME, 189
Laminin, 186, 243, 244
Lead zirconate titante, 85
Ligament transection, 226
Ligand-gated channels, 251
LIGAND software, 262
Limb lengthening, 46
Lipopolysaccharide (LPS), 193
Load bearing, 99–100, 101, 104
Load shielding, 34
Loading
    biophysical input during, 143
    compressive, 193
    connective tissue metabolism and, 185–200
    connective tissues, 186–187
    functional, 62
    intracellular signaling and, 193–194
    of joints, *121*
    mechanical regimen, 82, 189–191, 212
    skeletal, 173
    time-dependent changes in, 80–81
    tissue hydration and, 226
    ulnar, 250
Low-density lipoprotein receptor-related protein-5 (LRP-5), 209
Lubricin, 152

## M

Macrophages, 144
Marrow cells, 89–90
Matrix metalloproteinases (MMPs), 179
    effects of compression, 124
    MMP-3, 127
    MMP-13, 127
    MMP-13 genes, 89, *91*
Mechanical deformation, 3, 17. *See also* Deformation
Mechanical signals, low-level
    application in clinics, 70–71
    bone tissue response to, 65
    inhibition of disuse osteopenia, 67–69, 68
    noninvasive introduction of, 65–67
    physiologic relevance to, 62–64
Mechanical stimulation
    articular cartilage metabolism, 191–192
    calcium signaling and, 247–257
    external, 82–83
Mechanical strain, growth factors and, 173
Mechanogrowth factor (MGF), 175
Mechanosensors, 133, 134–135

Mechanotransduction, 125
    biophysical signals, 269–274
    cellular level, 185–186, *242,* 247
    integrins and, 241
    intracellular calcium in, 247–248, *248*
    intracellular calcium release and, 250–251
    intracellular pathways, 146–147
    mechanisms, 21–22
    signaling pathways, 191, 241–245
    skeletal, 209–216
Megakaryocyte-stimulating factor, 152
MEK-1, 92, *93*
Meniscectomy, 226
Metabotropic channels, 251
Metatarsal fractures, *87*
Microgravity, effects of, 241
Micromotion, 20, 80
Microtubules, 124, 229
Mineralization, *105, 106,* 190
Mitogen-activated protein kinases (MAPKs), 125, 146, *148,* 174, 180–181, 231
Mitogenesis, 244
Mitogenic effects, 243
MMPs. *See* Matrix metalloproteinases (MMPs)
Mouse SNP database, 213
MTS Bionix 858, 100
MTS mechanical testing machine, 100
Muscle, attenuation coefficient, *87*
Muscle spindles, 64
Musculoskeletal tissues, 119–120

## N

NECA, 265–266
Neurofibromatosis, 42
Neuron action potentials, 126
Neutrophils
    adenosine receptors in, 259–268
    cAMP levels in, 261
    cell suspension, 260
    membranes, 261
    PEMF response specificity, 266
    superoxide anion production, 261
Nifedipine, 249, 250
Nitric oxide (NO)
    antagonists, 189
    blockade of, 148
    compression and, 227
    production, 134, 135
    RANKL and, 147

# Index

release of, 188, 249
Nitric oxide synthase (NOS), 138
Nonunions
  combined magnetic fields in, 5
  decision trees, *48*
  electric stimulation, *42*
  European studies, *44*
  FDA-approved treatments, 4, *7*
  hypertrophic chronic, *203*
  hypertrophic model, 31
  PLIUS treatment for, 30, 34–36
  prospective controlled studies, 5–9
  reparative osteogenesis in, 42–44
  tibial, *6*
  ultrasound treatment, *87*
NS-398 blockade, 204
Nuclear factor κB (NF κB), 191, 244, 251, 252–253
Nuclear factor of activated T cells (NF-AT), 243
Nuclei, chondrocyte, *229*

## O

Opioid receptors, 267
Orthofix Spinal Stim Lite, *11*
Orthologic Spinalogic, *11*
OrthoPulse, *45*
Osmotic pressures, 125, 173
Osmotic stress, *230*
Osteoarthritis. *See also* Arthritis
  etiopathogenesis, 226, *227*
  guinea pig model, 179
  shear stress and, 189
Osteobit waveform, *45*
Osteoblasts
  calcium signaling in, 247–257
  differentiation, 90–91, 201
  growth factors, 201–207
  P2 receptor types, 252
  proliferation, 21
  recruitment, 77
  response to deformation, 18
  strain and, 243
  transduction pathways, 93–95
Osteocalcin, 132, 201, 203, *203, 204*
Osteoclast progenitor cells, 144
Osteoclastogenesis, 174, 252
Osteoclasts
  bone remodeling and, 135–139
  formation, 144–146
  P2 receptor types, 252
  repression, 143–150

response to deformation, 17
Osteocyte syncytium, 131–132
Osteocytes
  apoptotic, *136,* 137
  function, 133–139
  isolation, 132
  markers, 132–133
  mechanical regulation of, 131–142
  morphology, *132*
  nitric oxide release, 249
  nitric oxide synthesis, 138
  response to deformation, 17
Osteogenesis, reparative, 42, 44–47. *See also* Bone repair
Osteogenic protein 1 (OP-1), 55
Osteonal healing mechanisms, 77
Osteonectin, 132, 203, *203*
Osteons, 131, 136
Osteopenia, disuse, 67–69, *68*
Osteopontin, 132, 203, *203, 204*
Osteoporosis
  bone mineral density, 108
  genetic factors in, 209
  low-level mechanical signals and, 70–71
  vulnerability to, 69
Osteoporosis-pseudoglioma syndrome, 209
Osteosarcoma cell lines, 249
Osteotomies
  gap sizes, 19
  healing, 97–100, 107
  PEMF efficacy, *46*
  stimulation of reparative osteogenesis, 44–47
Oxytetracycline, 101

## P

P38, 124, 126, 193, 242
Parathyroid hormone (PTH), 144, 250
Paxillin, 92, 243
PD98059, 92, 93, *93,* 146
PEMFs. *See* Pulsed electromagnetic fields (PEMFs)
Pericarditis, 152
Pericellular matrix, 125
Periosteal cells, 90
PH, electromagnetic fields and, 205
Phosphatidylserine, 138, 189
Phospholipase $A_2$ ($PLA_2$), 204, 205
Phospholipase C (PLC), 242, 250, 251
Phospholipase D (PLD), 251
Piezoelectric materials, 85
Piezoelectric properties, 3

# Index

Plantar flexion, 81
Platelet-derived growth factors (PDGFs), 175
Pleural effusion, 152
PLIUS. *See* Pulsed low-intensity ultrasound
Polar moments of inertia (Ip), 210, 211
Potassium ions, 229
Preferred strain history, 61–76, *64, 72*
Prostaglandins
    P2 receptor function and, 252
    production, 134, 243
    prostaglandin E$_2$ (PGE$_2$), 176, 188, 205
        blockade of, 148
        compression and, 227
        PEMF and, 201, 202
        strain transduction pathways and, 21
Protein kinase C (PKC), 231, 242
Protein synthesis, 126
Proteoglycan 4 (PRG4)
    chondrocyte expression, 153
    immunolocalization, 154–155, 156–158, *157*
    immunoreactivity, 152
    regulation of, 151–161
    secretion of, 154, *155,* 155–156
Proteoglycans, 120
    in articular cartilage, 151
    deposition, 121
    hydrostatic pressure and, 192
    synthesis of, 88
Pulsed electromagnetic fields (PEMFs)
    adenosine receptors and, 260
    bone repair and, 39
    bone turnover and, 97–100
    devices, 4
    efficacy trials, *8*
    European experience, 41–47
    FDA summary data, *7*
    field characteristics, 260
    growth factors and, 177, *177,* 201–203, *203*
    in nonunion of the tibia, 42
    osteotomy healing, *46,* 97–100
    prospective, controlled studies, 4–5
    response specificity, 266
    in spinal fusion, *10, 11*
Pulsed low-intensity ultrasound (PLIUS)
    bone quality and, 30–31
    in fracture healing, 27–38
    fracture healing and, 85–96
    fractures, *33*
    initial studies of, 29–30
    retinoic acid-responsive genes and, 93
    tibial fractures, 32, *33*
    ultrasound signals, 85
Puringergic (P2) receptors, 251–253, *252*
P2Y receptors, 251

## Q

Quantitative autoradiography, 121, 122
Quantitative trait loci (QTL), 209, 210, *210*

## R

Radial fractures
    cancellous, 29
    distal aspect, *31*
    nonunion, *87*
Radiographic analyses, 101, 103
Radius model, 21
RANKL (receptor activator of NFκB ligand), 145–148, 174
Rehabilitation times, 32
Resveratrol, 204
RGD peptide, 92
Rho stress fiber formation, 242
Runx2, 175
Ryanodyne, 250

## S

SaOS-2, 175
Saturation assays, 262, *263, 264*
Scaphoid fractures, 32, *87*
Second messenger cascades, 231
Shear, dynamic, 121–122
Shear deformation
    biosynthetic response to, 121–122
    of the ECM, 120
    gastrointestinal tract, 241
Shear movement, 79–80
Shear stresses
    aggrecan synthesis and, 230
    connective tissue loading and, 186
    cytokine expression and, 188
    intermittent hydrostatic pressure and, 193
Signal transducers and activators of transcription (STATs), 194
Signal transduction, 179–181, 225–239
Single nucleotide polymorphism (SNPs), 213
Skeletal architecture
    deformation and, 17
    mechanotransduction, 209–216
Skeletal repair, 3–16, 17–26

Skeleton, mechanical stimulation of, 241
Skin, attenuation coefficient, *87*
Smoking, heal time and, 30
Soft tissues
    attenuation coefficient, *87*
    stabilizers, 226
Sonic Hedgehog (SHH) protein, 190
SOX-9, 194
Spinal fusion, 4, 9–12
Spongiosa, primary, 77
Statistical analysis
    binding assays, 262
    cartilage culture data, 155
    osteotomy healing, 101
    saturation assays, 262
Stra-8 genes, 89, *90*
Strain
    cyclical, 21
    distribution, 18
    histories, *64*
    recording, *63*
Streaming potentials, 230
Stress-activated proliferation factor (SAPF), 174
Stress-activated protein kinases, 179–181
Stress fibers, 229
Stress fractures, 41
Stress relaxation, waveforms, *123*
Stresses, 133–134. *See also* specific stresses
Stretch-induced matrix deformation, 174–175
Stryker saws, 98
Subcellular structures, 228–231
Subchondral bone remodeling, 226
Superficial zone proteins (SZPs), 151
Superoxide anions, 259, 261
Synovial fluids, osteoarthritis and, 226
Synovitis, hypertrophic, 152

## T

Technovit 9100, 100
Tenascin-C, 188
Tendons, attenuation coefficient, *87*
Tetracyclines, *40*
3-A-4 monoclonal antibody, 154–155, *157*
Tibia
    bending, 250
    fractures, *29, 31, 33,* 47
    nonunions, *6,* 42, *87*
    osteotomies, 44
    shaft fractures, 81
    strain recording, *63*
    ultrasound wave effects, *86*
Tibial osteotomy external fixation model, 20–21
Tissue inhibitors of matrix metalloproteinases (TIMPs), 127, 188
Torsional stiffness, 103, *104,* 107
Trabeculae
    spacing, 66
    volume, 66
Trabecular bone, 69–70, 136. *See also* specific bones
Trabecular bone pattern factor, 66
Trabecular bridging, 32
Transcription factors, activation, 241
Transforming growth factor-α (TGF-α), 92
Transforming growth factor-β (TGF-β), 153, 178–179
    blockade of, 148
    calcium-dependent pathways, 205
    cell metabolism and, 187–188
    cyclical strain and, 21
    mineralization and, 190
    PEMF and, 201
    preoperative application of, 22
    PRG4 regulation, 158
    upregulation of, *174*
Transforming growth factor-$β_1$ (TGF-$β_1$), 151–161
Transient receptor potential vanilloid (TRPV), 231
Tumor necrosis factor-α (TNF-α), 176
Turkey ulna model, *66*

## U

Ulnae
    fluorochrome labeling, *212*
    loading, 250
Ultrasound
    attenuation coefficients, 86–87
    biologic response to, 88–91
    continuous wave, 28
    fresh fracture healing, 8–9
    interaction with biologic materials, 85–86
    modeling wave effects, *86*
    pulsed low-intensity, 27–38, 29–30
    signal transduction processes and, 91–95
    stimulation, 4
    studies of, 5
    transmission in tissues, 175–176

Index

**V**
Vascular endothelial growth factors (VEGFs), 94
Venous ulcers, 12
Verapamil, 249, 250
Vibration, whole body, 65–66
Vitamin D, 144, 250

**W**
Weight bearing, 80–81, *102*

Whole body vibration, 65–66
Wnt proteins, 190
Wolff's law, 3, 71, 138
Wound healing, 126

**X**
Xylenol orange, 100